THE COMPLETE GUIDE TO
LOWERING HIGH
BLOOD PRESSURE
NATURALLY

THE COMPLETE GUIDE TO
LOWERING HIGH
BLOOD PRESSURE
NATURALLY

Deborah Mitchell

A Lynn Sonberg Book

St. Martin's Paperbacks

Notice: This book is intended as a reference volume only, not as a medical manual. The information given here is designed to help you make informed decisions about your health. It is not intended as a substitute for any treatment that may have been prescribed by your doctor. If you suspect that you have a medical problem, we urge you to seek competent medical help.

Mention of specific companies, organizations, or authorities in this book does not imply endorsement by the author or publisher, nor does mention of specific companies, organizations, or authorities imply that they endorse this book, its author or the publisher.

Internet addresses given in this book were accurate at the time it went to press.

THE COMPLETE GUIDE TO LOWERING HIGH BLOOD PRESSURE NATURALLY

Copyright © 2014 by Lynn Sonberg.

All rights reserved.

For information address St. Martin's Press, 175 Fifth Avenue, New York, NY 10010.

EAN: 978-1-250-02630-9

Printed in the United States of America

St. Martin's Paperbacks edition / September 2014

St. Martin's Paperbacks are published by St. Martin's Press, 175 Fifth Avenue, New York, NY 10010.

10 9 8 7 6 5 4 3 2 1

To Jobim and Abbey—
my furry four-legged feline blood
pressure "medication."

CONTENTS

INTRODUCTION: WHY YOU NEED THIS BOOK AND HOW TO USE IT

"I've got high blood pressure." "My doctor says my blood pressure is a little high." "I should do something about my high blood pressure."

If either of the first two statements is true for you, then this book can help you with the third one and the best time to start taking action is now.

High blood pressure is a silent, insidious disease with the power to completely change your life in seconds or slowly and relentlessly over time . . . and not for the better. This book offers you and your loved ones who may have high blood pressure ways to take control of hypertension on your own terms, using effective, natural solutions that involve lifestyle modifications as the main course of action, with use of medications only if necessary.

High blood pressure can place you at risk for or accompany other major health problems, including heart disease, stroke, kidney disease, diabetes, obesity, and congestive heart failure. These are health consequences you can avoid if you take action now, and this book can help you take those steps.

Have you or a loved one been prescribed drugs to help lower your or his or her blood pressure? If so, you are among the majority of people with high blood pressure who have been advised to take medications to manage their blood pressure. The good news is that you have other treatment choices, and ones with few or no side effects.

In the confusing and ever-changing health-care environment, including the complexities of health insurance, Medicare, and doctor shortages, it is even more important for you to take control of your health needs. Since high blood pressure is largely a condition associated with lifestyle, it is one of the health issues you can tackle with confidence by modifying habits and activities in your daily life and making new choices.

This book introduces those choices and explains how you can incorporate them into your life conveniently and safely. Of course, you should consult your health-care provider when making any lifestyle changes that can affect your blood pressure and other aspects of your health.

The power of diet and nutrition, physical activity, stress management, herbal and other natural supplements, and a variety of other lifestyle changes is much underappreciated when it comes to managing high blood pressure. Your health-care provider may not emphasize the potential benefits of these factors in managing high blood pressure, but rest assured they are potent if you use them as described in this book.

Individuals who are better informed about their treatment choices—be they lifestyle changes, complementary or alternative methods, or prescription medications—may be more likely to adhere to a management plan, especially when they have a hand in putting that plan together. That's exactly what this book can help you do:

devise your own treatment program for high blood pressure that fits your lifestyle.

The first part of the book discusses the different types of high blood pressure, its causes, symptoms, risk factors, and complications and provides a brief introduction to treatment options. How is blood pressure measured, what does it mean, and how can you check your own blood pressure at home? All these questions are answered in part 1 of the book. This section also addresses the rising prevalence of high blood pressure in children and adolescents, information that is critical for all parents to consider. Another important topic discussed is the intimate relationship between high blood pressure and so many other critical health issues and organ systems in your body.

Part 2 explores in detail the different active steps you and your family can take to prevent and treat high blood pressure efficiently and safely. Does high blood pressure run in your family? That's no excuse to throw up your hands and think there's nothing you can do about it: in fact, there are plenty of steps you can take immediately, and the majority of them involve convenient lifestyle changes. That's why in part 2 you will learn how to choose and incorporate the changes that most suit your lifestyle, including:

- Diet, with a look at three different dietary approaches (with recipes)

- Physical activity

- Lifestyle factors (e.g., weight loss and healthy weight control, sleep, alcohol use, smoking)

- Nutritional and herbal remedies

- Stress management techniques for your body and mind, including methods such as acupressure, biofeedback, laughter, and meditation

- Medications for high blood pressure, including risks and benefits

Each chapter will provide you with enough detailed information so you can try the different prevention and treatment options (with your health-care professional's knowledge, of course) or have the steps at your fingertips so you can take action now. The descriptions of each therapy or activity will include its benefits and risks, how to use it (as applicable), and scientific evidence that backs up its use.

High blood pressure may be silent, but its effects can hit you loud and clear. Are you ready to take control of your blood pressure and enjoy the healthy life you deserve?

PART I

Introducing High Blood Pressure

CHAPTER ONE

High Blood Pressure Basics

You walk into your doctor's office and hop up on the examining table, and a nurse or physician's assistant comes in and takes your blood pressure. He or she than scribbles a few numbers on a sheet of paper (or enters them into a computer) and prepares to leave the room. Before the health-care individual leaves, you might inquire, "How's my blood pressure?"

But what exactly do you know about blood pressure? Do you understand the significance of the figures your health-care professional tells you? What is considered to be a "healthy" blood pressure for someone of your age, health status, and weight? Do the figures really represent your blood pressure, or are there some factors that have influenced or distorted your pressure that day? How many times and how often should you have your blood pressure checked?

HIGH BLOOD PRESSURE: BY THE NUMBERS

More than 73 million men and women in the United States—about three times the number who have diabetes and about one-third of the adult population—have high blood pressure. Unfortunately, an estimated 20 to

30 percent of people are unaware their blood pressure is high. In addition, many people with hypertension do not fully appreciate the seriousness of high blood pressure. Ignorance, in this case, is not bliss.

One reason for this lackadaisical attitude is obvious . . . or should I say not obvious, since high blood pressure is a silent, invisible disease. Everyone with high blood pressure would likely be better off if every time their pressure rose above a certain point their nose lit up or their ears started to flap. Then it might get their attention!

And there's more. An additional 25 percent of adults have prehypertension, which means they are at risk for developing high blood pressure. These figures do not take into consideration the growing number of children and adolescents who have hypertension as well. Along with the incredible challenge to personal health, hypertension also costs the United States more than $76 billion in health-care services, medications, and missed workdays per year.

While these numbers are frightening enough, there is more:

- In growing numbers, high blood pressure is being diagnosed in younger and younger folks, including elementary-school–aged children. The long-term implications and health consequences of developing high blood pressure at a young age are enormous, and it is one of the concerns covered in this chapter and this entire book.

- About 66 percent of people older than age 65 have high blood pressure. Since many people in this age group are already dealing with other health problems and likely taking at least one medication, hypertension is a serious consideration.

- Even people who don't have high blood pressure at age 55 have a 90 percent chance of developing it within their lifetime. Thus the bottom line is, *nearly everyone can expect to have high blood pressure at some time during their lives.*

- Since high blood pressure is invisible and without symptoms, people tend to adopt the old "out of sight, out of mind" approach, but unfortunately, hypertension is not out of body. In fact, the impact of high blood pressure on the entire body is so significant, I dedicate an entire chapter to it.

None of this means, however, that you can't take steps to reduce and, dare I say, even prevent high blood pressure. Healthy management of hypertension is entirely possible and you can conveniently make it a part of your lifestyle.

Awareness of and knowledge about high blood pressure is of paramount concern among adults, however, not only because more men and women have this silent disease but also because they are the ones responsible for helping prevent the disease in children and adolescents and ensuring treatment if it does occur. Yes, high blood pressure can be a family affair.

So if you or a loved one can make the statement, "I have high blood pressure," let's help you better understand what's behind those words before exploring the many ways you can manage the disease.

WHAT IS HIGH BLOOD PRESSURE?

High blood pressure, or hypertension, is a condition in which the force of the blood on the artery walls as it travels throughout the body is greater than values that have been determined to be healthful. Those values are known as systolic and diastolic blood pressure. When a doctor tells you your blood pressure is 130/80 mmHg, it means your systolic pressure is 130 and your diastolic pressure is 80 millimeters of mercury (more on measuring blood pressure in chapter 2). One or both values can be too high, normal, or too low.

- Normal blood pressure is defined as 120/80 mmHg or lower.

- Prehypertension is defined as readings of greater than 120/80 mmHg to 139/89 mmHg.

- Stage 1 blood pressure is defined as 140 to 150 mmHg systolic or 90 to 99 mmHg diastolic.

- High blood pressure is defined as 140/90 mmHg or higher. However, high blood pressure is subdivided into stages: 140 to 159 mmHg systolic or 90 to 99 diastolic is stage 1; 160 mmHg systolic or higher or 100 mmHg diastolic or higher is stage 2.

- Systolic pressure is the force of the blood on the artery walls when the heart contracts

- Diastolic pressure is the pressure on the artery walls when the heart is relaxing, between beats

Blood pressure is a very fluid phenomenon, because it changes to meet your body's needs. Thus your blood pressure while you are propped up on the couch and reading a novel on your tablet will be different from your blood pressure when you are preparing dinner or racing up the stairs because you are late for a meeting at work. All of these changes in blood pressure are normal.

However, if your blood pressure remains in a high or abnormal range even when you are relaxing and then goes even higher to meet other situations in your life, then you have high blood pressure. But not all high blood pressure is the same, so let's look at the different types before going any further.

Essential Hypertension

Two other terms with which you should become familiar are "essential" or "primary hypertension" and "secondary hypertension." Essential hypertension is by far the most common type of high blood pressure, accounting for about 90 percent of all cases. This type of hypertension is also referred to as idiopathic because its cause is unknown, although it is generally associated with lifestyle factors (e.g., diet, overweight, lack of exercise, stress) and genetics. If you are wondering why experts do not know *exactly* what causes a condition as common as high blood pressure, the best I can say is that they are zeroing in on understanding the cause. In the meantime, they are gaining a much better understanding of the contributing factors, which you can read about in this chapter under "Why People Get High Blood Pressure."

WHY PEOPLE GET HIGH BLOOD PRESSURE

I have already mentioned that experts do not know exactly what causes high blood pressure. However, that does not mean they have not come up with a list of potential and likely suspects that have been shown to contribute to or be associated with its development. The list consists of <u>two major categories</u>: things people cannot change and things they can change. Obviously you want to focus on the factors you can change, but it's also good to know that even though there are some things you can't change, you *can still have an effect on them.* For example, you can't change the fact that high blood pressure runs in your family, but you can take steps toward modifying or eliminating certain lifestyle risk factors and significantly improve your chances of resisting high blood pressure.

The following list is not complete—scientists are continuously researching the origins, prevention, and treatment of high blood pressure, so there may be more factors to come. However, it represents what researchers have discovered thus far about high blood pressure. Do any of the following risk factors for high blood pressure apply to you?

Factors You Can't Change—but Can Influence

- **Ethnicity.** High on the list of risk factors you cannot change is your ethnicity. In the United States, African Americans are twice as likely as whites to have high blood pressure. That percentage declines somewhat around age 44, but the risk among blacks still remains higher than among whites. Among older adults (older than

65), black women have the highest incidence of hypertension.

- **Age.** The older you get, the greater your risk of developing high blood pressure. That's because aging is associated with more wear and tear on your blood vessels, more opportunity for the negative effects of other risk factors (e.g., poor diet, smoking, alcohol, and so on) to do their damage, and the like. So, as you can see, while getting older is a risk factor, you can still influence the degree to which it has an impact. Unfortunately, there is another angle to age and hypertension. An increasing number of young people—children and adolescents—have high blood pressure. According to a study in *BMC Pediatrics,* 21 percent of schoolchildren ages 8 to 13 had high blood pressure. The prevalence was especially high among overweight and obese children and Hispanic youngsters.[1] Another unfortunate situation is that many of these cases are not diagnosed because people generally don't associate hypertension with children. The topic of high blood pressure in children is important especially for parents to understand, and it is addressed in more detail in chapter 2.

- **Genetics.** If your mom, dad, grandparents, and/or siblings have high blood pressure, your chances are increased. Research suggests that about 25 to 30 percent of cases of essential hypertension are associated with genetic factors. So far, however, experts have not identified which genes are responsible for high blood pressure.

- **Gender.** A greater percentage of men than women develop high blood pressure up to about age 45. Both women and men have similar chances of developing high blood pressure between the ages of 45 and 64, after which time a greater percentage of women develop hypertension.

Factors You Can Change

- **Salt.** A high-salt diet can cause the body to retain excess water, which in turn causes the blood volume to expand, which then causes blood pressure to rise. Although everyone is not equally sensitive to salt, most people who have high blood pressure have some sensitivity to the sodium in salt. The association between high salt intake and high blood pressure can be seen especially among a group of people who live on the northern islands of Japan. These individuals consume more salt than people anywhere else in the world, and they also have the highest incidence of essential hypertension in the world. Salt is discussed in chapter 3 on diet.

- **Stress.** Stress plays a complicated role in blood pressure and heart health. One way it has an impact is that it activates the sympathetic nervous system, which results in more rigid arteries and thus a rise in blood pressure. You can learn to manage stress . . . before it manages you and your blood pressure.

- **Alcohol.** Experts say it doesn't take much alcohol to send your blood pressure higher, as well as increase your risk of irregular heartbeats, stroke, and heart failure. Intake in excess of one drink daily for women and two drinks for men can contribute to hypertension. Excess alcohol also can raise triglyceride levels.

• **Overweight/obesity.** Being overweight or obese is a significant risk factor for high blood pressure. If your body mass index (BMI) is between 25 and 30, you are considered overweight. A BMI greater than 30 is considered obesity. People who carry excess weight may have elevated production of insulin and higher blood volume, and the burden of extra pounds can make the heart work harder. Being overweight or obese also raises cholesterol and triglyceride levels while lowering levels of good cholesterol (HDL cholesterol) and raising the risk of developing diabetes.

• **Diet low in calcium, magnesium, and potassium.** These three minerals have an intimate relationship when it comes to blood pressure, and maintaining a healthy balance between them goes a long way toward avoiding high blood pressure. Thus it is critical to adopt eating habits that provide a balance of calcium, magnesium, and potassium.

• **Lack of physical exercise.** Engaging in regular physical activity promotes healthy blood circulation and heart muscle, both of which support a healthy blood pressure. Inactivity also contributes to obesity, another risk factor for hypertension.

- **Insulin resistance/diabetes.** Insulin resistance is when the body does not respond properly to insulin. Because the body cannot respond normally, the pancreas secretes more insulin, which results in high levels of insulin in the blood. Over time, people with insulin resistance can develop high levels of glucose (sugar) in the blood and thus diabetes. Insulin resistance can cause blood pressure to rise as a result of the inflammation associated with diabetes.

- **Smoking.** If you smoke, you not only temporarily raise your blood pressure every time you light up; you also damage your blood vessels. Even if you don't smoke, exposure to secondhand smoke can increase your risk of heart disease. It seems clear that smoking at any level is a health risk!

- **Elevated C-reactive protein.** You may be wondering how you can change a factor you know nothing about and perhaps never heard of until now. C-reactive protein is a substance in the blood that indicates the presence of inflammation, and inflammation is a predictor of the development of high blood pressure, as well as cardiovascular disease, in some people. Levels of C-reactive protein can be reduced by making dietary changes, and so it is a risk factor that you can influence.

- **Obstructive sleep apnea.** Do you snore, breathe with stops and starts, and wake up feeling like you didn't sleep well? You may have obstructive sleep apnea, a common condition in which people stop breathing for several seconds or longer while sleeping. It's estimated that nearly 20 percent of adults in the United States have some degree of sleep apnea, yet only about 10 percent have been diagnosed. In obstructive sleep apnea, the airways become blocked or narrowed and people do not get enough oxygen, which in turn causes damage to the blood vessel walls. This sleep disorder is a risk factor for both high blood pressure and heart disease. Sleep apnea also stimulates the nervous system to release chemicals that can cause blood pressure to rise.

And the Result Is . . .

Most people who have essential hypertension have stiff or inelastic arterioles, which are the tiny peripheral arteries the farthest away from the heart. Arterioles may be small, but they play a critical role in your health and in blood pressure. Specifically, arterioles transport oxygen-rich blood and nutrients to all the tissues in the body via even smaller blood vessels called capillaries. Once the oxygen has been delivered, veins carry the oxygen-depleted blood to the lungs and heart.

This brings us back to the basic question as to what exactly causes high blood pressure. Although scientists know these peripheral arteries get stiff and thus cause blood pressure to rise, they don't know exactly what makes the arterioles become stiff. That's where the risk factors come into the picture, because people with essential hypertension tend to have several of these factors, including genetic influences.

ENERGY DRINKS AND HIGH BLOOD PRESSURE

Energy drinks such as Red Bull, Monster, and 5-Hour Energy, for example, may do more than give you a shot of energy: they also can cause your blood pressure to spike and have a negative effect on your heart's natural rhythm. Research presented at the American Heart Association's Epidemiology and Prevention/Nutrition, Physical Activity, and Metabolism 2013 Scientific Sessions revealed that among 132 healthy adults tested, those who drank one to three energy drinks experienced an average rise in systolic blood pressure of 3.5 points. In a subgroup of 93 individuals, the QT interval was 10 milliseconds longer. The "QT interval" refers to a portion of the heart's rhythm on an electrocardiogram. When it is prolonged, it can cause sudden cardiac death or serious irregular heartbeats. While this study was done in healthy adults, the impact on people who already have high blood pressure and/or a heart condition could be more pronounced and hazardous.[2]

OTHER TYPES OF HYPERTENSION

Since essential hypertension makes up the majority of cases of high blood pressure, it is the focus of this book. However, there are several other types of high blood pressure that, although much less common, are still important. In fact, these lesser-known types of high blood pressure can develop as complications of essential high blood pressure, so it is helpful for patients and physicians to be aware of their existence and how to recognize them. With that in mind, let's take a brief look at these "other" types of high blood pressure.

Secondary Hypertension

Secondary hypertension makes up about 5 percent of all cases of hypertension. Like essential hypertension, secondary hypertension typically has no symptoms and so may be present without a person's knowledge. Secondary hypertension gets its name from the fact that it develops as a result of (secondary to) an underlying health problem or use of medications that affect different organs or systems in the body, including the heart, arteries, endocrine system, and kidneys.

The following is a list of conditions that are frequently associated with secondary hypertension. If you have any of these conditions, be sure to have your blood pressure checked regularly:

- **Diabetes.** Although you can have essential high blood pressure prior to or along with diabetes, secondary hypertension may develop in individuals who have a diabetic complication known as diabetic nephropathy (kidney damage). When high blood sugar levels damage the kidneys' ability to filter blood and toxins, secondary high blood pressure can result.

- **Pregnancy.** Being pregnant can have two effects on blood pressure. One, it can worsen hypertension among women who already have high blood pressure. Therefore, any woman who has high blood pressure and then gets pregnant needs to discuss safe treatment approaches with her doctor. Two, some pregnant women develop hypertension during pregnancy. This is called preeclampsia, a condition in which a pregnant woman develops high blood pressure

- **Cushing's syndrome.** This condition causes the pituitary gland to manufacture too much cortisol, a stress hormone. Elevated cortisol levels can in turn raise blood pressure.

- **Glomerular disease.** This kidney condition is characterized by swollen glomeruli, which are minute filters in the kidneys. Swollen glomeruli malfunction, which in turn can result in high blood pressure.

- **Aldosteronism.** This is a condition in which a tumor or other factors cause the adrenal glands, which are located on top of the kidneys, to produce too much of the hormone aldosterone. This excess amount of aldosterone in turn causes the kidneys to hold on to water and salt while giving up too much potassium. The combination of these events raises blood pressure.

- **Hypothyroidism and hyperthyroidism.** Whenever the thyroid gland, which resides in the neck, doesn't function the way it should, high blood pressure can result. Therefore, if the thyroid gland makes too much thyroid hormone (hyperthyroidism) or too little (hypothyroidism), hypertension can result.

- **Hyperparathyroidism.** The four tiny parathyroid glands, located behind the thyroid in the neck, are responsible for regulating levels of calcium and phosphorus in the body. If these glands release too much parathyroid hormone, calcium levels in the blood rise, which results in high blood pressure.

- **Obstructive sleep apnea.** This condition has already been mentioned as a risk factor for essential hypertension, but it also may present as the primary disorder. Your doctor can help make that determination. Obstructive sleep apnea is also discussed in chapter 5.

- **Obesity.** Being overweight or obese is a risk factor for essential hypertension, but it also may be the primary underlying condition behind hypertension.

- **Drug and supplement use.** Both prescription and over-the-counter medications—as well as illegal drugs such as cocaine and methamphetamine—can lead to high blood pressure. Hypertension can be associated with the use of antidepressants, pain relievers, birth control pills, decongestants, and some herbal remedies such as ginseng and St. John's wort. (See "Medications That Can Raise Blood Pressure" in chapter 8.)

More Types of High Blood Pressure

Several other types of hypertension are much less common, but they are still worth mentioning, especially since they can occur as complications of essential high blood pressure and have a negative impact on your health.

One of these special types of high blood pressure is commonly referred to as "white-coat hypertension." You may be familiar with this phenomenon: your blood pressure spikes or rises when you are in the doctor's office. Your blood pressure may rise because you are anxious or worried about what the doctor will tell you or perhaps because you are tired of waiting a long time to see the doctor. Whatever the reason, visiting the doctor is stressful for many people and can cause a temporary increase in a person's blood pressure. But there may be more to the story.

Now some experts believe that while white-coat hypertension may be nothing serious, it also may shine a light on individuals who are susceptible to a variety of stressors. That is, if visiting the doctor elevates blood pressure, so may a multitude of other events or situations the individual finds stressful. That means stress could play a significant role in that individual's problem with hypertension and this risk factor should be explored further. Therefore, both you and your doctor should not simply dismiss elevated blood pressure that appears to be associated with a doctor's office visit.

Some other less common types of hypertension include the following:

- **Malignant hypertension.** This is a potentially deadly condition that usually develops rapidly and quickly leads to organ damage, such as liver failure, brain damage, and bleeding in the eyes. People with malignant hypertension typically have a diastolic blood pressure value of 130 mmHg or higher. This type of hypertension affects about 1 percent of people who have high blood pressure and can affect both children and adults. In fact, it is more likely to occur in younger adults, especially if they are black men. It also can occur in individuals who have kidney conditions or collagen vascular disorder or women who have toxemia of pregnancy. Unlike essential hypertension, malignant hypertension has symptoms that can include blurry vision, fatigue, chest pain, cough, headache, confusion, nausea or vomiting, seizures, shortness of breath, and weakness of the limbs, face, or other areas of the body.

• **Pseudohypertension.** When is high blood pressure technically not *really* high? When it is pseudohypertension, also known as Osler's sign. Pseudohypertension is a condition in which the blood pressure reading on the sphygmomanometer (device that gives the blood pressure reading) is elevated, but the reason is because the person had calcified blood vessels. Because calcified blood vessels are physically incapable of compressing with pressure they technically do not indicate high blood pressure. In fact, if people with pseudohypertension are treated for high blood pressure, they can experience low blood pressure and symptoms such as fainting, dizziness, and confusion. Although pseudohypertension is not common, the risk increases with age.

• **Pulmonary hypertension.** This is a special type of high blood pressure because it affects only one part of the circulatory system: the arteries that carry oxygen-poor blood from the heart to the lungs become narrow and hard. Pulmonary hypertension is a chronic condition that interferes with both the ability of the lungs to carry oxygen and the heart's ability to pump blood, which makes it especially dangerous. In fact, untreated pulmonary hypertension can result in right heart failure. Symptoms include shortness of breath, fatigue, and dizziness. Pulmonary hypertension can affect people of any age, including children. Although it can be treated, there is no cure for pulmonary hypertension.

• **Resistant hypertension.** This type of high blood pressure initially appears as regular hypertension, but then it does not respond to treatment that typically helps most patients. In fact, the 2008 American Heart Association scientific statement regarding resistant hypertension notes that anyone who has high blood pressure despite treatment with three antihypertensive agents from different drug classes is said to have resistant hypertension.[3] Experts are concerned about resistant hypertension for several reasons, one of which is the rapidly aging population and the rise in obesity. These are the strongest risk factors for uncontrolled high blood pressure. Anyone who has resistant hypertension is at significant risk of cardiovascular disease, especially if the condition is not managed as soon as possible. In addition, people with resistant hypertension typically have other cardiovascular risk factors, such as sleep apnea, kidney problems, and diabetes, all of which also need attention. Most people with resistant hypertension usually have isolated systolic hypertension as well.

- **Labile hypertension.** You may hear the term "labile hypertension," which many physicians say is an inappropriate phrase used to describe individuals whose blood pressure is abnormally variable, because they claim nearly everyone has some degree of labile blood pressure. However, the presence of unusually variable blood pressure may indicate that something serious is going on, such as a brain tumor, although this is extremely rare. Since the nature of labile hypertension is uncertainty, doctors are hesitant to prescribe any medications to treat it because the drugs may cause blood pressure to go too low. Anyone with labile hypertension who suffers with anxiety should be treated for the anxiety, which may then cause blood pressure to return to normal. Otherwise, following the natural approaches to managing high blood pressure in this book can help make any fluctuations in blood pressure less severe.

DIASTOLIC AND SYSTOLIC PRESSURES

Both systolic and diastolic blood pressure values are important, but they mean different things and provide different clues to a person's health. For example, among people who are 50 and older systolic pressure values provide a more realistic picture of high blood pressure. In fact, diastolic pressure does not need to be in a high range for people to be diagnosed with high blood pressure. But when systolic pressure is high, as is common among people of middle age and older, this is known as isolated systolic hypertension.

Isolated systolic high blood pressure is the most common form of hypertension among older adults in the United States. Although both systolic and diastolic blood pressures tend to rise with age, around age 55 diastolic pressure begins to decline. This leaves about 65 percent or so of older Americans with isolated systolic high blood pressure, which is a risk factor for heart attack, stroke, kidney damage, blindness, and other serious health conditions.

Isolated systolic high blood pressure is characterized by a systolic pressure that is greater than 140 mmHg but a diastolic pressure that is less than 90 mmHg. The wide gap between the two figures places people who have isolated systolic hypertension at increased risk of a heart attack, stroke, enlarged heart, and death from heart disease.

The case of isolated systolic high blood pressure is good news/bad news. The good news is that you can manage this form of high blood pressure with lifestyle changes and medications (if necessary). Research has shown that treating isolated systolic hypertension can significantly improve quality of life and reduce the risk of developing other health problems.

Even though there is no cure for this form of high blood pressure, effective management is completely possible. However, most adults with isolated systolic hypertension do not have it under control. If you fall into this latter category, then it's time to talk to your health-care provider about the steps you can take, both complementary and conventional, to change it, and the suggestions in this book are a good place to start.

Diastolic pressure has its own special features, especially for younger individuals. The higher the diastolic blood pressure, the greater is a person's risk for heart attack, kidney failure, and stroke. As people get older, their diastolic pressure begins to decline while the systolic pressure rises.

DIAGNOSING HIGH BLOOD PRESSURE

High blood pressure is not only silent (i.e., typically has no symptoms); it is also sly and sneaky. Here's why I say that: You are probably thinking, "It's easy to diagnose high blood pressure: a nurse or doctor takes your blood pressure, and if it's high, then you have high blood pressure. What's so hard about that?"

But not so fast! Remember I mentioned something called white-coat hypertension? That could give your doctor a false reading. There also is secondary hypertension, so you could have high blood pressure that is associated with a disease that you may or may not have had diagnosed. Your blood pressure also depends on other factors, such as your age, current level of emotional stress, activity level, presence of heart disease, and the use of any over-the-counter or prescription medications or supplements you are taking. Do you regularly consume energy drinks or lots of coffee? These beverages could raise your blood pressure as well.

How Doctors Diagnose Hypertension

Blood pressure is measured using a device called a sphygmomanometer, which consists of an arm cuff, gauge, pump, valve, and stethoscope. You can have your blood pressure checked in your arm by a doctor or nurse during an office visit or at a pharmacy, clinic, or health fair, or you can do it yourself using a blood pressure monitor for home use, available from a pharmacy or online (see "DIY Blood Pressure Monitoring").

To make a diagnosis of high blood pressure, you should have your blood pressure checked at least three different times. Before each reading, you should have spent at least five minutes resting comfortably, and you should have your pressure taken while you are seated. Why?

Quite simply, it's the way the original clinical trials on blood pressure were conducted and the information from those trials provides the gold standard for measuring blood pressure today. Yes, blood pressure readings are often taken while people are lying down or even while standing. However, there can be significant changes in people's blood pressure when they change position from lying to sitting or standing.

Typically, the systolic value tends to be lower when you are sitting than when you are lying down, while the diastolic value tends to be somewhat higher when you are sitting than when you are lying down. These fluctuations in blood pressure are associated with the sympathetic nervous system responding to your posture changes. For some people, the fluctuations are minor, but for others, they can be significant. All of this is important information for a doctor to know when deciding how to treat someone who has high blood pressure.

Three elevated readings (see "What is High Blood Pressure?") are usually necessary before a doctor will declare that you have high blood pressure. Along with taking blood pressure readings, your doctor will ask about your personal and family medical history (especially past or current heart problems or blood pressure issues) and the presence of risk factors for high blood pressure, such as smoking and alcohol use.

A physical examination should include the doctor listening to your heart through a stethoscope to determine if there are any sounds that suggest a blockage.

Your doctor should also check the pulses in your ankles and arm.

If there are indications you have high blood pressure, the next step may be additional tests, especially if there are any indications of cardiovascular problems. Those tests may include any of the following:

- An electrocardiogram (EKG or ECG), which measures the electrical activity of your heart. Information from this test can help doctors determine if there is any damage to the heart muscle, which is a common complication of hypertension.

- An echocardiogram, which uses ultrasound waves to provide images of the heart's valves and chambers so the heart's pumping activity can be observed and the thickness of the heart's walls can be measured.

- Blood tests to determine levels of electrolytes, blood urea, and creatine. These are all substances that can help your doctor assess kidney function.

- Urine tests for electrolytes and hormone levels.

- Lipid profiles, which includes measurement of all the types of cholesterol as well as triglycerides.

- An eye examination by an ophthalmologist to look for any damage in the eyes, which can occur with high blood pressure. Be sure to check out "Blood Pressure and Your Eyes" in chapter 2.

• Doppler ultrasound, which checks blood flow through the arteries to areas farthest from the heart: arms, legs, hands, and feet. This test can help detect peripheral vascular disease, which is common among people who have high blood pressure.

Measuring Blood Pressure in the Ankles

Another way to measure blood pressure is in the ankles. Doctors occasionally take an ankle pressure to compare pressure in the legs to that in the arms, which is helpful in detecting peripheral artery disease (blocked arteries). Sometimes a person's upper arm is too large to place a blood pressure cuff comfortably or there may be an injury to the upper arm that makes taking a blood pressure painful.

The ankle brachial index (ABI) is the ratio of the blood pressure taken in the lower legs to the blood pressure in the arms. If the blood pressure in your lower leg is lower than that in your arm, this indicates peripheral vascular disease. A doctor determines the ABI by dividing the systolic blood pressure at the ankle by the systolic blood pressure in the arm.

You should be lying down when having your blood pressure taken in the ankles. The blood pressure cuff should be wrapped around the ankle so that the cuff is one inch above the bony part that sticks out from either side of the ankle, and it should not be placed over clothing. The stethoscope is placed against the front of the ankle and on the artery, just below the bottom of the cuff.

Getting accurate readings on the ABI can be challenging, so it typically is done by a skilled health-care provider. For that reason, individuals usually do not do ankle blood pressure readings at home (see "DIY Blood

Pressure Monitoring"). However, if your doctor wants you to check your ankle pressure, be sure to get some professional guidance and practice.

Ambulatory Monitoring

Sometimes a doctor orders ambulatory blood pressure monitoring, which provides a twenty-four-hour record of blood pressure levels recorded every fifteen to thirty minutes. Ambulatory blood pressure monitoring is frequently used for individuals who have severe hypertension or for those who have white-coat hypertension, and it is also helpful for identifying how well medications are working and to detect morning spikes in blood pressure. The regular readings from ambulatory monitoring can provide doctors with an accurate look at a patient's average blood pressure during the day.

DIY BLOOD PRESSURE MONITORING

The American Heart Association (AHA) and other medical associations recommend that people who have high blood pressure purchase a blood pressure monitor for home use. In addition, the AHA and various other medical associations recommend people purchase an automatic, cuff-style, upper-arm monitor, as both the wrist and finger monitors are not as accurate.

Home blood pressure monitors can be a great tool to have in just about anyone's home, but they are especially good for certain populations. Older people, whose blood pressure often varies because of health reasons and/or medications they are taking, can benefit from having a monitor at their fingertips. People with diabetes also should test their blood pressure at home, since tight control of hypertension is important. Home testing machines are also helpful for anyone monitoring his or her use of blood pressure treatments (be it medications, natural supplements, lifestyle changes, or a combination) as well as for any people who have difficulty getting to a doctor or facility to have blood pressure checked often.

Home testing of blood pressure allows you to take some control of your health care and monitor your pressure over time in the comfort of your own home. Home testing of blood pressure can actually provide more accurate readings than those you get at a doctor's office (but that doesn't mean you should forego professional readings!). Why? One reason is white-coat hypertension; another is you have the luxury of taking your time to get several readings rather than being rushed in a doctor's office.

Getting a Home Blood Pressure Monitor

When preparing to buy a home blood pressure monitor, take your time. Consult with your health-care provider before choosing a home blood pressure device. You now get to choose from both conventional home blood pressure monitoring machines as well as those designed to work with apps with your iPad or iPhone. These latter monitors may present a challenge until you get used to them. Some of the blood pressure systems for use with your iPad or iPhone allow your readings to be shared on Twitter and Facebook or to connect with health records sites such as myMediConnect. Your doctor also may be able to tell you which apps provide the most accurate readings.

Home testing devices for blood pressure are available at pharmacies and medical supply facilities and online. When shopping for a home blood pressure monitor, be sure to choose one with a cuff that fits your upper arm. It's not always true that one size fits all! If you buy a wrist or finger model, they are designed as one size fits all. (Remember, these types of blood pressure monitors are less accurate than an arm model.) Be sure you can read the display on the gauge or monitor and that you understand how to apply the cuff and operate the monitor.

Some home blood pressure monitors offer extra features, such as an ability to store your readings or to record your heart rate as well as your blood pressure. You may be tempted to buy your home blood pressure monitor online, and if you do be sure you have seen and tested the product in a store or elsewhere before making your purchase. Also, in some cases, insurance plans cover the cost of blood pressure monitors.

Last, be sure your monitor has been tested, validated, and approved by the Association for the Advancement of Medical Instrumentation. Other approved organizations include the British Hypertension Society and the European Society of Hypertension, which offers an International Protocol for the Validation of Automated BP Measuring Devices.

Please don't hesitate to ask your doctor, pharmacist, or other health professional how to use any home monitoring device if you are uncertain. After all, you are trying to keep your blood pressure down, not cause it to rise by getting stressed over trying to figure out how the monitor works!

Using a Home Blood Pressure Monitor

Once you are comfortable using your home blood pressure monitor, remember a few guidelines.

One is to always follow the five-minute rule: rest for at least five minutes before you take your blood pressure.

Therefore, if you are dashing around the pharmacy picking up needed items and you see a DIY blood pressure machine sitting in the corner you should rest for five minutes before you use it to take your blood pressure.

Similarly, do not use your home blood pressure monitor within thirty minutes of exercising, smoking, or drinking coffee.

Sit properly. The best position for taking blood pressure is while sitting in a chair with your back straight, your feet flat on the floor, your arms supported on a table so the upper part of your testing arm is at the level of your heart.

Place the cuff properly. The middle of the cuff should be directly above the crook of your elbow. Ask your health-care provider or pharmacist to show you how to position the cuff on your upper arm.

Take several readings. At every measuring session, take two or three readings at least one minute apart.

Measure at the same time every day. Ask your doctor which time of the day you should always check your blood pressure and do it the same time each day.

Keep records. Don't forget to record the time, date, and blood pressure readings for each session in a notebook. You can take this information with you on your office visits. If you use an app with an iPad or iPhone for blood pressure, this information can be sent to your computer and to your doctor. The AHA also has a blood pressure tracking tool online. Called Heart360, it allows you to track your blood pressure and which steps you are taking to manage it online. There is also a feature that lets you share the information with your doctor electronically.

CHAPTER TWO

High Blood Pressure and Your Body

You already know high blood pressure is a sneaky condition, but are you aware of all the incredible effects it can have on your body? Even more important is the fact that you have the power to make sure those effects and any related complications are minimized and even eliminated by taking a number of steps, as discussed in part 2 of this book.

For now, however, it's helpful for you to appreciate the relationship high blood pressure has with various critical organ systems, serious diseases, and other health situations. Why? Foremost, I hope this knowledge will impress upon you the importance of managing a condition that is virtually invisible. Out of sight, out of mind, right? This is not a good saying to follow when it comes to your blood pressure. The fact is, blood pressure is a whole-body condition, because blood—and thus blood pressure—reaches every part of your body, from your head to your toes. If you read through this chapter—and I highly suggest that you do—you will realize the *truly intimate and intense relationship between high blood pressure and many other serious and important health conditions.* In addition, if you successfully reduce your high blood pressure you will have a beneficial impact on your cardiovascular health and your risk of diabetes, dementia, kidney disease, obesity, high cholesterol, and vision problems. What a bonus!

Another reason it's crucial to appreciate high blood pressure is the impact it can have on young people. If you are a parent, grandparent, or other adult who cares for any children at all, you have the power to help prevent the development of high blood pressure and its future consequences in young people, because, unfortunately, hypertension is a growing problem among young children and adolescents.

High blood pressure can cause damage throughout your body and mind, and the consequences can be life threatening and long lasting. However, as you read through this chapter, keep in mind that while these relationships between high blood pressure and other health issues are hazardous, you *do* have the power to prevent them.

ENDOTHELIAL FUNCTION

A term you will see in this book is "endothelial function," so here's a quick and simple explanation of what it means and why you should know about it: The endothelium is the inner lining of blood vessels, and a healthy endothelium is critical for healthy blood flow. When the endothelium is functioning properly, it helps to regulate blood clotting, regulates the volume of fluid and the amount of electrolytes and other substances that pass from the blood into the body's tissues, assists with the immune system, and produces the dilation or constriction of the blood vessels.

If the endothelium is compromised in any way and thus unable to perform any of these functions at an optimal level, the condition is referred to as endothelial dysfunction. This condition is believed to play a major role in the development of atherosclerosis, or hardening of the arteries, and can be caused by several factors, including high blood pressure, diabetes, smoking, and lack of physical activity. In other words, endothelial dysfunction is just one of many players in the world of high blood pressure and the various related conditions.

HIGH BLOOD PRESSURE AND CARDIOVASCULAR DISEASE

Perhaps the relationship that is easiest to appreciate is the one between high blood pressure and cardiovascular disease, which includes heart-related conditions (e.g., heart failure, heart attack, congestive heart failure, coronary heart disease, angina) and stroke. Hypertension is one of the most common and powerful risk factors for cardiovascular disease. An estimated 25 percent of adults have cardiovascular disease, resulting in about 7.1 million deaths per year.

It's no secret that hypertension places excessive tension on the heart and blood vessels. Indeed, it's a fact that leads some people to envision high blood pressure causing a blood vessel to erupt in the brain, causing a stroke. Although a blood vessel certainly can burst and cause this cardiovascular event, it's not the main problem people encounter when they have high blood pressure. In fact, the impact of hypertension on the heart and cardiovascular system is more subtle yet pervasive: it contributes to a heart that needs to work harder to pump blood throughout the body.

The higher your blood pressure, the more damage occurs to the inner lining of your arteries and other blood vessels. This damage triggers events that leave your artery walls stiff and thick (a condition called arteriosclerosis). This damage sets up your arteries to attract cholesterol and other fats (see "High Blood Pressure and Cholesterol"). Other cardiovascular events also can develop, including heart failure, coronary artery disease, enlarged heart, angina, stroke, peripheral arterial disease, and heart attack. In some individuals, the persistent high pressure against the arteries can cause a bulge (aneurysm) in the arterial wall. If this aneurysm ruptures, it can cause life-threatening internal bleeding.

Don't forget that stroke is considered to be a cardiovascular event, and so the risks of transient ischemic attack (TIA) and stroke are associated with heart and blood vessel events when we talk about hypertension. A transient ischemic attack, or ministroke, is a temporary interruption of blood supply to the brain. A TIA can be caused by atherosclerosis or a blood clot, both of which can result from high blood pressure. A stroke occurs when your brain does not receive oxygen and nutrients, which in turn causes brain cells to die. Hypertension can contribute to stroke in two ways, one of which is its part in the formation of blood clots that can travel to the brain and the other of which is by causing damage to the blood vessels in the brain.

Women, Hypertension, and Cardiovascular Disease

Even though cardiovascular disease is the number one killer of both men and women, the seriousness of this fact seems to escape many women. Breast cancer will be the cause of death for about 16 percent of women, while cardiovascular disease will claim the lives of about 50 percent of women. Yet women are much more aware and afraid of breast cancer.

That's one reason why I am taking some time to emphasize the importance of women taking charge of their hypertension. Most women are unaware that high blood pressure has a greater impact on them than it does on men. For one thing, women's risk of having a repeat heart attack, stroke, or other cardiovascular episode increases as their blood pressure rises. A study conducted at Brigham and Women's Hospital found that a woman's risk of experiencing a cardiovascular event rose 28 percent when her systolic blood pressure was between 130 and 139 compared to a systolic pressure of 120 to 129.[1]

Women face some unique challenges when it comes to high blood pressure. One challenge is pregnancy, which is discussed separately later in this chapter. Another challenge is the use of birth control pills. Taking oral contraceptives is associated with elevated blood pressure in some women, especially those who are overweight and/or those who smoke.

Yet another challenge women sometimes face when it comes to hypertension is obesity. Women, more than men, tend to gain weight as they age, and this tendency is largely associated with menopause. The added weight increases the risk and dangers of high blood pressure.

HIGH BLOOD PRESSURE AND DIABETES

The combination of high blood pressure and diabetes is an especially volatile situation. According to the Third National Health and Nutrition Survey, 71 percent of all people with diabetes in the United States have high blood pressure, yet 29 percent of them don't even know it. Another 43 percent are not being treated for hypertension. What do blood sugar levels have to do with blood pressure? Plenty. For one, hypertension is an important risk factor for the development and the progression of diabetes, including complications associated with the metabolic disease. Among the many complications of diabetes are conditions also associated with high blood pressure, such as vision problems, heart disease, and kidney disease.

Another factor is that most people with diabetes develop hypertension at some point during their life. Why? Because diabetes is associated with high levels of sugar in the blood, which damages the blood vessels and increases the risk of developing hypertension and other cardiovascular problems. Because of this increased risk, anyone who has diabetes should attempt to achieve a blood pressure of less than 130/80 mmHg, as compared with 140/80 mmHg for people with the disease, since having diabetes is an additional stress on the body.

That stress can be significant. For example, research shows that people with diabetes are five times more likely to experience a stroke. After an initial stroke, they are two to four times more likely to have a second stroke.

Study after study has shown that the combination of diabetes and hypertension places individuals at great risk of cardiovascular events such as stroke or heart attack. For example, a University of Oklahoma study (*Hypertension*, 2006) evaluated people who participated in the Strong Heart Study. Over a twelve-year period, they followed more than twenty-six hundred adults and found that those with diabetes and prehypertension had nearly four times the risk of experiencing a cardiovascular

event as did nondiabetic individuals who had normal
blood pressure.[2]

The good news is that if you follow the suggestions
outlined in this book you can not only lower your blood
pressure but also reduce your risk of diabetes or, if you
have diabetes, improve your ability to manage the disease.
That's because the recommended ways to manage diabetes include attention to diet, regular exercise, achieving
and maintaining a healthy weight, stress management,
and other lifestyle modifications. If you follow these suggestions, you may even "cure" your diabetes and your
high blood pressure.

One other thing that closely links hypertension with
diabetes is the balance of calcium, magnesium, and potassium in the body. As you will learn in chapters 3
and 6, these minerals play a critical role in high blood
pressure. It also happens that these minerals, but especially magnesium, have an important role in diabetes as
well. Research has shown that people who have more
magnesium in their diet are less likely to develop diabetes
and hypertension.

Scientists then took the relationship even one step
further. They also found that low magnesium is associated with metabolic syndrome, a condition that includes
hypertension, overweight, insulin resistance (an inability
to properly utilize insulin), high triglyceride levels, and
lower than optimal levels of high-density lipoprotein
(HDL) cholesterol. People with metabolic syndrome frequently go on to develop type 2 diabetes. Magnesium has
been shown to lower triglyceride levels and to boost
HDL. As I mentioned earlier in this chapter, the inter-
relationship between hypertension and other health
conditions, such as diabetes, is pervasive.

If you have high blood pressure and either prediabetes

(a condition in which your blood sugar levels are not quite at the level recognized as diabetes) or diabetes, be sure to take action to combat both of these life-altering conditions. The chapters that follow provide a good launching point for that effort, and you are urged to consult a knowledgeable health-care provider to help you with your efforts.

HIGH BLOOD PRESSURE AND CHOLESTEROL

The relationship between high blood pressure and cholesterol is intimate at several levels. One is the fact that over time high blood pressure can speed up the deposition of cholesterol plaque in your arteries. Cholesterol is a waxy, soft lipid or fat that has many beneficial functions in the body, such as helping form cell membranes and various tissues. However, it also can accumulate in your arteries and other blood vessels, especially those damaged by high blood pressure, which can then lead to heart disease.

High blood pressure can also cause cholesterol to build up in other areas of the body, including the brain (which can lead to stroke), the kidneys (kidney failure), and the legs and feet (intermittent claudication, which is characterized by severe pain while walking). Thus, as you can see, high blood pressure and cholesterol have a relationship that ranges from head to toes.

Having high cholesterol is like having high blood pressure: there are no symptoms. Given that about two-thirds of people have high cholesterol (defined as a reading of 200 mg/dL or higher), there are lots of people walking around with this known risk factor for cardiovascular disease. The only way to know if you have high cholesterol is to take a blood test, which is recommended every five years for everyone age 20 and older. If you have high cholesterol and are taking steps to reduce it, you should have your levels checked more often to be sure you are on track.

The suggestions in this book, especially those on diet and exercise, are critical not only for lowering blood pressure but for helping reduce your cholesterol as well. That's right: when you lower your blood pressure, your cholesterol levels will likely decline as well. Conversely, as your blood pressure rises, so do the chances your cholesterol is inching up as well. So although this volume is not about how to lower your cholesterol, you may enjoy that benefit as well. If you need to address a high-cholesterol problem, there are many excellent natural options from which to choose and much online and print information to guide you through the process (see appendix).

HIGH BLOOD PRESSURE AND OBESITY

Overweight and obesity are caused by a number of factors, including genetic, metabolic, psychological, socio-cultural, and lifestyle (diet and exercise). Obesity is also a proven cause of hypertension. Nearly two-thirds of people who are obese are at risk of high blood pressure, as well as sleep apnea (which is also a risk factor for hypertension), coronary heart disease, and congestive heart failure.

Although experts are not entirely certain how obesity causes hypertension, they have a number of important clues, including the relationship between obesity and neuroendocrine activities. Any number of these activities can have a detrimental effect on blood pressure. Specifically, obesity affects what is known as the renin-angiotensin-aldosterone (RAA) system. The RAA system is responsible for several factors involved in hypertension, including blood volume, control of the sympathetic nervous system (which is involved in the body's internal organ function), sodium (salt) levels, and the amount of water retained by the body. All of these factors have a significant role in blood pressure, and since obesity disrupts each of them, the result can be high blood pressure. In addition, the accumulation of fatty tissue can result in kidney dysfunction, which can lead to hypertension.

The relationship between obesity and hypertension goes even further, as obesity is also associated with metabolic syndrome, a condition that often ultimately leads to type 2 diabetes, which is also associated with hypertension. So as you can see, several different conditions are closely related to high blood pressure and working to resolve one can help resolve others.

It's time for me to point out that losing weight is an important step toward managing high blood pressure and also for preventing cardiovascular disease, diabetes, and other related conditions. Help with weight loss is discussed in chapter 5 on lifestyle.

HIGH BLOOD PRESSURE AND KIDNEY DISEASE

High blood pressure and the health of your kidneys are closely related. In fact, hypertension is a leading cause of kidney disease and kidney failure. That's because high blood pressure causes damage to both the arteries that go to your kidneys and the minute blood vessels (glomeruli) that make up the filtering system in the kidneys, which makes it difficult for the organs to properly filter toxins from your body. Scarring of the glomeruli can result in glomerulosclerosis, which then leads to kidney failure and the need for either dialysis or a kidney transplant.

Like hypertension, kidney disease can be a bit sneaky, but there are some signs and symptoms of which to be aware. One is the presence of high blood pressure, but others include a change in your urination habits (e.g., it is more difficult to urinate or you are not urinating as much as you used to), fluid retention in your lower legs (e.g., swollen ankles or calves), and the need to urinate more often, especially during the night.

Along with having hypertension, there are other risk factors for kidney disease you should know. Therefore, if you are African American, Hispanic, or Native American and/or if you have diabetes or a family history of high blood pressure and kidney disease, you are at greater risk of developing kidney disease yourself. You and your doctor should discuss being tested for kidney disease, which includes lab tests that measure serum creatinine, protein in the urine, and blood urea nitrogen levels.

You can help prevent kidney damage associated with high blood pressure by keeping your blood pressure under control using the natural approaches discussed throughout this book. If your doctor has prescribed medication, discuss the risks and benefits of the drug and how you might reduce or eliminate your need for the medication.

HIGH BLOOD PRESSURE AND ALZHEIMER'S DISEASE

High blood pressure can have a detrimental effect on your brain, and that includes the possibility of mild cognitive impairment and dementia, including the most common type of dementia, Alzheimer's disease. For many years, experts have known that high blood pressure is associated with vascular dementia, a type of dementia that develops when individuals have a series of small strokes. Now increasing evidence indicates that hypertension is linked to Alzheimer's disease as well.

Mild cognitive impairment is a transition stage between a person's brain changes' effect on memory and understanding on a mild level and the more serious impact associated with Alzheimer's disease. Not everyone who has mild cognitive impairment goes on to develop Alzheimer's disease, but nearly everyone who has Alzheimer's disease first experienced mild cognitive impairment. Both mild cognitive impairment and dementia/ Alzheimer's disease can result from blockage of blood flow to the brain when hypertension damages the blood vessels. High blood pressure that appears in early life can increase a person's risk of dementia in later years.

A March 2013 study that appeared in *JAMA Neurology* indicated that people who control or prevent high blood pressure earlier in life may limit or delay the changes that occur in the brain associated with Alzheimer's disease and other dementias. Among those brain changes is the accumulation of a protein called beta-amyloid. The buildup of beta-amyloid has been implicated as a potential cause of Alzheimer's disease.

About 20 percent of the population has a specific type of gene called an APOE4, which makes these individuals more likely to have elevated levels of beta-amyloid. In this study, Dr. Karen Rodrigue, assistant professor at the University of Texas at Dallas Center for Vital Longevity, and her team found that people with APOE4 as well as high blood pressure were at greater risk of accumulation of beta-amyloid—and therefore at higher risk of developing Alzheimer's disease—than individuals without APOE4 or hypertension.[3]

Scientists have noted a link between high blood pressure and Alzheimer's disease regarding something called white-matter lesions. When high blood pressure damages the arteries, it causes a type of scarring called white-matter lesions. In the brain, white matter is involved in cell communication. When the blood vessels in the brain are impacted by white-matter lesions, it can affect memory and cognitive functioning.

In a Johns Hopkins study involving nearly one thousand adults, researchers found that the longer middle-aged people with high blood pressure did not adequately control their hypertension, the more white-matter damage they incurred. Evidence of the damage was seen on brain scans. One argument for managing high blood pressure as quickly as possible is that a rapid response lowers your risk of developing dementia or Alzheimer's disease in the future. In fact, a National Institute on Aging study discovered that patients in a study who were treated for twelve years or longer for high blood pressure had 60 percent less dementia risk than people who were never treated for hypertension.

Hypertension can silently take its toll on your brain and your cognitive functioning. To protect yourself against the possibility of dementia and Alzheimer's disease, it's critical to take control of your high blood pressure now.

HIGH BLOOD PRESSURE AND CHILDREN

Children are eating more fast food, getting heavier, and spending more time being inactive than ever before. The result has been a growing population of young people who are overweight or obese and who are developing serious health problems traditionally viewed as diseases of adulthood: hypertension, heart disease, stroke, and type 2 diabetes. As this chapter shows, high blood pressure is intimately associated with all of these serious health conditions. When children and adolescents develop hypertension or any of these other health conditions at a young age, they expose themselves to an increased risk of dying sooner of these or related health problems as well as experiencing years of symptoms and complications from these diseases.

For all of these reasons and more, it's critical for parents and other responsible adults to ensure young children and adolescents avoid high blood pressure. Yet at this time, approximately 30 percent of all overweight children have elevated blood pressure and children who are eligible for kindergarten are showing up in doctors' offices with hypertension. The time to do something about hypertension in children is now!

Managing High Blood Pressure in Children

Do you know one good thing about hypertension in young people? More than half of young children and adolescents who have high blood pressure have symptoms, such as frequent headaches, problems with sleep, tiredness during the day, and chest pains. If you have a child with any of these symptoms, and especially if he or she is overweight, be sure to have blood pressure checked as soon as possible. Check it several times over a period of a few days. You can use an at-home monitor to take these readings. High blood pressure that is caught early in children can typically be managed with weight control and exercise and no drugs. Therefore, the suggestions offered in this book can be helpful.

A healthy blood pressure for children is lower than that for adults. Generally, the systolic blood pressure among children ages 8 to 12 increases by 0.44 mmHg per year and by 2.90 mmHg between the ages of 13 and 17. For diastolic blood pressure, the average rise is 0.33 mmHg from ages 8 to 12 and 1.81 mmHg from ages 13 to 17. As a guideline, a healthy blood pressure for a child age 8 years is 100/57 mmHg, while that of a 17-year-old is 117/66 mmHg. Every parent and guardian should know what their children's blood pressure is and it should be checked during every doctor visit. Young children and adolescents who are overweight and/or who have health conditions such as asthma, heart problems, or behavioral disorders or who are experiencing sleep problems especially should be checked regularly.

HIGH BLOOD PRESSURE AND PREGNANCY

Pregnancy can be a time of joy, but for a significant number of women health challenges are part of the experience, and high blood pressure is one of them. Women can experience high blood pressure three different ways during pregnancy:

- They may have high blood pressure before they get pregnant

- They may develop gestational hypertension, which is high blood pressure that presents itself during the pregnancy. This form of hypertension typically goes away after giving birth.

- They may develop preeclampsia, a condition that typically develops around week 20 of pregnancy and is characterized by high blood pressure and the presence of protein in the urine. Women with preeclampsia may also develop persistent headache, vision changes, pain in the upper abdominal region, swelling of the hands or face, and sudden weight gain.

The one thing all three types of hypertension during pregnancy have in common is that they need to be treated with care, for both the sake of the mother's health and that of her unborn child. Hypertension during pregnancy is associated with the following problems:

• Reduced blood flow to the placenta, which in turn limits the supply of nutrients and oxygen to the baby and places the child at risk for low birth weight and numerous medical problems

• The placenta's separating from the uterus prematurely, which can deprive the infant of oxygen and cause heavy bleeding in the mother

• The need for premature delivery if blood pressure cannot be controlled adequately and there are life-threatening complications present

• The presence of preeclampsia increasing a woman's risk of developing cardiovascular disease later in life, even when her blood pressure returns to normal levels after giving birth

High blood pressure during pregnancy can be treated with natural approaches. However, if these measures do not work or if a woman develops preeclampsia there are several blood pressure medications that have been found to be safe when taken during pregnancy (see chapter 8).

BLOOD PRESSURE AND YOUR EYES

The eyes are truly the window to the soul, as well as a number of health issues. One of them is the effect of hypertension. High blood pressure can have a significant impact on your eyes, especially since they are the home of delicate blood vessels that are highly sensitive to changes in blood pressure. Some of the ways hypertension can affect your eyes are listed here:

- **Retinopathy.** High blood pressure can damage the blood vessels that supply blood to the retina, resulting in a condition known as retinopathy. This condition is characterized by blurry vision, bleeding in the eye, and even complete vision loss.

- **Choroidopathy.** In this condition, fluid accumulates under the retina and can cause distorted vision or scars that impair vision.

- **Optic neuropathy.** If your optic nerve experiences damage associated with high blood pressure, this condition is known as optic neuropathy. This condition may cause bleeding in the eye and loss of vision.

- **Glaucoma.** Hypertension is associated with glaucoma, a common eye disease that is the leading cause of irreversible blindness around the world. More than 2.2 million people in the United States have glaucoma. The combination of hypertension and diabetes is associated with an increased risk of glaucoma: people with hypertension alone have a 17 percent increased risk for glaucoma, while those with diabetes alone have a 35 percent increased risk. People with both diabetes and hypertension have a 48 percent increased risk of developing open-angle glaucoma, the most common form of the eye disease.[4] Like hypertension, open-angle glaucoma is a condition that typically does not show symptoms, at least not until the disease has progressed. Therefore, if you have high blood pressure it's important to have your eyes examined regularly and tested for glaucoma by an eye specialist.

PART II

How to Prevent and Treat
High Blood Pressure

CHAPTER THREE

Eat Your Way to a Healthy Blood Pressure

One of the most proactive and effective ways to both prevent and manage high blood pressure is through your food choices. Food can be your medicine, and medicine can be your food, to paraphrase Hippocrates, and the great thing about this medicine is that it can not only taste great, but it also can make you feel wonderful and vital. However, like medicines and supplements, not all foods are equally effective or healthful, and moderation is key. Fortunately, the list of exciting and delicious foods that can help you achieve and support a healthy blood pressure and cardiovascular health is long and diversified, so you should never be bored or at a loss to find convenient, appropriate choices.

A well-researched and well-known diet for reducing the risk of hypertension as well as helping in managing the condition is DASH, or Dietary Approaches to Stop Hypertension. However, DASH is not the only dietary approach you can take to accomplish these goals, so for individuals who like to have options in life there are two more related diets discussed in this chapter: vegetarian and vegan. All three share some basic characteristics—emphasis on fruits and vegetables, low amounts of saturated fat, richness in fiber, and low (or no) amounts of cholesterol—although there are some differences, which

I explain. All of these diets also offer a wealth of tasty options. (I have even included some easy recipes to prove it!) So let's get started on that menu and shopping list for fighting high blood pressure!

A DASHING APPROACH TO HIGH BLOOD PRESSURE

Doctors who are worth their salt (pun intended) will recommended DASH to their patients who are at risk for or who already have high blood pressure for one simple reason: it has been proven to work, and quickly—as rapidly as two weeks. Indeed, the U.S. Guidelines for Treatment of High Blood Pressure state that all doctors should recommend the DASH diet for anyone who has just been diagnosed with hypertension. DASH can be especially helpful for people who have prehypertension or mild to moderate high blood pressure. Individuals with severe hypertension can significantly reduce their need for medication if they follow the diet, while patients with mild to moderate high blood pressure often can stop taking their antihypertensive drugs altogether.

DASH also can improve cholesterol levels and is associated with reducing the risk for developing type 2 diabetes. For three years in a row (2011, 2012, 2013), DASH was rated the number one diet by *U.S. News & World Report,* and it is endorsed by the National Heart, Lung, and Blood Institute, the American Heart Association, the 2010 Dietary Guidelines for Americans, and doctors everywhere. But the only one who *really* matters when it comes to embracing DASH is you, because if you don't follow it, it can't help you achieve your goals of lower blood pressure and overall better health.

What Is DASH?

DASH is a way of eating that evolved out of research from the National Institutes of Health, in which investigators tested the impact of various nutrients in food on blood pressure. They found that elevated blood pressure could be safely and effectively reduced when people followed an eating plan that focused on fruits, vegetables, whole grains, and low-fat dairy products, as well as poultry, fish, lean meats, and nuts. In addition, the overall approach of DASH is low in total fat and saturated fat (no more than 6 percent of total calories from saturated fat and no more than 27 percent from total fat), cholesterol, sodium, sugar, and red meats.

Why DASH Lowers Blood Pressure

When the elements of DASH are evaluated, numerous features stand out as being important players in the lowering of blood pressure. One is believed to be the high levels of electrolytes—potassium, calcium, and magnesium—in the diet, which are largely associated with the focus on fruits and vegetables. Potassium in particular has been shown to have an ability to lower blood pressure. However, other research shows that taking supplements of these minerals doesn't yield the same benefits, so foods with these nutrients seem to have other qualities that are important for lowering blood pressure, which helps support the argument for choosing food over supplements for your nutritional needs.

DASH is effective at lowering blood pressure for other reasons as well. For example, the emphasis on whole grains, fruits, and vegetables in the diet increases the amount of fiber, which helps lower cholesterol (important for blood pressure) and makes it easier to drop excess pounds. The focus on lower-fat foods (both dairy and meats) also helps lower blood pressure, cholesterol, and weight, while the plan also follows U.S. guidelines for salt content (see "Salt").

Yet another reason why DASH can reduce blood pressure levels may be linked to the amount of plant protein in the diet rather than animal protein. DASH emphasizes plant-based more than animal-based foods, although it is not a vegetarian diet. According to the *INTERMAP* study, which involved nearly forty-seven hundred men and women from the United States, the United Kingdom, Japan, and China, eating animal protein did not have an impact on blood pressure. However, consumption of plant protein was significantly associated with lower blood pressure. (Now you can see why both vegetarian and vegan diets can be effective in lowering blood pressure!) So this means if you are a meat lover there is no reason you can't include moderate portions of lean beef, lamb or pork in your diet, in addition to poultry and fish.

Toss in the fact that there's plenty of variety in DASH and that it contains all the foods you'll find in the popular Mediterranean diet and you have a plan for success, if you choose to follow it.

What Does DASH Look Like?

DASH is good for the entire family and not just people with high blood pressure or anyone who wants to avoid it. Yes, a number of studies have shown that a DASH approach is effective in reducing, preventing, and managing high blood pressure in young children and adolescents as well. With all this in mind, here are the recommended numbers of daily servings for different food categories of DASH based on average calorie intake ranging from 1,600 to 3,100 calories per day. You can make adjustments based on your or your family member's average recommended calorie intake per day:

Grains and related products: 6–12 servings, including at least 3 whole grains
Fruits: 4–6 servings
Vegetables: 3–6 servings
Low-fat or no-fat dairy: 2–4 servings
Lean meats, fish, poultry: 1–2 servings
Nuts, seeds, legumes: 3–6 servings per week
Fats and oils: 2–3 servings
Sugars/Sweets: less than 5 servings per week

How Big is a Serving?

Based on the DASH eating plan, here are standard serving sizes. Some of these serving sizes differ slightly from those of other plans, but they are basically similar.

Grains: 1 slice bread, ¼ bagel, ½ English muffin, ½ cup cooked rice, barley, couscous, or other grains, ½ cup cooked pasta. Typically, one serving equals 1 ounce (dry weight for grains that need to be cooked).
Fruits: 1 small apple, banana, orange, 1 medium peach, ½ grapefruit, 1 cup fresh berries or melon cubes, 4 ounces unsweetened juice
Vegetables: 1 cup raw and/or salad greens, ½ cup cooked, ½ cup vegetable juice
Dairy: 1 ounce no-fat, low-fat cheese, 1 cup no-fat, low-fat milk or yogurt
Meats, fish, poultry: 3 ounces (about the size of your palm)

Nuts, seeds, legumes: 1.5 ounce dry roasted or raw nuts, 2 tablespoons nut butter, 2 tablespoons (0.5 ounce) seeds, ½ cup cooked legumes/beans

Fats: 1 teaspoon butter, mayonnaise, margarine; 1 tablespoon reduced-fat margarine or mayonnaise

Sugars/sweets: 1 tablespoon sugar, jelly, or jam

VEGETARIAN DIET APPROACH

A vegetarian diet approach for high blood pressure is similar to DASH except it excludes flesh foods, which includes meats, fish, and poultry. Not all vegetarian diets are the same: for example, some people eat eggs but not dairy (ovo vegetarians), others eat dairy but not eggs (lacto vegetarians), while yet others avoid both eggs and dairy (ovo-lacto vegetarians). Individuals who make these choices do so because of ethical and/or health reasons. Regardless of which type of vegetarian diet you may want to choose, it is easy to make adjustments to your menus to ensure you get balanced and varied nutrition that supports your desire to lower blood pressure and experience other health benefits as a bonus!

For example, people who are new to a vegetarian diet often worry about getting enough protein. "If I don't eat meat or chicken, where will I get my protein?" is a common question. Vegetarians who eat dairy and/or eggs can get some of their protein from these sources, as well as from substituting beans, seeds, and nuts for meat protein.

The DASH diet recommends consuming only small amounts of meat, fish, and poultry, so it is not difficult to find delicious substitutes for these protein foods if you choose a vegetarian route. For example, bean or veggie burgers, no-meat chili, grilled seitan (a high-protein wheat protein food), split-pea soup, scrambled eggs and mushrooms, marinated tofu, cashew butter on whole wheat toast, hummus and brown rice, macaroni and cheese, and stir-fried mock chicken and vegetables are all excellent alternatives to animal-flesh protein sources. If you have decided to opt out of dairy, try soy dairy foods such as soy yogurt, soy beverages (including vanilla and chocolate flavors), and soy- and grain-based cheeses.

Is a vegetarian diet healthy? Absolutely! The mainstream American Dietetic Association reported in its 2009 position paper: "Vegetarians also appear to have lower low-density lipoprotein cholesterol levels, lower blood pressure, and lower rates of hypertension and type 2 diabetes than nonvegetarians." It credited these health benefits to certain features of a vegetarian diet, such as lower intake of saturated fat and cholesterol and greater intakes of fruits, vegetables, whole grains, fiber, soy foods, nuts, and phytochemicals (see "Daily Servings for Vegetarian and Vegan Diets").

Numerous studies show that people who follow a vegetarian diet have a lower risk and a lower prevalence of high blood pressure, as well as related conditions. Among the many studies conducted, a critical review from Loma Linda University and published in the *American Journal of Clinical Nutrition* explored the evidence on the health effects of a vegetarian diet. The author explained that there is "convincing evidence that vegetarians have lower rates of coronary heart disease, largely explained by low LDL cholesterol, probable lower rate of hypertension and diabetes mellitus, and lower prevalence of obesity."

A vegetarian diet also tends to involve greater consumption of folate, potassium, vitamin C, and flavonoids, largely because of the increased consumption of fruits and vegetables. Potassium in particular is associated with a reduction in blood pressure, and both fruits and vegetables are major sources of this mineral and electrolyte. Vegetarians also tend to consume a healthy amount of L-arginine, an amino acid that is involved in the production of nitric oxide, a substance that helps dilate blood vessels and thus improve blood flow.

Another advantage of a vegetarian diet is the lack of saturated fat from meats. Saturated fat appears to have a negative impact on blood viscosity, which in turn worsens blood pressure. Fats from nonanimal sources (polyunsaturated fats such as linoleic acid and alpha-linolenic acids) are associated with a lower risk of developing high blood pressure.

VEGAN DIET APPROACH

A vegan diet approach is rich in fruits, vegetables, whole grains, legumes, seeds, and nuts and excludes meats, fish, poultry, eggs, and dairy foods. A major advantage of a vegan diet for high blood pressure is the lack of cholesterol and a very low amount of saturated fat and, typically, total fat as well. However, don't be fooled into thinking a vegan diet is always a low-fat diet. If you tend to eat a lot of French fries, onion rings, and pasta and skip the fruits and veggies, then you can quickly pack on the pounds and the fat. There are ways to eat smart and not so smart regardless of which dietary approach you choose!

Admittedly, following a vegan diet can be a challenge for many people who are used to eating animal-based foods and who feel this dietary approach is too restrictive. However, another way to look at a vegan approach is that it can open the door for opportunities to try foods you may never have considered before, including the ever-growing selection of mock meat, poultry, fish, and dairy foods now available in many mainstream supermarkets. Most of these selections have been improved to the point where texture, taste, and aroma are similar and, in many cases, barely discernible from the "real" thing. (See "Vegetarian and Vegan Food Manufacturers" in the appendix.)

If you choose to try a vegan approach to high blood pressure, you will need to make some adjustments to the recommended servings in the various categories of the DASH diet. Here are some guidelines for those who choose a vegetarian or vegan diet for prevention and management of high blood pressure.

DAILY SERVINGS FOR VEGETARIAN AND VEGAN DIETS

Note: Compare the number of servings here with those of DASH. You will notice that the numbers of servings for legumes, nuts, and seeds are more than double, as they take the place of meat, fish, poultry, and (for vegans) dairy and eggs.

Grains: 5–12 servings of whole grains
Fruits: 3–4 servings
Vegetables: 6–9 servings
Nuts, seeds, legumes: 2–5 servings daily (not 3–6 per week as in the DASH diet)
Oils, dairy, eggs: 1–2 servings daily; eliminate dairy and eggs for vegans

Vegetarians and especially vegans need to be mindful of certain nutrients that are more difficult to get when following a plant-based diet. Vitamin B_{12}, for example, is found only in animal foods. Therefore, be sure to eat foods that have been fortified with B_{12} (such as some cereals, tofu, and other soy products, including soy beverages) or take a supplement that provides this necessary nutrient. Other nutrients that may be consumed in insufficient amounts, depending on your food choices, include calcium, iron, zinc, and vitamin D. Members of the legume family tend to be good sources of the first three of these nutrients, so be sure to make beans, split peas, lentils, and other legumes a significant part of your diet. Again, foods fortified with these vitamins and minerals and/or supplements are recommended.

BASIC ELEMENTS OF A HIGH BLOOD PRESSURE DIET

DASH, vegetarian, and vegan diets for the prevention and management of high blood pressure all share some common elements, and the healthful characteristics of those elements are important for you to appreciate so you can better realize just how much food impacts your blood pressure and related health issues.

Grains

Grains are an important source of carbohydrates (energy food), fiber, and nutrients, while also being low in fat. The 2010 Dietary Guidelines for Americans recommend that everyone include whole grains in at least half of their grain choices. Why? Whole grains and cereals retain nutrients that are stripped away during processing. Unrefined grains keep their bran and germ and at the same time are a better source of fiber and minerals that are important for high blood pressure, including potassium and magnesium. Therefore, choose brown rice over white rice, unmilled oatmeal over processed brands, and whole wheat pasta over white pasta.

What about fortified or enriched grains? This means the food manufacturer has added back some of the nutrients—but not the fiber—that were lost during processing. The added nutrients also are not the natural ones found in the unrefined food. Enriched grains can be important for people who choose a vegetarian or vegan diet, but if you eat whole grains you don't need to worry about enriched foods.

How should you shop for grains? Don't let the marketing terminology fool you. The words "stone-ground" and "seven grain" sound impressive, right? But what do they mean? The only way to know if you are buying a whole grain product is to check the ingredient panel on the food. If the first ingredient is whole grain (such as "whole wheat" or "whole barley"), stone-ground whole (grain or cereal name), whole (grain or cereal name), oats, oatmeal, or brown rice, then you probably have a whole grain product. But if the label says "enriched flour" or "fortified flour" or "bran," then you don't.

Here are some tips on how to boost the amount of whole grains in your diet:

- Look for whole grain products when you shop: brown rice rather than white rice, whole wheat bread rather than white bread, whole wheat pasta rather than white pasta.

- Order brown instead of white rice at a restaurant.

- Add barley, buckwheat, or couscous to your recipes or use as a side dish instead of white rice.

- Choose unmilled oatmeal or whole grain cereals for breakfast.

- Select whole grain flours and mixes for pancakes and muffins when shopping.

- Try air-popped popcorn for a snack (skip the butter and salt and try spray-on oil and powdered herbs).

- Choose whole grain breads, pitas, bagels, and rolls.

Low-Fat, No-Fat Dairy

If dairy is part of your dietary plan, choose fat-free (skim) or low-fat (1 percent) milk, buttermilk, cheeses, and yogurt. While dairy foods are a major source of protein and calcium, vegans and vegetarians who choose to skip dairy foods can still get plenty of protein and calcium from fortified soy- and grain-based dairy alternatives. Dairy foods also are often fortified with vitamin D, and since many people are deficient in this vitamin, fortified foods can help.

Meats, Fish, and Poultry

The inclusion of meat and poultry in the DASH approach emphasizes lean meats. You should trim off any visible fat, remove the skin from poultry, and prepare meats, fish, and poultry by broiling, roasting, or poaching. Meats and poultry are a significant source of protein and magnesium, which are important for blood pressure.

Eggs are also included in this category. Because egg

yolks are high in cholesterol, DASH recommends limiting intake to no more than four yolks per week, but your doctor may have a different recommendation.

Those who choose a vegetarian or vegan eating plan could probably include any plant-based faux meats in this category, such as the many "fake" burgers, hot dogs, chicken strips, ground beef, and other plant-based faux meat products. These foods are typically moderate to high in protein, low in fat, and free of cholesterol and provide fiber and a variety of nutrients. Whether you want to classify such foods as "meat" or consider them to be in the legume category (which is where they are usually placed), be sure to give them a try!

One advantage of eating fish (at least certain fish) is their omega-3 content. Omega-3 fatty acids are a type of polyunsaturated fatty acid that has been shown to protect the heart and help lower blood pressure, cholesterol, and triglycerides. The two main omega-3 fatty acids are eicosapentanoic acid (EPA) and docohexaenoic acid (DHA), which are found primarily in cold-water fatty fish, such as salmon, tuna, mackerel, herring, and sardines. These omega-3s appear to reduce blood pressure by lowering the resistance to blood flow surges, which in turn promotes healthy, flexible arteries and a better blood pressure. In addition, omega-3s help prevent the development of blood clots, lower heart rate, and reduce triglyceride levels, all of which benefit the cardiovascular system.

The American Heart Association recommends, and numerous research studies support, eating fish rich in omega-3s twice a week. This fits in nicely with the DASH diet but obviously not with a vegetarian or vegan approach. However, omega-3 fatty acid supplements (see chapter 6) can be added to these diets to promote better blood pressure management. If you want to avoid fish oils altogether, there are DHA supplements prepared from algae shown to be effective as well.

Nuts and Seeds

If you choose a vegetarian or vegan eating plan, you will likely depend on this category more than if you select DASH. However, in either case, both nuts and seeds tend to be nutrient dense but also a bit high in calories. Therefore, you should choose wisely from this category, picking dry roasted and unsalted varieties. Among some of those healthful choices are the following:

- **Pistachios:** 1 ounce of unsalted pistachios contains only 3 mg of sodium, 295 mg of potassium, 34 mg of magnesium, 3 grams of fiber, and a mere 1.5 grams of saturated fat.

- **Almonds:** 1 ounce provides only 1 gram of saturated fat, 200 mg of potassium, 76 mg of magnesium, and 4 grams of fiber.

- **Hazelnuts** (also called filberts): Although these nuts are a bit higher in total fat, only 1.5 g per ounce is saturated fat. One ounce of hazelnuts also provides 46 mg of magnesium, 193 mg of potassium, and 3 g of fiber.

Legumes

Legumes include beans, soybeans, peas, lentils, and peanuts. These high-protein foods are a great alternative for meat in the DASH diet, and they also provide an excellent amount of fiber and are low to moderate in fat and free of cholesterol, unlike most animal protein sources. Other nutrients in legumes include calcium, folate, iron, selenium, and zinc. If you also have diabetes, legumes are low on the glycemic index and have a low glycemic load. Other benefits of legumes are low cost, ease of preparation, the lots of different ways to enjoy them, ranging from soups to sandwich spreads, salads, burgers, casseroles, and sauces.

Here are some tips on how to include more legumes in your diet.

- Substitute beans and other legumes for meat or dairy whenever possible. For example, try a three-bean chili (no meat), add lentils instead of meat-balls to pasta sauce, make a bean spread instead of egg salad for a sandwich or pita stuffing, or try a bean burger instead of a beef burger.

- Learn to love legumes by trying them in soups. Either add lentils, peas, or beans to one of your favorite soups (e.g., minestrone, tomato) or make a bean soup. (Note: if you use a canned soup, look for low-sodium varieties)

- Make bean dips or hummus and eat them with fresh-cut veggies.

- Keep a variety of canned (low-sodium) beans on hand for a quick meal (see "Thirty-Minute Bean Lover Recipe").

- Try a variety of beans. Different beans have different textures and flavors. A chili with chickpeas and black beans will taste different from one that contains lentils and kidney beans.

• Experiment with a new legume every week.

Fruits and Vegetables

Fruits and vegetables harbor a class of nutrients known as polyphenols, which are known, among other things, for their antioxidant properties. Among the many different types of polyphenols found in fruits and vegetables are flavanols, flavonols, stilbenes, catechins, and isoflavones, among others, which have been shown to have a positive effect on blood pressure. Some of these polyphenols are also found in herbal remedies, which I discuss in chapter 6.

While it is possible to extract specific polyphenols from foods and nicely package them in tablets, powders, teas, extracts, and capsules, the optimal way to get your vitamins, minerals, polyphenols, and other nutrients is from whole, natural foods. One reason is that whole fruits and vegetables provide the whole enchilada: a natural package of nutrients that work synergistically in ways that often still baffle scientists.

However, researchers are hot on the trail of discovering how and why the basic chemical factors of polyphenols and other phytonutrients ("phyto" means "plant") have an impact on blood pressure and other bodily functions. Among the hypotheses being considered is one that says polyphenols regulate the body's ability to access and use (a characteristic known as bioavailability) nitric oxide. Nitric oxide is an important substance to remember when talking about blood pressure, because it has an impact on endothelial function, which in turn affects blood pressure.

Vegetables and fruits are also rich in potassium, which has already been mentioned as having a significant role in reducing blood pressure. Another important nutrient in fruits and vegetables is folic acid. The Nurses' Health Study found that women who ate the greatest amounts of folate from their diet and from supplements (at least 1,000 micrograms daily) had only one-third the risk for developing high blood pressure as did women who consumed less than 200 micrograms daily.

Fats and Oils

This category includes butter, margarine, salad dressings, and vegetable oils. These foods certainly can be a part of your menu, but choose the healthier options and use them in limited amounts. Suggested vegetable oils include those highest in monounsaturated fat, including olive, safflower, canola, almond, and soybean oils. If you like salad dressings, select low-fat, low-sodium brands and use them sparingly. Along with your healthy oils, choose fresh and dried herbs and spices to perk up your salads, vegetables, and other dishes.

Sugar and High Blood Pressure

Lots of other diets warn you to limit or avoid intake of sugar and sugary foods, and so similar advice can be levied concerning the prevention and management of high blood pressure. Let's back it up with a few examples, with one coming from the University of Colorado Health Sciences Center concerning fructose. Fructose is a sugar and a component of all major sweeteners that have calories, including sucrose, honey, fruit juice concentrates, and high-fructose corn syrup. Since people in industrialized nations have been consuming an increasing amount of fructose in recent years and blood pressures have been rising as well, a research team decided to explore the possibility of a relationship between the two. Here's what they found.

First they analyzed data from 4,528 adults without a history of hypertension, and part of that data included dietary information about soft drink consumption. After the team made adjustments for factors such as physical activity, total calorie intake, use of vitamin C, and the presence of health conditions, they determined that people who consumed 74 grams or more of fructose daily in the form of added sugar (e.g., soft drinks, candy) had a significantly greater chance of developing high blood pressure.

Experts also suggest sucrose (common table sugar) may cause a rise in blood pressure because it increases the production of adrenaline, which in turn causes blood vessels to constrict and the retention of sodium.

Then there is the concept of the "fructose hypothesis," which is basically the idea that fructose plays a role in high blood pressure, cardiovascular disease, diabetes, and cancer. The debate is ongoing, as is the research, but face it: while a small amount of sugar is likely not going to cause any significant health problems, the healthiest route is to avoid or limit added sugars and enjoy the natural sweetness of whole foods.

Salt

I have already mentioned that salt (sodium) intake is associated with high blood pressure. Although everyone has his or her own level of salt sensitivity, the bottom line is that most people consume more sodium than the body needs to function optimally. According to the guidelines released by the U.S. Department of Agriculture in 2011, no one should consume more than 2,300 milligrams of salt per day. Anyone who is 51 years or older, is African-American, or has high blood pressure, chronic kidney disease, or diabetes should not take in more than 1,500 milligrams daily.

The organs responsible for balancing salt content in the body are the kidneys. If your sodium levels drop too low (e.g., if you are sweating excessively or you have been vomiting), the kidneys retain sodium. When sodium levels are high, the kidneys eliminate sodium in urine.

That's what should happen, but sometimes the kidneys can't get rid of enough sodium, so it builds up in the blood. Sodium attracts water from the blood, which then causes blood volume to increase and triggers the heart to work harder, which then increases blood pressure.

One teaspoon of salt contains 2,325 milligrams of sodium, which is the limit for many people and far too much for many others. It's the hidden sodium in processed foods that can be most worrisome, so the best ways to monitor your salt intake are to:

• Eat natural, fresh foods as much as possible.

• Read food labels for the sodium content. Pay attention to the amount of mg of sodium per serving. Foods are considered to be "low sodium" if they contain 140 mg or less sodium per servings. "No sodium" means less than 5 mg per serving.

• If you do eat processed foods, look for those marked as "low" or "no sodium," but always check the ingredient panel to be sure.

- Rinse your food. If you can't find a low-sodium version of a canned vegetable or beans, you can rinse the food with water before using it. Naturally, this does not work with all canned foods!

- Try seasoning alternatives. Instead of salt, try fresh or dried herbs or spices, lemon juice, or salt substitutes.

- Taste before you season. Some people tend to put salt on their food even before they taste it. Taste your food, especially items you have not prepared yourself, before you season it.

- When eating out, ask how food has been prepared. You will want items that are made without added salt. The same goes for condiments, dressings, and sauces. Ask the waitstaff for no-salt or low-salt condiments or bring your own from home with you.

SALT ALTERNATIVES

How can you jazz up your food without adding salt? Here are some suggestions. A few of them are low-sodium versions of typically high-salt items.

- Monounsaturated oils, such as olive oil and canola oil
- White, red wine, balsamic, and flavored vinegars
- Low-sodium salsas
- Mrs. Dash

- Mustards
- Lemon pepper
- Pepper
- A wide variety of fresh and dried herbs and spices
- Garlic
- Tabasco sauce
- Lemon or lime juice
- Brown mustard sauce (see recipe at end of chapter)

Natural, fresh fruits and vegetables, legumes, nuts, seeds, and grains contain very little sodium. Nature has packaged these foods with just the right amount of salt. However, refined and processed foods are typically brimming with added salt, both for taste and for preservation purposes. For example, an apple and a banana each contain about 1 milligram sodium, while one ounce of American cheese contains more than 400 milligrams and one cup of low-fat cottage cheese contains more than 900 milligrams. When shopping for groceries, always read the labels for sodium content.

RECIPES

Here are a few simple low-sodium, low-fat, delicious recipes you can enjoy as part of an eating plan to prevent or manage high blood pressure. All the ingredients are readily available, the recipes are easy to prepare, and the nutritional values are high.

Quick and Easy Minestrone

46 ounces of low-sodium tomato juice
2 cups water
1 tsp. each dried basil, cilantro, and oregano
6 cloves garlic, minced
1½ cups canned low- or no-sodium kidney or
    white beans (rinsed)
1 zucchini, sliced into small pieces
2 cups green beans, sliced
1 cup carrots, chopped
1 small red onion, chopped
2 stalks celery, chopped
1 small potato, chopped
1 cup spinach, chopped

Combine all the ingredients except the spinach in a large
electric cooking pot and cook on low for 8 to 10 hours.
Ten minutes before serving, add the spinach and stir
well, allowing the greens to wilt completely. Serves 8.

Thirty-Minute Bean Lover Recipe

If you used canned beans (rinse the beans to remove
the salt and reduce the tendency to develop gas), you
can have this recipe ready in about 30 minutes.

1 tbs. vegetable oil
2 green and 2 red bell peppers, chopped
2 white potatoes, cut into 1-inch cubes
1 red onion, chopped
5 cloves garlic, minced
¼ tsp. cinnamon
½ cup water
2 cups chopped fresh tomatoes

3 cups cooked beans—your choice. Feel free to
   mix them up. If you used canned beans, be
   sure to rinse them and drain
1 tbs. minced jalapeno peppers
½ tsp. dried oregano

In a large Dutch oven or soup pot, heat oil and sauté the
bell peppers, potatoes, onion, garlic, and cinnamon for
about 5 minutes. Add ½ cup of water, cover, and simmer
for 8 minutes. Add all the remaining ingredients, reduce
heat, cover, and simmer for about 15 minutes. Serves 4.

Too-Busy-for-Breakfast Smoothie

This smoothie provides lots of potassium and magnesium, as well as calcium, which are critical for managing high blood pressure. At less than 350 calories, it's
also a low-calorie treat.

8 ounces of nonfat milk or soy milk (nonfat
   vanilla soy milk tastes great!)
2 ounces egg substitute
1 medium banana
2 cups frozen berries (your choice, all the same
   or mix them up)

Combine all ingredients in a blender. You can make
two or more times the amount and keep the extra in the
refrigerator for about two days. Serves 1.

Simple Salmon

This recipe allows you to make your salmon and
vegetables all in the same baking dish, and it takes only
15 minutes to bake.

4 fillets of salmon, 4 ounces each
1 zucchini, cut into 1-inch slices
2 tomatoes, cut into quarters
1 cup button mushrooms
1 green or red bell pepper, seeded and cut into
    eighths
1 red onion, sliced
1 lemon
1 tsp. dried oregano
Black pepper to taste
¼ cup fresh cilantro

Rinse and pat dry the fish. Place the fish on a baking
dish lined with aluminum foil. Arrange all the vegetables in the dish, squeeze lemon on each piece of fish,
and season them with black pepper and oregano.
Sprinkle the cilantro over the entire mixture. Cover
with a lid and bake in a preheated oven (400 degrees F)
for 15 to 20 minutes. Check the doneness of the fish at
15 minutes. Serves 4.

Can't Be Beet Salad

Research shows that beets and beet juice can significantly
lower blood pressure. That's because beets are a rich
source of nitrates, substances that your body converts
into nitrites once you consume them. Nitrites are
involved in nitric oxide synthesis, and nitric oxide helps
widen blood vessels, which can reduce blood pressure.
So be sure to include beets in your diet as much as
possible. Here's an easy recipe to get you started.

2 apples, washed and cored, thinly sliced
2 cups sliced beets. If you used canned beets, buy
    salt-free or rinse the beets before adding to the

salad. If using fresh beets, steam or boil until tender, cool, peel, and slice or cut into bite-sized chunks.

2 cups celery, sliced thin
½ cup red onion, diced
¼ cup chopped raisins
3 tbs. chopped pecans or walnuts
2 tbs. olive oil
2 tbs. balsamic vinegar
Lemon juice to taste
Black pepper to taste

Combine the apples, beets, celery, onion, raisins, and nuts. Mix the oil, vinegar, lemon juice, and black pepper in a small shaker and add to the salad mixture. Toss well and refrigerate. Serves 4.

Brown Mustard Sauce

Here's a no-salt-added recipe for a flavorful sauce/dressing you can use to jazz up vegetables, grains, potatoes, and legumes.

¾ cup balsamic vinegar
¼ cup olive oil
⅛ cup water
4 tbs. prepared Dijon mustard
4 garlic cloves, minced
½ tsp. ground black pepper
1 tsp. ground cumin
2 tbs. minced red onion
Few hot pepper flakes (if desired)

Place all ingredients in a container with a lid, shake well, and refrigerate until ready to use.

CHAPTER FOUR

Be on the Move

Let's not mince words here: regular physical activity is a key factor in the prevention and management of high blood pressure and associated cardiovascular health. If the *e* word conjures up visions of sweaty, grunting bodies in a gym or tortuous weight and running machines, then perhaps a fitness club is not the best idea for you. But I'm not necessarily talking about that type of physical activity; that is, unless that's what you enjoy, and if so, fantastic! Go for it. In fact, exercising in a gym or fitness club can be an exciting change of pace.

In this chapter, however, the focus is not so much on where you move but simply that you *do* move, how to make physical activity more pleasurable, and how critical it is for preventing and managing high blood pressure. Keeping physically active on a regular basis can take many forms and be incorporated into your daily life in various ways that are convenient and enjoyable, and exploring new ways to stay active can be an enlightening learning experience as well.

HOW PHYSICAL ACTIVITY LOWERS
BLOOD PRESSURE

Let's cut to the chase and tell you how exercise can reduce your blood pressure. Although there's a lot happening on a biochemical level, the gist of it is, your heart is a muscle and regular exercise makes your heart stronger. A strong heart is capable of accomplishing more (pumping blood throughout the body) by doing less. When the heart doesn't have to work as hard, there is less pressure or force against the artery walls and blood pressure is lowered. How much can exercise improve your blood pressure?

- Regular physical activity can lower your blood pressure about as much as some antihypertensive medications can: an average of 4 to 9 mmHg systolic. That means if your doctor wants to prescribe a drug to bring your blood pressure down this amount, exercise may be the only prescription you need. At the very least, staying physically active can reduce the amount of medication you may need to take.

- Your blood pressure can improve with physical activity, but give it a little time. It takes about thirty to ninety days for the blood-pressure-lowering benefits of exercise to kick in.

- After thirty to ninety days, don't quit! If you want to continue enjoying the blood-pressure-lowering benefit of physical exercise, you need to keep going. Exercise is like an umbrella in the rain: it only protects you if you keep it up!

- Physical exercise can prevent the progression of blood vessel (vascular) changes that occur with hypertension, cardiovascular disease, diabetes, and obesity, such as endothelial dysfunction and stiff arteries. In fact, exercise improves the availability of nitric oxide, which is essential for opening up blood vessels so blood can flow more smoothly.

- If your blood pressure is already in a healthy range, less than 120/80 mmHg, regular exercise can help maintain that level as you get older and help prevent hypertension.

Doesn't Exercise Raise Blood Pressure?

The answer to this question is "yes": physical activity does cause blood pressure to rise. So why on earth do experts recommend exercise for people who have high blood pressure? Isn't it dangerous? Well, you're not going to use this argument as an excuse not to exercise! Although it is true that exercise will cause your blood pressure to rise for a short time, once you stop the activity your blood pressure should return to its normal level. The faster your blood pressure returns to its resting rate (resting heart rate, or RHR, which I discuss later in this chapter), the more physically fit you probably are.

In fact, most people who have hypertension are able to increase their physical activity levels without any cause for alarm. According to the Blood Pressure Association, it is safe for people who have a blood pressure of 90/60 mmHg to 140/90 mmHg to increase their activity level. For those with a blood pressure of 140/90 mmHg to 179/99 mm Hg, it should be safe to begin increasing exercise levels. Anyone with a blood pressure reading greater than 179/99 mmHg should definitely talk to his or her doctor before exercising. As a general rule, however, it is always best to first consult your doctor before starting an exercise program, trying new types of exercises, or participating in sports, regardless of your blood pressure levels.

"I Can't Exercise Because" Antidotes

Okay, so your blood pressure is moderately high and I just eliminated one excuse you might want to use to avoid exercise. Here are a few more "I can't exercise because" reasons and antidotes for each one.

- **I don't have enough time.** Sure you do, and the antidotes to this excuse are twofold. One is time management and the other is perspective. If you schedule in physical activity as part of your day *and* you view it as a positive experience, you may be surprised how the time issue disappears. For example: I have already discussed the fact that you can break up your activity into smaller segments, so incorporate your exercise into convenient ten- to twenty-minute slots throughout the day. These opportunities may include walking to the train or bus stop, a brisk walk during lunch, raking leaves while dinner is cooking, spinning or using a treadmill while watching television, using hand weights while on the phone, or parking a few blocks away from an errand. On days when you have bigger slots of time, choose to do something with a friend, go to an aerobics or yoga class, or go dancing.

- **I'm too tired.** Yes, the first step is the most difficult one to take, but you know deep down that

once you get moving you will feel more ener-
gized. Do you need some incentive? Plug in your
iPod while you walk or jog or crank up the stereo
while you do aerobics or yoga to a DVD at home.

- **I don't want to exercise alone.** Lots of people
feel the same way, so all you need to do is find
one of them! Seriously, hook up with your partner, kids, other family member, neighbor, friend,
and/or coworker and be active together. Kids
have play dates, so why don't you? Engaging in
physical activities with others also is a good way
to motivate yourself and your exercise partner
not only to keep moving but perhaps to also even
try new things, such as a zumba class, roller
skating, or ballroom dancing.

- **Exercise is boring.** The reason exercise may be
boring is because you haven't introduced a way
to spice it up. What would make your activities
more exciting? Do them with friends? Add music?
Try something completely new? It's up to you to
add some spice to your sessions.

WHAT TYPE OF EXERCISE IS BEST FOR BLOOD PRESSURE?

If you raised your hand and answered, "Aerobic exercise," to the preceding question, you would be only partly
correct, at least according to the results of several important studies. It used to be that aerobic exercise (e.g.,
activity that involves large muscle groups working continuously and rhythmically, such as walking, jogging,
bicycling, inline skating, jumping rope, swimming) was

believed to be the best exercise for fighting high blood pressure. However, not all studies have come to that conclusion. For example, let's look at a large review and meta-analysis of ninety-three trials that involved more than five thousand healthy adults and four types of exercise: endurance (e.g., running, biking, swimming, rowing), dynamic resistance (e.g., lifting weights, using exercise bands; also known as strength training), isometric resistance, and combination. All the studies reviewed involved trials that lasted at least four weeks.

Overall, this is what the reviewers found:

- Systolic blood pressure declined after endurance (range: 4.6–2.3 mmHg), dynamic resistance (3.7–0.011 mmHg), and isometric resistance (14.5–7.4 mmHg) but not after combination training.

- Diastolic blood pressure declined after endurance (range: 3.2–1.7 mmHg), dynamic resistance (4.5–2.0 mmHg), isometric resistance (10.3–2.0 mmHg), and combination (3.9–0.48 mmHg) training.

- Individuals with hypertension who participated in endurance training experienced a better reduction in blood pressure than did people with prehypertension or without high blood pressure.

- Improvement in blood pressure after dynamic resistance training was best in prehypertensive patients rather than in those with high blood pressure or normal blood pressure.

The conclusion from this large study is that endurance, dynamic resistance, and isometric resistance exercise

lowered both systolic and diastolic blood pressure and
that the largest drop in systolic blood pressure was among
those who participated in isometric resistance exercise.
Surprised? Don't throw away your aerobic walking shoes
yet, however.

A study of healthy elderly men (average age range
67.0–71.7 years) looked at the impact of aerobic training
alone, combined (aerobic and resistance) training, and
no training (controls) on hypertension, obesity, and lipid
levels. The two training programs involved moderate to
vigorous activity for three days a week for nine months.
The researchers found that the combination of aerobic
and resistance training was more effective in improving
blood pressure and lipid levels than was aerobic exercise
or no exercise.

What if you have resistant hypertension? Can physical activity help? A randomized controlled trial conducted in Germany involving fifty adults with resistant
high blood pressure sought to answer that question. The
participants were assigned to an eight- to twelve-week
treadmill exercise program or to no program. Those in
the exercise program experienced a significant decline
in both systolic and diastolic blood pressures and also
improved physical performance.

There's more. An Indiana University study looked at
the impact of exercise on people classified as prehypertensive and hypertensive. The authors found that participating in four ten-minute brisk walks daily reduced
systolic blood pressure by 6.6 points in prehypertensive
individuals and by 12.9 points in people with high blood
pressure.

And here is the good news for those who say they
don't have time to exercise: the authors found that these
brief walks were more effective than taking one long walk
when it came to reducing blood pressure. Therefore, if

you can put on those walking shoes and take a short brisk walk and/or some time on an exercise bike or jumping rope before work, at break, during lunch, and before or after dinner you can have a positive impact on your blood pressure without putting a significant disruptive dent in your busy day. Added benefits of such workouts can include better sleep, raised metabolism (and possibly help with weight loss), and stress reduction, all great advantages for people who have high blood pressure as well as those who want to prevent it.

Aerobic Exercise—Not What It Used to Be

Walking, brisk walking, jogging, bicycling, rowing, and jumping rope are all great aerobic exercises, but let's face it: aerobic exercise isn't what it used to be. There's certainly nothing wrong with traditional aerobic physical activity such as jogging, bicycling, and brisk walking—it works great. However, there are other ways to pump up the blood flow, such as Jazzercise, Rollerblading, kickboxing, salsa dancing, and Zumba. And don't forget the scores of aerobic videos on the market that can help you burn those calories and improve blood flow using innovative moves. It's important to enjoy your physical activities, because then you will be more likely to continue doing them and thus enjoying the health benefits.

Resistance Exercise

Now let's get back to resistance exercise. Is it really beneficial for people with high blood pressure? Let's choose a group for whom this type of exercise may seem least likely to benefit: elderly women. The study involved elderly women with high blood pressure who participated in resistance exercises (e.g., leg presses, pull-ups, biceps curls, and machine bench presses). The women performed three sets of exercises with eight to ten repetitions at two-minute intervals.

During the sixty minutes after they completed the resistance exercises, there was a significant difference in both systolic and diastolic blood pressures. The authors concluded that resistance exercises "may be prescribed safely to this group of patients" and that the improvement in blood pressure "appears to be influenced by the rest that occurred after the protocols and not by exercise."

Resistance or strength training can be done easily at home using home gym equipment, inexpensive hand weights or exercise bands, or even free equipment. Free hand weights are probably already in your house. For example, you can make your own hand weights using plastic bottles (with handles, such as milk or laundry detergent bottles) filled with sand, or you can use one- or two-pound bags of rice or beans! Or you may prefer going to a fitness club or gym, where you can learn how to use various strengthening equipment.

Here are a few resistance exercises that can be done at home or at the gym using hand weights.

Shoulder Exercise

• Stand up straight and place your feet slightly apart. Hold hand weights in your hands and place your arms comfortably at your sides.

• Inhale and shrug your shoulders up toward your ears as high as you can. Hold this position for up to five seconds, then exhale while you roll your shoulders back and squeeze your shoulder blades together.

• Hold the squeeze for up to 5 seconds, then relax your shoulders back to your starting position. Do the entire sequence 10 times.

Upper Arm Exercise

• Stand up straight and place your feet slightly apart and your knees slightly bent.

• Hold hand weights in your hands with your palms up and your arms comfortably at your sides.

• Inhale slowly as you tighten your abdominal muscles and curl the hand weights up toward your shoulders. Twist your palms so they are facing you when your hands reach your shoulders.

• Hold the hand weights at shoulder level for a second and then exhale slowly as you gradually lower the weights to your starting position.

• Repeat this exercise 10 times. Over time, you may increase the weight that you lift.

Upper Leg Exercise

• Stand up straight with your feet slightly wider than your shoulder width and your toes pointed slightly out. Bend your knees slightly.

• Hold hand weights in your hands with your arms at your sides and your palms facing inward.

- Inhale slowly as you tighten your abdominal muscles and bend your knees, slowly lowering your body as if you were going to sit in a chair. The goal is to reach a position where your thighs are almost parallel with the floor. However, only go down as far as is comfortable.

- Hold the lowest position for a few seconds, then exhale slowly as you push up with your heels and rise to your starting position.

- Repeat the exercise 8 to 10 times.

Isometric Resistance Exercise

Would you like to exercise without moving? That's basically how isometric resistance exercises look on the outside, although on the inside there is some muscle action going on. Isometric exercises involve contracting one or more muscles, although the muscles don't noticeably change length. The main goal of isometric resistance exercises is to help maintain muscle strength. Isometric resistance exercises are especially helpful for people who are recovering from an injury or who have arthritis or another condition that makes movement painful or limited. In fact, isometrics are typically prescribed as part of rehabilitation or recovery from an injury to help stabilize muscles.

Although isometrics can cause an increase in blood pressure, increasingly research is showing that they can actually lower blood pressure. In fact, a large, important study published in April 2013 in *Hypertension* revealed some interesting results. The authors reviewed about one thousand studies on nondrug approaches to treating high blood pressure, including exercise, diet, and behavioral therapies. When they looked at the effects of isometric resistance exercises, they were somewhat surprised.

They found, for example, that four weeks of isometric hand grip exercises resulted in significant improvements in blood pressure: a 10 percent decline in both systolic and diastolic blood pressures. One of the studies reviewed appeared in *Current Hypertension Reviews,* where the authors reported on the use of isometric exercise using a handgrip device. They noted that "in patients recommended for traditional exercise therapies, low intensity isometric exercise . . . is well tolerated and acceptable."

Individuals who have severely uncontrolled high blood pressure, defined as 180/110 mmHg or higher, should avoid isometric exercises. However, research is showing that use of isometric resistance exercises may have an important role in the physical activity program of many people who have hypertension. Just be sure you consult your doctor or physical therapist before you dive into doing isometrics.

Here are a few examples of isometric resistance exercises, including the handgrip exercise that has been shown to help lower blood pressure:

• The handgrip exercise can be done in several ways. One way involves using a tennis ball or other small ball or object that has some give when it is squeezed. Such objects are often handed out for free at health fairs that have booths offering information on blood pressure and heart health. Hold the ball or object in one hand and squeeze it for 60 to 90 seconds. Then switch hands. Repeat the exercise 3 to 5 times with each hand. (Bonus: this exercise can also help reduce stress!)

You also can use an athletic gripper device, which can be found in sporting goods stores and department stores. Grippers are available in different resistances, so choose one that suits you. Hold the athletic gripper in one hand and squeeze it for 2 minutes; then switch hands. Repeat the exercise 2 to 3 times with each hand.

• Sit on the floor, an exercise bench, or a table and extend one leg in front of you. Squeeze your thigh muscle, which allows you to fully straighten your leg. At the same time, flex your ankle and lift your toes up. Hold this position for 5 seconds; then rest for 3 seconds. Repeat this exercise 10 times; then switch and do the other leg. Over time, increase the number of contractions to 50 for each leg. This exercise can strengthen your knees.

• Sit on the edge of a chair, exercise bench, or table. Place a small exercise ball, rolled-up towel, or pillow between your knees. Squeeze your knees together and hold the contraction for 10 seconds. Release, relax for 5 seconds, and repeat this exercise 20 times. Over time, increase the number of contractions up to 50. This exercise can strengthen your hips.

HOW MUCH EXERCISE DO YOU NEED?

How much exercise do you need to help lower your blood pressure and strengthen your heart? According to the American Heart Association, you should aim for at least 150 minutes of moderate exercise, 75 minutes of vigorous exercise, or a combination of both every week. You can split up that time into segments that are convenient for you, as I already mentioned. Perhaps on the weekends you have time for a thirty- to forty-minute bicycle ride or cross-country ski outing, but during the week your schedule permits two fifteen-minute brisk walks: one before work and one during lunch.

Finding time to engage in physical activity is also about time management. You might jump rope or do some resistance training while watching a favorite TV show or waiting for dinner to cook. You can also multitask: do some bicep curls and other arm resistance exercises using light hand weights while taking a walk or using a treadmill.

One question that usually arises when talking about exercise is the definition of "moderate" and "vigorous" intensity. What's moderate for one person may be considered mild for some people yet vigorous for others. So how can you decide for yourself?

Be warned: there's a bit of math involved here, but it's worth knowing so you can determine what constitutes your optimal exercise heart rate (EHR).

A moderate exercise rate is one that means you are exercising at between 50 and 80 percent of your maximum capacity. Generally, this is a rate that is comfortable but somewhat challenging. You need to know your resting heart rate (RHR) before you can do the math. To take your resting pulse rate, rest quietly for at least five minutes. Place the tips of two fingers on the pulse in your wrist and count the number of beats during one minute. (Use a watch with a second hand or any accurate timepiece that counts off seconds.) You can also count the number of beats in 10 seconds and multiple by 6 or the number of beats in 30 seconds and multiple by 2. Now let's do the math to discover your exercise heart rate.

Here's an example of how to determine your EHR. Let's pretend you are 50 years old and your RHR is 80. (Use your age and RHR in the formula to figure your EHR.)

STEP 1: (220 – age) – RHR; therefore:
(220 – 50) – 80 = 90
STEP 2: 90 × % (50–80% for moderate exercise); therefore:
90 × 50% = 45; 90 × 75% = 67.
STEP 3: Add your RHR to each resulting number; therefore:
90 + 45 = 135; 90 + 67 = 157.

Therefore, your target exercise heart rate is between 135 and 157 beats per minute. When you are physically active and your heart rate falls in this range, you should feel slightly short of breath but still able to carry on a conversation.

PUTTING IT TOGETHER: EXERCISE FOR REDUCING HIGH BLOOD PRESSURE

Here are some general guidelines to consider when choosing and participating in physical activities to help prevent and manage high blood pressure:

• Aerobic, dynamic resistance, and isometric resistance exercises can help you lower blood pressure. However, you should consult your health-care provider before starting any physical activity program

• Since different types of physical activity can help with hypertension, be sure to enjoy a wide variety of choices, from dancing, jogging, brisk walking, raking leaves, and skating to lifting hand weights, using weight machines, and practicing isometrics.

• Be sure to include physical activities that you truly enjoy. Not only will you feel more motivated to keep doing them; you also will continue to reap their physical, emotional, and stress-reducing benefits.

• Keep track of your heart rate and your progress. Do you have a daily planner, calendar, or wall chart? How about an app like LivNow? These are convenient ways to keep track of your heart rate, minutes spent at each activity, and any other goals, such as weight loss. It can be very motivating to have a visual account of your activities and progress.

• Pat yourself on the back. Everyone likes to be recognized for a job well done, and you are no exception. Before you pat yourself on the back, however, set realistic yet challenging goals and reward yourself only when you reach those goals. For example, say your weekly goal is thirty minutes of moderate aerobic activity three days a week and fifteen minutes of strength training twice a week. When you complete this goal for four weeks in a row, reward yourself with a professional pedicure, a massage, or a leisurely afternoon with a great book and no interruptions!

The bottom line concerning exercise and high blood pressure is the sticky factor: you need to stick to it and make it a regular part of your lifestyle. Sure, you may miss a few days if you become ill, but as you return to your other normal activities exercise should be part of that return. Follow the suggestions in this chapter and also inject some of your own ways to stay motivated. If you take control of your exercise program and integrate it into your lifestyle, it will become second nature.

TAI CHI

Someday soon, your doctor may hand you a prescription for tai chi to help manage your high blood pressure. Tai chi is a gentle yet powerful and enjoyable way to exercise. The ancient Chinese discipline of tai chi goes back at least twenty-five hundred years and has its roots in martial arts, though today it is largely used to promote inner peace, reduce stress, and improve balance. However, it also has been found to have aerobic benefits, so I have included it in the physical activity chapter. You might say practicing tai chi is an excellent example of good time management (for all of you who say you don't have time to exercise), since it reduces stress and helps with cardiovascular health at the same time.

Types of Tai Chi

The three most popular styles of tai chi are Yang, Wu, and tai chi chih, and each one has its own special features. All of them involve slow, graceful movements and practiced breathing, yet you may want to select the style that best suits your abilities and fancy. The simple Yang style includes twenty-four movements and involves keeping your knees bent for most of the moves. The Wu style includes twenty-four to thirty-six movements, and you don't need to bend your knees as much. If you choose the tai chi chih form, there are twenty movements that don't require much knee bending and you don't shift your weight from one leg to the other as much as you do in the wu style.

Tai chi is for people of all levels of physical ability. When exploring tai chi sessions, you may want to talk to the teachers or instructors about your needs and what you wish to accomplish with the lessons. Once you learn the basics of tai chi, you can practice at home on your own, at your leisure. Daily practice is recommended for effective management of high blood pressure and overall health.

Tai Chi Studies

Even though tai chi is performed in slow motion, it can provide significant health benefits for preventing and managing high blood pressure. For example, a Stanford University study examined the impact of tai chi on thirty-nine adults age 45 and older, all of whom (except one) had high blood pressure. The study volunteers participated in community-based tai chi sessions three times a week for twelve weeks. By the end of the study, blood pressure had declined from an average of 150/86 mmHg to 131/77 mmHg and participants showed an improvement in aerobic endurance.

In a meta-analysis, researchers evaluated seven studies that explored the effects of tai chi on aerobic capacity in middle-aged adults. The experts found that people who participated in tai chi for one year (in this case the advanced Yang style that involves 108 movements) had greater aerobic capacity than did their peers who were sedentary.

In another study, fifty-eight individuals with high blood

pressure were assigned to participate in Yang form tai chi three times a week for eight weeks or to practice routine care for hypertension but no tai chi. At the end of eight weeks, those in the tai chi group showed a significant reduction in both systolic and diastolic blood pressures compared with the placebo group.

In a review of seven studies involving 947 middle-aged subjects, the authors evaluated the results concerning the impact of tai chi on blood pressure, blood lipid levels, and blood glucose. They found that tai chi had a "significant and positive effect on blood pressure and lipid levels."

Some other advantages of practicing tai chi are an improvement in upper and lower body flexibility, better balance, and improvement in muscular strength and endurance. All in all, frequent practice of tai chi appears to be an excellent addition to your physical activity (and stress reduction) program.

PHYSICAL ACTIVITY GUIDELINES

Whether you want to help prevent the development of high blood pressure or you already have been diagnosed with some level of hypertension, you should check with your health-care provider before starting any type of exercise program. Your doctor should be able to help you determine which aerobic, resistance, and other types and degrees of physical activities are best for you.

Be sure to tell your health-care provider about any and all supplements and over-the-counter and prescription drugs you may be using, your current level of physical activity, smoking and alcohol use, and any health or medical problems you are experiencing about which your doctor may not be aware. You want your exercise experiences to be as enjoyable, safe, and effective as possible!

Here are some other guidelines to consider once you begin your activity program:

- Do not exercise outdoors if the weather is too hot or too cold or the humidity is high. These extremes in weather conditions can increase your level of fatigue, make it difficult to breathe, and stress your heart. Plan some alternative activities. For example, if the weather is too cold you might stay indoors and exercise with an aerobics DVD, jump rope, or take a brisk walk at an indoor mall.

- Do not use a sauna, steam room, hot tub, or extremely hot or cold shower after an exercise session.

- If you ever feel short of breath or extremely fatigued, stop your activity and relax by resting in a seated position. If you experience heart palpitations or an irregular heartbeat, check your pulse. If your pulse is irregular or greater than one hundred beats per minute or you continue to experience shortness of breath after you have rested quietly for five to ten minutes, contact your doctor.

- If you need to miss several days of activity because of illness, injury, or other reasons, be sure to ease back into your previous level of activity.

- Do not exercise if you have a fever, have cold or flu symptoms, or otherwise do not feel well.

- Forget "no pain no gain." If you experience pain anywhere in your body, and especially chest pain, stop the activity. If the pain continues, contact your physician.

CHAPTER FIVE

Lose Weight, Sleep Better, and Other Lifestyle Matters

There's no doubt about it: the choices you make every day, from the time you get out of bed in the morning until you climb back in at night—and all night long, too!—have an impact on your blood pressure. In this chapter I discuss some of those lifestyle choices and how you can take control of those that apply to you and that will improve your blood pressure.

For example, if you are carrying around some extra pounds, then it's time to take action to lose a few. Being overweight or obese predisposes you to high blood pressure and also places undue burden on your heart and blood vessels. This chapter provides self-help tips on how to lose and maintain a healthy weight.

How well do you sleep? Did you know that sleep has a significant impact on your blood pressure? You will learn how to be proactive about any sleep issues and help improve your blood pressure in the process.

Still smoking? How many alcoholic beverages do you regularly consume? Does your coffee or cola habit have an impact on your blood pressure? It's time to review your use of substances that may have a dramatic effect on your blood pressure and help you make different choices.

Are you game to improve your blood pressure by making some lifestyle changes? Then let's go.

DROP THE WEIGHT, DROP THE PRESSURE

If you are reading this section, then you probably realize you need to lose weight, so let's skip the small talk. Losing excess weight can improve your health in numerous ways, and one of those benefits is a lowering of your blood pressure. If you are more than 10 percent over your ideal weight, then you can likely significantly lower your blood pressure once you drop those excess pounds. In fact, the *Seventh Report of the Joint National Committee on Prevention, Detection, Evaluation, and Treatment of High Blood Pressure* (*JNC 7* for short) noted that individuals can reduce their systolic blood pressure by 1 mmHg for every two pounds they lose. That sounds like an impressive benefit from losing weight! For those unfamiliar with the *JNC 7,* it was released in 2003 and provides practice guidelines for clinicians and patients when making decisions about the most appropriate health care.

What is your ideal weight? You can go to your doctor and have him or her help you make that determination, or you can do it yourself, using the accompanying chart as a guide. Find your height in the far-left column of the chart and then move your finger across the row until you come to the column that shows your current weight. At the top of that column is a number—your body mass index (BMI) number. What does it mean?

A BMI of 19 to 24 places you in the healthy category, while a BMI of 25 to 29 is considered overweight. Anyone with a BMI of 30 or greater is considered to be obese. There is some wiggle room in these figures, how-

BODY MASS INDEX (BMI), kg/m²

weight (pounds)	5'0"	5'3"	5'6"	5'9"	6'0"	6'3"
			Height (feet, inches)			
140	27	25	23	21	19	18
150	29	27	24	22	20	19
160	31	28	26	24	22	20
170	33	30	28	25	23	21
180	35	32	29	27	25	23
190	37	34	31	28	26	24
200	39	36	32	30	27	25
210	41	37	34	31	29	26
220	43	39	36	33	30	28
230	45	41	37	34	31	29
240	47	43	39	36	33	30
250	49	44	40	37	34	31

ever, because an athlete may have a lot of lean muscle weight and low body fat yet show as being overweight. Generally, however, the BMI value you get from this chart is an accurate representation of whether you are normal weight, overweight, or obese. (Download this chart for free at www.nhlbi.nih.gov/guidelines/obesity /bmi_tbl.htm)

Which Fad Diet Is Best?

Okay, I got your attention. The answer is "none." To lose weight, you need to burn more calories than you take in. You can reduce your caloric intake, boost your exercise (and thus calorie-burning power), include a natural weight loss aid, or do all three.

Diet and exercise are a must for several reasons. One, it gives you two ways to achieve success. If you choose to do just one approach, you will need to dedicate a lot of effort into that one activity and your chances of failure increase. Two, it's better to go for a balanced approach and dividing your efforts between reduced calories and extra activity provides that balance. Three, a healthier diet and regular exercise are super for heart health and overall health as well, so you will be accomplishing a great deal with your joint efforts. And four, it's always better to have some flexibility and tackling weight loss from two angles gives you some latitude. Did you enjoy too much chocolate cake yesterday? Then boost your brisk walking time by twenty minutes.

You can give your weight loss efforts a boost if you add a natural dietary aid, which are discussed in "Natural Weight Loss Aids." These are not magic bullets—they are substances shown to *assist* in weight loss efforts when used along with diet and exercise. Prescription weight loss drugs, which included Xenical and Belviq as of this writing, also require you to follow a healthy diet and to exercise if you want to experience any weight loss. In addition, these drugs are associated with significant side effects and have been shown to provide only modest assistance in weight loss. Therefore, your best bet is to go the natural route—diet, exercise, and supplements.

Tips on Losing Weight

One pound of extra body fat is equal to about thirty-five hundred calories that you consumed and did not burn. Therefore, to lose one pound of body fat you need to decrease your caloric intake by about thirty-five hundred calories. Experts typically recommend losing about one pound per week, so to lose that pound you would need to reduce your calorie intake by about five hundred calories per day.

Sure, you've seen lots of diets that say you can drop seven pounds in seven days or twenty pounds the first month. What the promoters of these diets fail to tell you is that these plans are unhealthy and that you will probably gain all the weight back—and more. In fact, if you have high blood pressure and need to lose weight, you don't need a diet—you need a healthy eating plan that you can live with for the rest of your life, because you need to stay on top of your blood pressure. As I mentioned in chapter 4 on exercise, you need to *keep* moving and exercising to manage your blood pressure. So, like exercise, weight management is a lifelong process.

Here are some tips to help you not only achieve a healthy weight to help lower your blood pressure but also improve your chances of keeping those extra pounds off:

- **Use one of the eating plans in chapter 3 as your guide.** DASH, vegetarian, and vegan eating choices include the types of foods that can help you drop pounds as well as lower blood pressure.

- **Beware of how foods are prepared.** Even the healthiest foods can turn into calorie- and fat-laden horrors if they are prepared in unhealthy ways. For example, avoid fried foods and foods served with butter, cream, cheese or cheese sauces, or gravies. Steam your vegetables, broil, bake, stir-fry, or poach your low-fat meats and fish, and bake your potatoes, squash, and yams.

- **If you eat out, always ask how an item is prepared, including the method used and the ingredients that are added to the preparation process.** If they cannot prepare it to your specifications, order something else.

- **Use spray-on oils for cooking.** A light coat of these oils allow you to "fry" without the added calories.

- **Choose whole grain and high-fiber foods rather than processed or refined foods.** Whole grain breads, pastas, and cereals not only provide more fiber and nutrients; they also fill you up faster, making you want to eat less.

- **Add foods to your diet.** Yes, I said *add*. Remember, you need to make a lifestyle change in your eating habits to keep your blood pressure at a healthy level, so think about tasty foods you can add to your menu instead of those you may need to avoid. How about fresh raspberries or peaches dipped in no-fat yogurt? Have you tried black bean and fresh tomato dip with cilantro with fresh veggies? How about a low-fat, low-calorie version of chocolate-chip cookies? All of these foods, and more, are available. Remember, millions of people who have high blood pressure and other health issues can benefit from low-fat, low-calorie choices and the recipes and food items are out there, waiting for you to try them.

- **Choose lighter versions of favorites.** If you feel like you absolutely can't live without eating chocolate pudding several times a week, then find low-fat, low-calorie versions or recipes for that pudding. Many recipes can be modified to reflect lower fat, cholesterol, and calories. You don't have to give up anything . . . just modify it!

- **Use smaller dishes.** Did you know researchers found that using smaller dinner plates helped people eat less food and less calories? Investigators from the Georgia Institute of Technology and Cornell University found that the bigger the dinner bowl or plate, the bigger the portion of food people ate. In fact, you could eat 9 to 31 percent more food if you chose a bigger serving container.

- **Don't get hungry.** Eat small, nutrition-dense foods throughout the day. Forget the three-meal-a-day routine. You may find it better to eat a small breakfast, a mini mid-morning snack (say a piece of fruit or a small container of low-fat yogurt), a small lunch, a mid-afternoon snack, and a small dinner. If you hear the refrigerator or pantry calling you after dinner, reach for a high-fiber, nutrient-rich snack, such as an apple or dried apricots.

- **Write down what you eat.** And I mean *everything*. You may be surprised when you look at your food diary and see what you eat while watching television, sitting in front of the computer, cooking dinner, at your desk at work, and before you go to bed. Having a visual reminder of what you actually consume can help you make changes to your eating habits and establish healthier goals.

- **Get some support.** Find friends, neighbors, family members, coworkers, or Internet friends to support and who can support you with your weight loss efforts and your goal to maintain a healthy eating program for the rest of your life. Fighting pounds can be a challenge, and surrounding yourself with a cheerleading team, of which you are also a member, can be a great help.

- **Stay active.** That means your mind as well as your body. If you get bored, you may begin to eat mindlessly, and that can mean consuming lots of extra calories, fat, and cholesterol that can be detrimental to your blood pressure. Be prepared for boredom by having a list of things you can do when life becomes a bit slow. Call friends, find something interesting on the Internet, take a walk, start a new project, watch some funny videos, or work on a puzzle. Basically, have an "activity box" available so you don't open the refrigerator or kitchen cabinet door instead.

NATURAL WEIGHT LOSS AIDS

If you walk into a health foods store or the weight loss section of a pharmacy or if you search on the Internet, you'll found countless numbers of supplements that claim they can help you lose weight. The trouble is, most of these supplements are not effective. However, some of them have been scientifically tested and shown to be beneficial, while others have demonstrated conflicting results, which means they probably aren't yet ready for prime time.

Let me also stress, however, that you should not depend on natural weight loss aids to help you lose weight. At best they can enhance your other *necessary* weight loss efforts, which include adopting healthy eating habits that focus on low-fat, high-fiber foods such as fruits, vegetables, grains, and plant-based proteins, as well as regular physical activity. There may be natural supplements other than those explained here that you want to try to help you lose weight. Research findings are always changing, and so you may find convincing evidence that supplements other than those included here may enhance your weight loss efforts. Whatever you do, you should consult a knowledgeable health-care provider before you take any supplements to be sure they will not interact negatively with anything else you are taking or with any health issues you have. Here are some supplements that may help you with your weight loss efforts.

Seaweed Supplements

The oceans offer a variety of seaweeds that contain components shown to help reduce body weight and body fat. Don't worry: the seaweed comes disguised in capsules or other unrecognizable forms so you won't even know what you're taking.

Among the seaweeds found to help with weight loss are brown seaweeds, including the edible brown seaweeds such as *hijiki* and wakame. These and other seaweeds contain a pigment and carotenoid (plant nutrient) called fucoxanthin, which has been shown to have anti-obesity properties. Basically, scientists believe fucoxanthin may help with weight loss by focusing its action on a protein called UCP1, which increases the rate at which the body burns abdominal fat.

Since you would need to eat an incredible amount of wakame and other brown seaweeds to get any possible weight loss benefits, seaweed supplements are an option. Several studies conducted in animals and people that have used seaweed supplements have shown some benefits.

For example, a twelve-week double-blind study involved eighty obese adults who were divided into two groups. Both groups were following a low-calorie diet, but one group also consumed a beverage that contained a seaweed-based supplement. The control group was given a beverage that did not contain the supplement.

By the end of the study, the participants who had taken the seaweed supplement had lost four pounds more than the subjects in the other group. Although four pounds may not sound like a lot, over a year that equals about sixteen pounds and you may reduce your systolic blood pressure by 1 mmHg for every two pounds you lose.

The types of seaweed used in the study supplement were *Laminaria digitata* and *L. hyperborea*. These are both large brown seaweeds and contain a natural fiber called alginate, which has been shown to significantly reduce the amount of fat the body absorbs. But the seaweeds were also effective in humans. When the researchers tested the seaweed by adding it to bread, the alginates significantly reduced the digestion of fat. In fact, the head of the study, Dr. Iain Brownlee, commented that their findings "suggest alginates could offer a very real solution in the battle against obesity."

Black Pepper

Did you know that the black pepper you sprinkle on your food could help you drop additional pounds? That is probably good news, especially if you like your food to pack a bite. The reason black pepper helps with weight and fat loss is because it contains an ingredient called piperine, which is also responsible for pepper's unique taste.

Beyond taste, however, research indicates that piperine increases metabolism, especially when the diet consists of high-fat, high-sugar foods. At least that's what investigators found when they gave black pepper to mice and studied its effects in computer models. Specifically, they discovered that piperine helps interfere with the formation of new fat cells, which in turn helps stop weight gain, and has potential as a treatment for overweight and obesity. Overall, the researchers noted that "our results suggest that piperine could be a lead natural compound for the treatment of fat-related disorders" and thus also help with weight loss for people who have high blood pressure.

In the laboratory, scientists have discovered that piperine has the ability to suppress activities that are involved with fat metabolism. This finding led one team of researchers to note in a *Journal of Agricultural and Food Chemistry* study that black pepper and piperine could be a "potential treatment for obesity-related diseases." The black pepper component also prevents the liver from immediately breaking down certain supplements and drugs, which in turn increases the body absorption of the substances and the effects they provide.

The pure form of piperine is BioPerine, which is extracted from the fruit of black pepper. A typical dose is 10 milligrams taken twice daily before meals. The most common side effects of piperine are nausea, vomiting, and diarrhea, but these tend to be mild. If you consume more piperine than recommended, you may experience some heartburn. Chronic inhalation of black pepper or piperine powder can irritate the lungs.

Green Coffee Bean Extract

You may have read about the excitement surrounding the use of green coffee bean extract as a weight loss aid. Green coffee beans are raw, unroasted coffee beans.

Based on a number of scientific studies, it appears that this supplement can help you drop pounds. But wait: What about the caffeine in coffee beans? Should you worry about the stimulating effect of caffeine if you have high blood pressure?

Let's address the concern about caffeine before looking at how green coffee bean extract may help with weight loss. Although it seems green coffee bean extract would cause an increase in blood pressure and heart rate, surprisingly researchers have found the opposite to be true.

For example, consider the results of a 2012 study published in *Diabetes, Metabolic Syndrome and Obesity* and conducted by researchers at the University of Scranton. The investigators enlisted sixteen overweight adults in a twenty-two-week crossover study, which means the subjects participated in both the treatment and the placebo segments of the study. In this case, the adults took either 1,050 mg or 700 mg of green coffee bean extract or a placebo for six weeks, with a two-week washout period in between each segment of the study.

All the participants lost weight (average: about seventeen pounds) and body fat (average: 4.44 percent) when they were taking green coffee bean extract, and all of them also had a reduction in body mass index. In addition, three had a reduction in systolic blood pressure and five had a reduction in diastolic blood pressure, while twelve had a decline in heart rate. The authors of the study concluded that green coffee bean extract may be an effective and inexpensive way to reduce weight and prevent obesity.

What's the secret ingredient in green coffee beans that helps people lose weight but does not necessarily cause their blood pressure to rise? As typically happens, scientists conduct their research and make their discoveries in animals before they perform testing in humans.

Therefore, in early studies researchers found that the blood-pressure-lowering effect of green coffee beans is due to the presence of chlorogenic acid. This acid is an antioxidant, which means it can help fight molecules that cause disease, aging, and other deteriorating events in the body. Clorogenic acid also breaks down when coffee beans are roasted, so any health benefits associated with the raw beans are lost.

Chlorogenic acid contains ferulic acid, which in turn has an effect on nitric oxide and the blood vessels. Thus chlorogenic acid has a positive effect on blood vessels and blood pressure. This benefit has been seen in human studies, including one in which twenty-eight adults with essential hypertension took part. Participants took either 140 milligrams per day of chlorogenic acid or placebo. Both systolic and diastolic blood pressures declined significantly among participants who took chlorogenic acid but not among those who took placebo.

Now let's get back to the ability of green coffee bean extract to help with weight loss. It appears that chlorogenic acid also has an ability to reduce the amount of fat people absorb from food while also stimulating the burning of fat. These weight loss benefits seem to be related to how chlorogenic acid interferes with the activity of an enzyme called glucose-6-phosphatase.

So there you have it: a brief but impressive story about green coffee bean extract, weight loss, and high blood pressure. I suggest you keep your eyes and ears open for continuing research on green coffee bean extract, as well as the other supplements discussed in this chapter, so you'll have the latest information on their effectiveness and safety.

If you decide to try a green coffee bean extract supplement, the suggested dose for weight loss is 400 to 500 milligrams twice a day taken about thirty minutes before a meal. Because green coffee bean extract contains a small amount of caffeine, it may bother you (e.g., cause jitteriness or insomnia) if you are sensitive to caffeine. Some green coffee bean extract supplements also contain other ingredients that are associated with weight loss, such as green tea extract, African mango, and kelp (seaweed). Look for green coffee bean extract supplements that are standardized for 45 percent chlorogenic acid.

SLEEP AND HIGH BLOOD PRESSURE

A good night's sleep is essential for everyone's health, but if you have high blood pressure quality sleep is especially critical. The American Heart Association's High Blood Pressure Research 2012 Scientific Sessions reported that people with high blood pressure who got six or fewer hours of sleep per night, as well as those who said they did not sleep well, were twice as likely to have resistant hypertension (that's the kind that doesn't respond well to three or more medications).

Women appear to face more of a challenge with sleep and high blood pressure than men do. In fact, the report from the same scientific sessions noted that women were more likely to say they suffered with poor sleep quality than were men and that women who had resistant hypertension were five times as likely to also experience poor sleep quality. Other research that same year from Henry Ford Hospital in Detroit reported that people who suffer with insomnia have an increased likelihood of developing hypertension.

Men don't escape the claws of sleep problems and hypertension, however. Hypertension in men has been associated with males who do not get sufficient deep sleep, and getting fewer than seven hours of sleep at night has been associated with high blood pressure in both men and women.

How Sleep Affects Blood Pressure

What's the relationship between sleep, insomnia, other sleep problems, and high blood pressure? The truth is, experts are not exactly sure and they admit more research is needed to identify all the factors involved and how they operate.

What experts do know is that insomnia, which is the inability to fall asleep or stay asleep, is the most common sleep problem reported by Americans. About 30 to 40 percent of adults have reported some symptoms of insomnia during any given year, and about 10 to 15 percent say they have chronic insomnia, according to the National Center on Sleep Disorders Research and the National Institutes of Health.

Sleep deprivation also has been linked to obesity. Yes, not getting enough sleep (less than six hours per night) can raise your risk of obesity, which as you know is a risk factor for high blood pressure. Did you ever realize sleep was so important?

Scientists have found that if you get too little sleep the cycle of certain hormones that are involved in regulating your appetite and metabolism are disrupted. In fact, scientists have identified two of the hormones: ghrelin, which triggers hunger; and leptin, a hormone that lets your brain know if you have eaten enough and should feel full. A lack of sufficient sleep also may promote an increase in how much food you eat and reduce insulin sensitivity, which then increases your blood pressure and your risk of type 2 diabetes.

Therefore, it is clear that sleep disturbances are a significant factor in high blood pressure. What can you do to improve sleep quality and thus your blood pressure? Quite a bit, actually, if you follow the tips provided here. Sleep is critical for achieving and maintaining a healthy blood pressure, so consider the following suggestions for preparing and using your sleep environment. Your sleep/wake cycle is regulated by an internal clock and your pineal gland, which is located deep in your brain. Light affects the pineal gland's production of hormones called melatonin and serotonin. Levels of melatonin and serotonin are highest at night, but exposure to light can disrupt those levels and thus your sleep.

Although these hormones play a critical role in your health and your sleep, other factors come into play as well. Therefore, here are some tips to help you get the most effective and beneficial sleep possible and to boost your efforts to lower your blood pressure naturally.

How to Sleep Better, Naturally

Bypass the sleeping pills and focus on these natural approaches to better sleep and, as a result, a healthier blood pressure:

- **Keep it dark.** Don't allow any light in your bedroom, as any hint of light can have an effect on your pineal gland and melatonin production. Therefore, keep the drapes closed, put up blackout shades, or wear an eye mask. Don't keep a night-light in your room, and cover up your alarm clock if it glows. Light signals your brain and disrupts your natural rhythms at night. Naturally, you want to be safe when you get up during the night, so use a low-voltage orange or amber-colored night-light that does not expose you to the short light wavelengths from regular bulbs.

• **Keep it cool.** Experts say the optimal sleeping temperature is between sixty and sixty-eight degrees. Because your internal body temperature drops to its lowest level about four hours into your sleep pattern, it's believed that a lower room temperature aids natural sleep.

• **Keep it quiet.** Do you like to be frightened awake? I didn't think so. A loud alarm clock can be stressful. Consider using an alarm that simulates sunrise by gradually increasing the amount of light in your room or one that slowly raises the sound of soothing music.

• **Hide the time.** If you wake up during the night, do you always check the alarm clock to see what time it is? Worrying about the time can add to your stress and make it more difficult to get quality sleep.

• **Choose your bed partners carefully.** Bed partners, both human and those of the four-legged variety, can interfere with your sleep if they are restless or snore. You may need to consider separate sleeping arrangements.

• **Reserve your bed for sleep and sex.** Avoid the habit of using your bed for working on your computer, watching television, eating, or reading (although reading something soothing, spiritual, or uplifting can be helpful). View your bed as your comfortable transportation vehicle for sleep.

• **Keep it comfortable.** Speaking of comfort, do you like your bed pillow(s)? Is your mattress

firm or soft enough (depending on your needs?)
Do your bed linens provide the right amount of
warmth?

• **Follow a regular routine.** Your body and blood
pressure will respond best if you establish and
follow a regular time to go to bed and get up
every day of the week. This will help your body
recognize a pattern, which will make it easier for
you to fall asleep, stay asleep, and wake up more
refreshed.

• **Relax before bedtime.** Turn off the horror
movie on television, put down the mystery thriller,
and get off the treadmill. Prepare for bedtime by
easing into sleep: meditate; listen to soothing
music; get a foot massage; use aromatherapy (a
diffuser, not candles!); practice guided visualization. You don't need to always use the same
routine, but have stress-relieving things you can
do before you go to bed each night.

• **Reduce your need for nighttime bathroom
trips.** That means don't drink any fluids within
two hours of going to bed and go to the bathroom immediately before getting into bed.

• **Choose a wise after-dinner snack.** If you feel
you need something to eat a few hours before
going to bed, choose something high in protein,
sugar-free or low in sugar, and low in fat. Foods
that contain L-tryptophan, an amino acid that
can help melatonin production and thus boost
sleep potential, are a good choice. A two-hundred-

calorie serving of the following foods provides a significant amount of tryptophan: cooked spinach (600 mg), turkey or chicken (400–500 mg), low-fat cottage cheese or low-fat cheddar cheese (330–400 mg), and tofu (400 mg).

• **Beware of electromagnetic fields.** Not everyone agrees with this idea, but some experts say that electromagnetic fields (EMFs), which radiate from high-power lines and electrical devices such as televisions, electric blankets, and refrigerators, can interfere with the production of melatonin and serotonin by the pineal gland. EMFs may reduce heart rate and disrupt electrical activity in the brain while you sleep.

• **Consider melatonin supplements.** Short-term use (no more than two months is recommended) of melatonin supplements may help with difficulty falling asleep or staying asleep. The most common side effects of melatonin are dizziness, daytime sleepiness, and headache. Be sure to talk to your doctor before taking melatonin. Although melatonin is typically a safe supplement, it can interact with blood-thinning medications, drugs to treat diabetes, birth control pills, and immunosuppressants. The suggested dose can range from 0.5 milligrams per day up to 3 to 5 milligrams, depending on your sleep problem and how you respond to the hormone. The best advice is to start low and slow.

• **Keep your feet warm.** Feet typically have the poorest circulation in the body, and so they tend to get cold. If you wear socks to bed and keep your tootsies warm, you can reduce your chances of waking up during the night.

- **Bring in the noise (white, that is).** Some people say they can fall asleep much better if they have white noise or nature sounds in the background. Scores of relaxation and sleep CDs are available, including those that involve guided visualization and meditation to help you drift into sleep within a few minutes. If you haven't tried it, borrow some nature sound CDs from the library and try them.

- **Avoid alcohol.** Although drinking alcohol may make you sleepy, you will likely wake up several hours later and be unable to go back to sleep. Drinking alcohol also prevents the brain from entering deep stages of sleep, which your body needs to rejuvenate.

- **Be cautious about caffeine.** Some people feel the effects of caffeine for many hours, while others seem to be able to have a cup of coffee and go right to sleep. If you are uncertain about how your body responds to caffeine, keep track of your coffee, cola, and other caffeine-containing liquid intake and how you sleep at night. You may need to make some adjustments.

- **Exercise.** Once again, physical activity can benefit your blood pressure, but be sure to do your exercising at least a few hours before you go to bed. Boosting your endorphins and heart rate right before bedtime can actually make falling asleep more difficult.

Sleep Apnea and Hypertension

Do you have obstructive sleep apnea? It's been estimated that up to 90 percent of people with sleep apnea
don't even know they have this sleep condition, and the
reason is simple: they are asleep when the symptoms
occur, so they need to have someone—typically their
sleep partner—tell them about the apnea. The reason
knowing about sleep apnea is especially important for
our purposes is that about 50 percent of people who
have essential hypertension have sleep apnea and about
50 percent of people with sleep apnea have essential hypertension.

Obstructive sleep apnea is defined as a condition in
which individuals experience at least ten occasions per
hour when the throat muscles relax and block the airway during sleep, causing the individual to stop breathing for about ten to twenty seconds or longer. This lack
of breathing reduces the amount of oxygen in your blood
and causes the brain to respond by briefly waking you
up so your airway will reopen. Fortunately, you will
rarely remember being awakened, but your body remem-
bers, because you will feel tired the next day. The most
apparent sign of obstructive sleep apnea is snoring,
while some people snort, gasp, or make choking sounds
as well. If you are middle-aged or older and are overweight, you are more likely to be affected by obstructive
sleep apnea, but it can affect people of any age.

In fact, many people who have this sleep disorder
don't even realize it because it requires that their sleep
partner tell them it is happening. Even then, many people
don't equate snoring or brief breathing stoppages with
sleep apnea.

However, if your doctor asks you whether you snore,
if you are excessively tired during the day, and if your

sleep partner has told you about interrupted breathing events and you answer "yes" to any of these questions, then you could have obstructive sleep apnea. It's true that not everyone who snores has obstructive sleep apnea. However, if your snoring is accompanied by periods of silence and not breathing it is likely sleep apnea. Other signs of obstructive sleep apnea is waking up with a sore throat or dry mouth, headache in the morning, and waking up abruptly accompanied by shortness of breath. If you also have high blood pressure, then this is important information you can use to help you improve both your sleep and your blood pressure.

The good news is that most studies that have looked at the impact of treatment for sleep apnea on blood pressure have found that it not only eliminates snoring, daytime tiredness, and interrupted breathing but also significantly lowered blood pressure. So how do you treat obstructive sleep apnea?

Treating Obstructive Sleep Apnea

If you suffer with obstructive sleep apnea and hypertension, relief could be as easy as a few lifestyle changes, depending on the severity of your problem. For example:

- **Don't sleep on your back.** People with obstructive sleep apnea and/or who snore tend to sleep on their back. Make an effort to sleep on your side, and ask your sleep partner to help you. You might also use pillows behind your back to prevent you from rolling over on your back.

- **Drop some pounds.** Being overweight is a significant risk factor for obstructive sleep apnea.

- **Limit your alcohol consumption.** In fact, avoid alcohol altogether if you can, but if you do drink, have only one or two and don't drink for about three or more hours before bedtime. Alcohol suppresses the nervous system, which can make it more difficult to breathe.

- **Stop smoking.** Smoking causes your upper airway to swell, which can make sleep apnea worse. See "Tips to Quit Smoking" in this chapter for help quitting.

- **Use a nasal decongestant.** Rather than an over-the-counter medication, you can choose a natural saline solution or use a neti pot to help clear your sinuses.

- **Use CPAP.** If your doctor diagnoses you with obstructive sleep apnea and natural treatments don't provide enough relief, then you may get help from a machine that delivers air pressure through a mask you wear at night while you sleep. Continuous positive airway pressure (CPAP) provides air through a mask with just enough pressure to keep your upper airway passages open, which can prevent snoring and obstructive sleep apnea. There are several different types of CPAP, so be sure to discuss the options with your doctor. If wearing a mask while you sleep doesn't work or is not acceptable, a dentist may fit you for an oral device that helps keep your throat open and/or your jaw forward while your sleep. Surgery is a last resort but can be arranged for severe obstructive sleep apnea or cases that involve enlarged tonsils or adenoids. One minimally invasive procedure for people with mild obstructive sleep apnea is the placement of implants in the soft palate. The implants help reduce the amount of collapse of the upper airway.

SMOKING

Most people understand the relationship between smoking cigarettes or cigars and lung cancer, but when you mention high blood pressure the association gets a big hazy. Researchers cleared the air on that topic when they measured blood pressure while people smoked and documented that within five minutes of taking the first drag systolic blood pressure rose an average of more than 20 mmHg. It then takes about thirty minutes for systolic blood pressure to gradually return to the presmoking level.

If you smoke one cigarette an hour during waking hours (assume you are awake sixteen hours), your blood pressure is higher than your normal level for about eight hours a day. If you are a heavy smoker (say two cigarettes per hour or thirty-two cigarettes), then your blood pressure barely reaches normal before it rises again. The only time your blood pressure returns to a nonsmoking level is when you sleep. If you have a habit of smoking a cigarette if you wake up during the night, you will send your blood pressure surging again.

Nicotine causes blood vessels to constrict, which hampers the flow of blood and makes the heart work harder. The result is a rise in blood pressure. Nicotine also increases the chance of blood clots, damages the cells that line the arteries and other blood vessels, and reduces the amount of oxygen that reaches the heart.

Are You Ready to Quit?

As a former smoker, I believe people will quit smoking only when they are truly ready to quit. Smokers also need one or more reasons to quit that mean something to them personally so they can stay motivated. For some it's the chance to see their grandchildren grow up; for others it may be a fear of dying before they reach certain goals or because they are tired of feeling ill and fatigued. Other cannot bear the expense any longer or they are plagued by smoking-related diseases such as high blood pressure, heart disease, cancer, gum disease, or emphysema. Whatever your reason is for quitting, know that you can achieve that goal if you plan ahead for the hurdles that you will face.

For most smokers, quitting is not easy, but it is completely doable. The following tips have been shown to help some smokers some of the time. Read through them, think about them carefully, and chose the ones that you believe will work for you. Then you need to do two things:

1. Get a calendar and choose the date you will stop smoking. Mark the date and put the calendar where you can see it clearly.
2. Make a list of the reasons why you are going to quit. You may have only one item on the list or you may have a dozen—it doesn't matter. What matters is that you write them down and read the list every day before the date you have chosen to quit and every day that follows until you don't feel the need to read the list anymore.

Tips to Quit Smoking

- **Identify your smoking triggers and write them down.** If you know what causes you to reach for a cigarette, you can hijack the desire and do something else or change how you think about that activity so you will feel less like smoking. For example, do you light up every time you get behind the wheel of your car or during your morning coffee break at work? Then it's time for you to do something different in these circumstances so you can help break the habit of reaching for the cigarette. For example, you could put a comedy CD into your player in the car or take a walk during your coffee break (and ask a coworker to join you!) to break up your routine.

- **Be prepared for some withdrawal symptoms.** The good news is that withdrawal symptoms are temporary—they usually fade and disappear after about two weeks. However, as your body adjusts to not being fed nicotine you may feel cranky and hungry and have difficulty concentrating. Many people experience headache, coughing, and even light tremors. All of these symptoms are a sign you are on your way to healing from the effects of smoking, so stay strong and tough it out!

- **Be prepared with a list of distracting activities.** Whenever you want to have a cigarette, you should be ready to do something else. Make a long list of options to cover lots of different circumstances. For example, your list might include the following: take a walk, do a crossword puzzle, call a friend, send an e-mail to a friend, read or watch something funny, visit a stop-smoking Web site for support, have some sugar-less gum or candy, practice deep-breathing exercises or meditate (see chapter 6), turn up the music and dance, squeeze a stress ball. A hobby that keeps your hands occupied, such as needle-work, jigsaw puzzles, playing an instrument, painting, or gardening, can be helpful.

• **Seek support.** Many people will help you with your efforts to quit smoking if you reach out. Be-yond friends and family, who can be extremely important in helping you quit, there are also stop-smoking helplines, programs offered by the Amer-ican Lung Association and the American Cancer Society, smoking cessation support groups, and online support forums and chat rooms.

• **Get an app.** It's true—there is an app for every-thing, and you can get apps that can assist you in your quit-smoking efforts.

• **Consider medications.** Temporary use of medi-cations that help fight nicotine cravings as well as nicotine substitutes (e.g., patches, gum) can provide additional support for smoking cessation. Be sure to talk to your doctor about these prod-ucts before you use them.

• **Avoid trigger situations whenever possible.** For example, if you used to hang out with fellow coworkers during break and have a cigarette take a walk during your break or watch a brief funny video on your smart phone or computer. Avoid venues that allow smoking and go to places that are smoke-free, such as movie theaters, libraries, and museums. Fortunately, the number of smoke-free facilities and environments is increasing every day, with many cities and towns banning smoking in public places, including parks and beaches.

- **Get rid of the evidence.** Eliminate all reminders of smoking from your home and workplace, such as lighters, matches, ashtrays, and even any stray cigarette butts.

- **Stay hydrated.** Drinking lots of fluids can help cut nicotine cravings, but limit intake of alcohol and caffeinated beverages, as they can increase the urge to smoke. Try herbal teas and sparkling flavored waters instead.

- **Eat healthy foods and snacks.** Weight gain is a major concern of people who want to quit smoking, but you can help prevent the encroachment of unwanted pounds by chewing sugar-free gum, sucking on sugar-free candies, and crunching on carrots and raw bell pepper sticks. Another popular substitute for smoking is air-popped popcorn (no butter or salt) sprinkled with powdered cayenne or even cinnamon.

- **Remind yourself every day why you quit.** Reread the list you made of why you wanted to quit smoking.

- **Calculate the savings.** How much were your spending on cigarettes before you quit? Take that amount of money and put it aside every day you don't smoke. Better yet, every time you crave a cigarette put the cost of one cigarette into a jar. At the end of every week (or every few days) check to see how much money you saved by not smoking. You can use that money to reward yourself or save it for a special occasion.

ALCOHOL AND HYPERTENSION

If you occasionally enjoy a glass of wine with dinner or a few cold beers over the weekend, the amount of alcohol in those drinks is unlikely to have a significant impact on your blood pressure. While the general recommendation is to avoid alcohol if you have high blood pressure, moderate drinking—one drink daily for women and two drinks daily for men younger than 65 (but one for those older than 65)—is the amount of alcohol usually suggested. For reference, one drink equals 12 ounces of beer, 5 ounces of wine, or 1.5 ounces of 80-proof distilled spirits.

Reasons to Avoid Alcohol Use

Drinking to excess can raise your blood pressure to unhealthy levels, and binge drinking can result in long-term and even dangerous blood pressure problems, including a greatly increased risk of heart attack and stroke. The exact way alcohol impacts blood pressure is not known, but it may contribute to hardening of the arteries by making the blood vessels more likely to form plaque or for the plaque to rupture.

If you are taking blood pressure medications or any other medications either over the counter or by prescription, use of alcohol can have devastating effects, including dangerous fluctuations in blood pressure and risk of bleeding. Even one or two drinks can cause these serious reactions, especially in people who are elderly or who have other health problems.

But alcohol consumption also has a positive side.

How Much Alcohol Is Good?

How much impact does light to moderate drinking have on blood pressure? Some research indicates that moderate drinking can lower your blood pressure by 2 to 4 mmHg while excessive consumption erases that benefit. Among the scientists who have wondered about alcohol's impact on blood pressure is a team of researchers at Harvard who looked at alcohol consumption reported by 28,848 women and 13,455 men from two different studies.

At the beginning of the studies, the participants in both groups were free of hypertension, cancer, and cardiovascular disease. The participants were followed up at an average of 10.9 years (women) and 21.8 years (men), and this is what the researchers found:

- Eight thousand, six hundred and eighty women and 6,012 men developed high blood pressure during the follow-up period.

- Light to moderate alcohol intake reduced the risk of hypertension in women but increased the risk in men.

- The threshold above which use of alcohol became a risk for high blood pressure was four or more drinks daily for women versus one or more drinks daily for men.

These findings seem to contradict what doctors typically advise when it comes to alcohol use, especially for women. However, moderation is still recommended, especially since excessive alcohol use has other detrimental effects, including weight gain, damage to the liver, increased risk of some cancers, worsening of depression, greater risk of falls, and more rapid aging.

You may also be familiar with studies stating that drinking red wine can help the heart and blood pressure. That's because red wine contains potent antioxidants such as resveratrol. However, beer and spirits also contain antioxidants, albeit not the same ones found in red wine. Alcohol also has a blood-thinning effect, which can be helpful in promoting blood circulation and thus assist with controlling hypertension.

All of these findings, however, are not an endorsement to start drinking alcohol if you don't drink or to drink more if you are a consumer already. Rather, they serve as a reminder that a little alcohol can go a long way when it comes to your blood pressure.

How to Reduce Alcohol Use

If you have an alcohol addiction or are a binge drinker and you have high blood pressure, you are at great risk of stroke and heart attack. While it is important for you to reduce or even eliminate your alcohol use, it's also critical to do so with professional guidance from a medical doctor or mental health provider. Alcohol withdrawal syndrome is a potentially deadly condition that can occur in anyone who has been drinking heavily for weeks or longer and who then stops or significantly cuts back on alcohol consumption.

If your alcohol use is not severe but you want some ideas on how to reduce your drinking, here are some tips:

- **Get rid of the evidence.** Don't keep alcohol in the house or, if you do, keep only a small amount and keep it out of sight. The same goes for items that remind you of drinking: beer mugs, wineglasses, and bar items.

- **Sip sparkling water.** When you go to a party or are out with friends, resist the alcohol and ask for sparkling water with a twist of lime or cranberry juice. Some people like sparkling cider, nonalcoholic beer, or alcohol-free wine.

- **Slow down.** When you do drink, sip your drink slowly. Start with a nonalcoholic beverage, then drink your wine or other alcoholic beverage, and finish off the night with another nonalcoholic drink.

- **Avoid salty foods when drinking.** Those salty nuts (which are not good for your blood pressure anyway!) encourage you to drink more, so avoid them.

- **Identify your triggers and avoid them.** Once you know what prompts you to want a drink, you can take steps to sidestep the triggers. If you always reach for the merlot as you prepare dinner after work, substitute a pitcher of iced tea with lemon for the wine bottle. If the gang always meets at a favorite bar on Fridays, suggest a new location or skip the venue until you feel confident you can beat the urge to drink.

- **Eat lots of fruits and vegetables.** What does this tip have to do with alcohol and hypertension? Remember that DASH and other diets discussed in this book stress the importance of fruits and vegetables, and one reason is because they are rich in potassium and calcium. Potassium and calcium are important because they work together to counteract the negative effects of alcohol and help moderate your blood pressure.

CAFFEINE AND HYPERTENSION

If you have high blood pressure, should you give up that morning cup of java or avoid those tall glasses of iced tea? Generally, research shows that consuming caffeine in the form of coffee, tea, cola, chocolate, or medications does not increase the risk of high blood pressure or heart-related events such as heart attack. Reviews of studies of the effect of caffeine on blood pressure and cardiovascular disease have shown that while caffeine and coffee intake can cause an increase in blood pressure (about 8 mmHg systolic and 5.7 mmHg diastolic), it is only temporary, lasting only a few hours. Research also shows no association between habitual use of caffeinated coffee and a higher risk of cardiovascular disease. In fact, the Joint National Committee on Prevention, Detection, Evaluation, and Treatment of High Blood Pressure has stated that there is no proof that coffee or tea consumption is linked to high blood pressure.

So why talk about caffeine and high blood pressure at all? There are several reasons. One is the misconception that coffee and tea, and the caffeine they contain, are detrimental if you have high blood pressure, and I have already explained that this is generally not true, but you should still consult your health-care provider. Another reason is that drinking coffee and tea may offer some health benefits regarding blood pressure, because they are a rich source of plant compounds called polyphenols.

Polyphenols is a broad category that includes thousands of different antioxidants, which are molecules that fight disease-causing and cell-damaging substances. In other words, they play an important role in your health, including help with hypertension and your heart. Among the benefits of polyphenols found in coffee and tea are the ability to reduce the formation of blood clots that can lead to stroke, lower the concentration of C-reactive protein, which is involved in inflammation, and reduce the risk of cardiovascular disease.

Although there is lots of scientific evidence showing that coffee and tea drinkers with high blood pressure should not worry about continuing their beverage habit, you can also be assured you don't need to start drinking coffee or tea just to get the polyphenols. Indeed, polyphenols are available in a wide variety of fruits, vegetables, legumes, and seeds. Therefore, if you follow the diets presented in this book you should consume plenty of polyphenols. Drinking cola beverages, however, which can contain significant amounts of caffeine, is not recommended not because of the caffeine content but because of the sugar, phosphorus, and empty calories.

If you want to add green tea to your menu, however, that would be a positive move, as I discuss in chapter 6 on supplements. Green tea and green tea extract have been shown to reduce blood pressure in people who are hypertensive. Green tea is naturally lower in caffeine than black tea and coffee and is an excellent source of the polyphenols called catechins.

Yet one more reason to discuss caffeine and hypertension is cola. If you are a big fan of colas, then you may want to rethink your consumption. A large study involving more than 155,000 women and spanning more than twelve years found that while habitual coffee consumption was not associated with an increased risk of hypertension, the same was not true of drinking cola beverages. Women who consumed colas had an increased risk of hypertension regardless of whether they drank sugared or diet colas. Because colas and other soft drinks are empty calories, they are best avoided and replaced with more nutritious and satisfying beverages.

So are you prepared to make some lifestyle changes to improve your blood pressure? Remember, improvements in your blood pressure will likely come as you combine your lifestyle modification efforts with diet, exercise, stress reduction, and supplements.

CHAPTER SIX

Try Nutritional and Herbal Remedies

The use of natural nutrients and herbal remedies can be an effective and safe complementary approach to help lower blood pressure when included as part of your overall prevention and management program. Although taking an herbal remedy, vitamin, or other natural supplement won't cure your high blood pressure, it may help reduce or even eliminate your need for harsh blood pressure medications, with their side effects, especially if you have adopted other lifestyle changes like those discussed in this book.

Naturally, you should always discuss your desire to use natural supplements with your health-care providers and ask them or other knowledgeable professionals to help you choose those that would be best for your needs. Many natural supplements for managing high blood pressure are also beneficial for related conditions, such as cardiovascular disease and diabetes, so you may want to choose supplements that can offer you the most advantages overall. Whatever you do, never start a supplement program without first consulting your doctor.

Why? Your doctor cannot accurately and effectively monitor your progress in lowering your blood pressure if he or she does not know all the substances you are taking that can have an impact on your pressure. This is true in all cases, and especially if you have other medical problems for which you are being treated. Nutrients and herbal remedies are not benign substances: they can have a significant and beneficial effect on your health. After all, that's why you take them, right?

If you have a doctor who resists or flat out refuses to discuss or consider supplements or other complementary approaches, you have several choices. One, you can look for another doctor who is open to complementary medicine. Fortunately, it is getting much easier to find such physicians, as more and more doctors integrate alternative treatments into their practices. Hopefully he or she will be part of your insurance plan if you have health insurance. Two, you can go outside of your insurance plan and consult another doctor. Or three, you can give up the battle. However, many patients find they can find satisfaction using either of the first two choices.

That said, let's take a look at the nutritional and herbal supplements that have been shown to have a positive impact on blood pressure. It's important to remember that just because a supplement is natural does not mean it is entirely safe. Nutritional and herbal supplements can have potent effects, and so respect their powers. Use them as directed by a knowledgeable professional, and make sure *all* your health-care providers (including any outside of your insurance plan) are aware of *all* the treatments you are using to lower your blood pressure or for any other health condition, because nutritional and herbal supplements can interact with each other, as they can with medications as well.

OLIVE LEAF EXTRACT

Olive leaf extract is one of the more promising natural supplements for lowering high blood pressure. The supplement is made from the leaves of the olive tree (*Olea europaea*) and is often marketed as an antiaging product as well as a natural way to help manage high blood pressure.

Several active ingredients have been identified in olive leaves, including oleacein, oleanolic acid, and oleuropein. The latter ingredient is the one you should especially look for on the product label when buying olive leaf extract. Oleuropein has been shown to have antioxidant and immune system boosting properties, as well as an ability to support blood flow and maintain normal blood pressure.

According to the renowned medicine hunter and ethnobotany instructor Chris Kilham, olive leaves have more antioxidant activity than green tea, which is well-known for its antioxidant powers.[1] Olive leaf is also an anti-inflammatory agent and a good source of apigenin and luteolin, which have anticancer capabilities.

Here's what the research says about olive leaf extract and high blood pressure. One study compared the supplement with captopril, which is a prescription drug commonly used to treat hypertension and congestive heart failure and to prevent kidney failure associated with high blood pressure and diabetes. The participants in the study all had moderately high blood pressure (140–159 mmHg over 90–99 mmHg).

In the double-blind study, the participants were given either 500 milligrams of olive leaf extract twice daily or 12.5 milligrams of captopril twice daily for eight weeks. Blood pressure was measured every week during the study. After eight weeks, patients in both groups had experienced significant reductions in both systolic (average decline: 12.6 mmHg) and diastolic (average: 5.6 mmHg) blood pressure. Patients who took olive leaf extract not only achieved a significant drop in blood pressure similar to that of captopril; they also did not experience side effects and had yet one more benefit not seen in the captopril group: lower triglyceride levels, which is important for cardiovascular health and diabetes.[2]

How to Use Olive Leaf Extract

Olive leaf extracts are available as capsules, powders, and a liquid concentrate. No side effects have been reported when using olive leaf extract, although anyone who has low blood pressure should not take the supplement because it can cause blood pressure to drop too low.

In a Swiss study, researchers explored the impact of olive leaf extract on forty sets of hypertensive monozygotic twins. The individuals in each pair were given either 500 or 1,000 milligrams per day of olive leaf extract for eight weeks or no treatment (controls). The average systolic and diastolic blood pressure by the end of the study had declined significantly (137/80 mmHg–126/76 mmHg) in individuals who took 1,000 milligrams daily but not the 500-milligram dose or among controls. Cholesterol levels also declined in both olive leaf groups.

GARLIC

Even if you don't love the smell or taste of garlic, you'll have to love the research that shows how garlic can help lower blood pressure, even in people whose hypertension is uncontrolled. But don't worry: you don't need to make garlic a part of every meal to enjoy the blood-pressure-lowering abilities of this herb, although feel free to enjoy it as much as you want.

Garlic (*Allium sativum*) has been valued both as a food and for its medicinal abilities since the time of the pharaohs. During World I and World War II, garlic was used to help prevent gangrene in injured soldiers. Aside from its reputation for warding off vampires, today garlic is used to help lower blood pressure and cholesterol levels, prevent or reduce symptoms of the common cold, and improve blood flow. Some research indicates it may also assist in the fight against certain cancers.

What's Special About Garlic?

Garlic is grown around the globe and is a rich source of antioxidants, which fight cell-damaging molecules. A number of plant chemicals in garlic are believed to be responsible for its health benefits, including the sulfur compounds allicin, alliin, and ajoene and polysulfides.

Without getting too technical, researchers have found that allicin (which is made from alliin in garlic) has the ability to block the activity of a protein called angiotensin II, which has a role in making blood vessels contract. Allicin can help prevent blood vessels from abnormal contractions and thus help prevent a rise in blood pressure.

Garlic also contains sulfur-containing molecules called polysulfides. When these polysulfides enter red blood cells, they can be transformed into a gas called hydrogen sulfide, which helps control blood pressure.

Other added bonuses from garlic are its ability to help prevent cardiovascular problems, which go hand in hand with hypertension. Garlic contains anti-inflammatory compounds, such as 1,2-vinyldithiin and thiacremonone, which appear to inhibit the actions of molecules that cause inflammation, a risk factor for cardiovascular disease.

In a 2013 Australian study, seventy-nine people with uncontrolled systolic hypertension were enrolled in a double-blind, placebo-controlled study that involved taking placebo or 240, 480, or 960 milligrams daily of an aged garlic extract. The treatment period lasted twelve weeks. By the end of the trial, the average systolic blood pressure had declined significantly (mean of 11.8 mmHg) in participants who had taken 480 milligrams garlic extract. Individuals who took 960 milligrams reached a significant decline in systolic blood pressure by week 8 (7.4 mmHg decline) of the study. People in the 240-milligrams and control groups did not experience a significant decline in blood pressure.

Other studies have had similar results. In a Japanese study from 2013, people with prehypertension and mild hypertension were given 300 milligrams of a Japanese garlic product daily for twelve weeks. The garlic was associated with a significant reduction in systolic blood pressure (between 6.6 and 7.5 mmHg) and diastolic blood pressure (between 4.6 and 5.2 mmHg) when compared with placebo.

How to Use Garlic

Garlic can be enjoyed either raw or cooked and added to a wide variety of foods, depending on your taste preferences. If garlic is not one of your favorite herbs or if you want to get the benefits of garlic supplements, they are available made from fresh, dried, or freeze-dried garlic and as capsules, tablets, gel caps, and aged garlic extracts. Many garlic supplements are now available in forms that do not leave you smelling like a loaf of garlic bread as well! However, the aging process necessary to make garlic nearly odorless also can make garlic less effective. Therefore, look for supplements that are enteric coated so they will dissolve in the intestinal tract rather than in the stomach.

GARLIC HINTS

• Boost the benefits of fresh garlic by allowing your garlic to "breathe" after you chop or mince it. If you are going to enjoy garlic raw, then you can add it to your food immediately. However, if you plan to cook the garlic, allowing it to sit for about five to ten minutes gives the alliinase enzymes time to do their "work" and boost the health advantages of garlic.

• If you heat or cook with garlic, remember that too much heat for too long will reduce the herb's health benefits. Tossing minced garlic into hot oil is a sure way to banish the benefits. Try to keep the cooking temperature around 250 degrees F or lower. That means the suggested temperature of 350 degrees F to roast garlic will leave you with nutrient-deficient bulbs.

When buying garlic supplements, look for those containing standardized alliin or allicin. Not all garlic contains the same amount of active ingredients. Some typical doses of garlic and garlic supplements include the following. However, always defer to the doses recommended by your health-care provider:

Fresh garlic: 2–4 grams daily. Each clove (not
bulb!) is about 1 gram.

Garlic tablets, freeze-dried: 400 mg three times
daily of standardized 1.3 percent alliin or 0.6
percent allicin. You may also see alliin and
allicin given in microgram amounts, such as
26,400 mcg alliin and 12,000 mcg allicin.

Aged garlic extract: 600 mg–1,200 mg daily in
divided doses

Fluid extract (1:1 weight/volume): 4 milliliters daily

Garlic can interact with certain medications, so beware. Birth control pills, for example, may be less effective in women who use garlic. Anyone who is taking
blood thinners such as warfarin, aspirin, and clopido-
grel or who is using nonsteroidal anti-inflammatory
drugs (NSAIDs) such as ibuprofen and naproxen should
talk to their doctor before starting garlic, because the
herb can increase the risk of bleeding.

HAWTHORN

It appears that our ancestors knew that hawthorn (*Crag-
aegus laevigata*) was good for the heart and heart conditions, even though they didn't have the technical skills
or knowledge to identify why it was so. People have been
using hawthorn since the first century to help treat heart
problems. During the early 1800s, doctors in America
were using hawthorn berries to treat high blood pressure,
chest pain, hardening of the arteries, and irregular heartbeat.

Even though the pharmaceutical industry has taken
over the treatment of many of these conditions, there is
still a place for hawthorn. In fact, today many practitio-

ners in the United Kingdom use hawthorn to help manage high blood pressure along with prescribed medications.

What's Special About Hawthorn?

Hawthorn is a member of the rose family that grows in wooded areas around the world. It has small red, pink, or white flowers from which sprout small red or black berries, called haws. The leaves, flowers, and berries are used for medicinal purposes. Studies show that hawthorn contains antioxidants, including quercetin and oligomeric proanthocyandins (OPCs), which are also found in grapes.

The antioxidants in hawthorn are believed to be responsible for its ability to benefit blood pressure and the heart. A number of studies in both animals and people indicate that hawthorn helps improve blood circulation and lowers blood pressure.

For example, in a study conducted among general practices in the United Kingdom seventy-nine individuals with type 2 diabetes were randomly assigned to take either 1,200 milligrams of hawthorn extract or placebo daily for sixteen weeks. Blood pressure and fasting blood samples were collected at the beginning of the study. Nearly three-quarters of the participants were also using medications to treat their high blood pressure.

By the end of the study, patients who took hawthorn had a greater reduction in diastolic blood pressure than did individuals who took placebo. Systolic blood pressure did not change significantly in either group. The authors did not observe any herb and drug interactions.

How to Use Hawthorn Supplements

A typical dose of hawthorn can range from 160 to 1,800 milligrams daily, which has been found to be safe. Side effects of hawthorn are rare, but some people have experienced headache, nausea, and palpitations.

Hawthorn can interact with other medications, including any you may be taking for high blood pressure or your heart. For example, hawthorn can make the effects of beta-blockers (e.g., atenolol, metoprolol, propranolol) and calcium channel blockers (e.g., amlodipine, diltiazem, nifedipine) stronger. (Read more about these medications in chapter 8.) If you take hawthorn and nitrates, you may experience dizziness. Men who are using phosphodiesterase-5 inhibitors for erectile dysfunction together with hawthorn may have a severe drop in blood pressure.

VITAMIN C

Vitamin C is often heralded for its possible role in fighting colds and boosting the immune system, but what about high blood pressure? Scientists were not about to pass up the opportunity to determine whether this popular antioxidant could help fight one of society's greatest health issues. Scores of studies have been conducted, and the consensus seems to be that vitamin C can help lower blood pressure, but not by a lot.

Let's consider the results of a meta-analysis conducted by a team from Johns Hopkins School of Medicine. They evaluated the findings from twenty-nine clinical trials that examined the effects of vitamin C supplementation on blood pressure. Overall, use of vitamin C supplements (average dose: 500 mg/day for 8 weeks) yielded a 4.85 mmHg drop in systolic and a 1.67 mmHg drop in diastolic blood pressures in people with high blood pressure.

Let's look at vitamin C and blood pressure from a

slightly different angle. This time let's consider a study of nearly twenty-one thousand adults who participated in the European Prospective Investigation into Cancer Norfolk Study, which reported on the association between plasma vitamin C concentrations and blood pressure. The authors discovered that people with high vitamin C concentrations had lower blood pressure and that "there appears to be a strong association between vitamin C concentrations, an indicator of fruit and vegetable consumption, and a lower level of blood pressure." These findings are supported by other studies as well.

Thus it appears that no matter how you slice or dice it, higher levels of vitamin C are associated with lower blood pressure. According to one of the study's researchers, Edgar R. Miller III, MD, PhD, "Although our review found only a moderate impact on blood pressure, if the entire US population lowered blood pressure by 3 [points], there would be a lot fewer strokes," and that can only be a good thing.

An Italian study added more support for the use of vitamin C in essential hypertension. The authors administered intravenous vitamin C or placebo to thirty-two untreated patients with essential hypertension and twenty individuals with normal blood pressure. Vitamin C significantly lowered blood pressure (mean of 4.9 mmHg) in the individuals who had hypertension but not in those with normal blood pressure.

How to Use Vitamin C

So how much vitamin C should you take as a supplement? Assuming you are getting a decent amount of vitamin C from your diet (see chapter 3), about 250 to 500 milligrams daily is suggested. (The RDA for women is 75 mg; and for men, 90 mg). According to Andrew Weil, MD, founder and director of the Arizona Center for Integrative Medicine and clinical professor of medicine and professor of public health and the Lovell-Jones Professor of Integrative Rheumatology at the University of Arizona Health Sciences Center, most healthy individuals can only retain and utilize about 250 milligrams of vitamin C each day, while any excess is eliminated in the urine. Researchers in a study published in the *American Journal of Therapy* note that 500 milligrams per day is a suggested dose and that higher dosing does not appear to provide any additional blood-pressure-lowering benefits.

VITAMIN D

The sunshine vitamin can be good for your blood pressure, bone strength, mood, and a whole lot more. Unfortunately, the majority of people don't get enough of this nutrient. One reason is there are few foods that are rich in vitamin D and the ones that are excellent sources tend not to make the top ten list of favorite foods for most people. (For example, that list includes fatty fish such as salmon and tuna, and beef liver. Fair sources are fortified orange juice, fortified cereals, and egg yolks.) Another reason is that few people get adequate, healthy exposure to the sun, which the body needs to manufacture vitamin D.

Vitamin D is unlike other vitamins because the body makes this nutrient when you expose your skin to sunlight regularly. When the skin is exposed to sunlight, it makes large amounts of vitamin D_3 (cholecalciferol) and sends it to the liver, where the organ transforms it into a substance called 25-hydroxyvitamin D, or 25(OH) D. This substance travels throughout the body, and some of it ends up in the kidneys, where 25(OH)D is changed into activated vitamin D, which is the form that performs its many functions, such as supporting bone health, enhancing the immune system, participating in calcium metabolism, and promoting heart health.

How Vitamin D Affects Blood Pressure

Although experts do not fully understand the relationship between vitamin D and hypertension, there are some things they do know. For example, vitamin D may help lower blood pressure in three ways:

1. It can modify the activity of an enzyme called renin, which is involved in constricting blood vessels and thus raising blood pressure.
2. It can increase insulin sensitivity. This is important because resistance to insulin is a risk factor for high blood pressure.
3. It can reduce hardening of the arteries. Vitamin D has a role in regulating the absorption and metabolism of calcium. Calcification that develops in the arteries can contribute to high blood pressure. However, if the body has an adequate amount of vitamin D, it can help ensure the calcium is sent to the bones and teeth rather than to the arteries.

Why is vitamin D important for high blood pressure? Investigators have made some observations. One is that people with lower vitamin D levels are at a greater risk of high blood pressure. For example, a review of the association between vitamin D intake and hypertension conducted at Massachusetts General Hospital and reported in 2012 noted that low levels of 25-hydroxy vitamin D was associated with higher systolic blood pressure levels as well as a higher incidence of high blood pressure. The 25(OH)D form of vitamin D is the one that is measured in the blood to determine your vitamin D levels and whether you are vitamin D deficient. A Harvard study of women found that those with vitamin D levels of 17 nanograms per milliliter (nm/mL) (42 nanomoles per liter, nmol/L) had a 67 percent increased risk of developing high blood pressure.

The Vitamin D Council, a nonprofit dedicated to educating the public about vitamin D, reports that the ideal level of vitamin D is 50 ng/mL. To learn what your vitamin D is, you will need to have a simple blood test (see "Testing for Vitamin D Levels"). If you have high blood pressure and low levels of vitamin D, then taking vitamin D supplements may be beneficial.

Another group of researchers observed the risk of developing systolic hypertension among premenopausal women over a fifteen-year period. At the beginning of the study in 1992 and annually thereafter, the 559 white women (ages 24–44) had their blood pressure checked. Vitamin D levels were measured in 1993 and in 2007. The investigators found that women who had vitamin D deficiency in 1993 had three times the risk of developing systolic hypertension fourteen years later than did women who had normal vitamin D levels.

If you are black, you should be especially mindful of your vitamin D intake. That's because research shows not only that African-American men and women tend to have lower levels of vitamin D than whites but also that lower vitamin D levels are associated with an increased risk of hypertension. The good news is that taking vitamin D supplements seems to help, as demonstrated in a 2013 study from Brigham and Women's Hospital researchers. They found that taking 4,000 International

Units (IUs) of vitamin D daily resulted in a 4.0 mmHg decline in systolic blood pressure compared with an increase of 1.7 mmHg among study participants who took a placebo. A dose of 2,000 IUs daily resulted in a 3.4 mmHg decline in systolic blood pressure.

TESTING FOR VITAMIN D LEVELS

Testing for your vitamin D level is relatively simple and nearly painless. A simple blood test, called a 25(OH)D blood test, is all you need. There are three ways you can have this test done:

1. **See your doctor.** He or she can take a blood sample and send it to a lab. You should check with your insurance company to see if it covers this test.
2. **Self-test.** There are in-home tests you can order online. These tests are accurate and easy to use: just prick your finger, place the sample on the material sent to you, and then mail it to the appropriate lab for testing.
3. **Have laboratory testing done.** Several Web sites offer the ability to skip going to your doctor and allow you to go straight to a testing laboratory. If you don't want to do an in-home test, you can purchase a test from healthcheckusa.com, mymedlab.com, or privatedmdlabs.com and then have the test done at a LabCorp location near you.

Taking Vitamin D

The best way to "take" your vitamin D is through regular exposure to sunlight and those all-important ultraviolet B (UVB) rays. You can get all the vitamin D for one day from just about fifteen minutes of exposure to the sun (without sunscreen) if you are fair skinned, but you will need more time in the sun if your skin is medium to dark. A general rule to follow, according to the Vitamin D Council, is to expose your skin to the sun for half the time it takes your skin to turn pink. Therefore, if you know your skin begins to turn pink after being in the sun for thirty minutes you have had your daily vitamin D "fix" from the sun after fifteen minutes.

Your body can produce 10,000 to 25,000 IUs of vitamin D in less time than it takes for your skin to turn pink. The more skin you expose to the sun, the more vitamin D your body can make. Naturally, you should be sure to put on sunscreen after the time you spend making vitamin D to protect your skin against cancer and aging.

Many people don't get enough sun exposure, especially during the winter months. Therefore, supplements are often necessary to boost vitamin D levels. However, before you take vitamin D supplements you should have your 25(OH)D levels checked. If you are significantly deficient in vitamin D, you may need to take higher doses of vitamin D supplements for a while, then taper back as your blood levels of vitamin D improve.

The recommended daily dose of vitamin D differs among experts. The U.S. government's Food and Nutrition Board recommends adults take 600 to 800 IUs, while the Endocrine Society more than doubles that amount to 1,500 to 2,000 IUs daily. The Vitamin D Society recommends adults take 5,000 IUs per day. More and more clinicians and researchers are finding that the 600-to-800-IU dose seems to be too low and are recommending their patients take higher amounts, depending on their blood vitamin D levels and amount of sun exposure.

Vitamin D is fat soluble, which means your body's fat cells hold on to the vitamin for a while. Therefore, you don't want to take too much vitamin D. The safe upper limit of vitamin D ranges from 4,000 to 10,000 IUs daily, depending on which experts you believe. However, unless you take more than the upper limit of vitamin D every day for several months you are unlikely to experience any side effects. Indications of an overdose of vitamin D include headache, weakness, fatigue, loss of appetite, dry mouth, nausea, vomiting, and a metallic taste.

When you are choosing a vitamin D supplement, experts recommend you take D_3 rather than D_2, because vitamin D_3 is the form of the nutrient your body makes. However, vitamin D_3 is typically made from lambs' wool, so if you are a vegetarian or vegan and have ethical reasons for not wanting to take vitamin D_3 you may choose vitamin D_2, which is made from plants (fungi). However, you should be aware that vitamin D_2 is not metabolized by the body in the same way as vitamin D_3 and also produces some substances that the body may have difficulty eliminating.

Vitamin D supplements are available as tablets, capsules, and liquid and can be taken with or without food. You often see supplements that contain both calcium and vitamin D because these two nutrients benefit bone health. Be sure the vitamin D in these supplements is D_3 and check the amount of vitamin D delivered per dose to be sure you are getting the recommended amount per day.

GREEN TEA

When was the last time you enjoyed a hot cup of green tea? How about iced green tea with mint or lemon? Green tea isn't everyone's, well, cup of tea, which is why green tea supplements can be an excellent alternative. What's important for our discussion of high blood pressure, however, isn't necessarily which form of green tea you choose to enjoy but that you give it a try. Why? Because green tea possesses some proven blood pressure and overall cardiovascular benefits that you might not want to pass up.

Consider the findings of a June 2012 study published in *Nutrition Research*. The authors randomly assigned fifty-six obese, hypertensive patients to take either one capsule containing 379 milligrams of green tea extract or a placebo daily for three months. At the end of three months, compared with individuals in the placebo group, those who took green tea extracted experienced all of the following benefits:

- Significant decline in blood pressure, both systolic and diastolic

- Considerable reduction in fasting glucose and insulin levels (good indicators for people with diabetes)

- Significant declines in both total and low-density lipoprotein (LDL, or bad) cholesterol

- Increase in high-density lipoprotein (HDL, good) cholesterol

- Significant decline in C-reactive protein levels

- Increase in total antioxidant status

The bottom line: green tea extract got an A+ when it came to blood pressure and cardiovascular risk factors. And this is not the only study that has shown green tea to benefit blood pressure.

If you are wondering about the caffeine in green tea, you have a right to be skeptical. Some studies have been done using decaffeinated green tea, including one that involved giving decaffeinated green tea extract to rats. In that study, the extract significantly lowered blood pressure and glucose and insulin levels and also improved endothelial function, which translated to better blood pressure.

It is recommended you use decaffeinated green tea supplements as well as drink a decaf version of green tea. At the same time, bear in mind that green tea contains substantially less caffeine than coffee and somewhat less than black tea. The exact amount of caffeine in each beverage depends on the brand, brewing time, and other factors, but here are some approximate amounts of caffeine in each eight-ounce serving:

- Brewed coffee: 95–200 mg

- Decaffeinated brewed coffee: 2–12 mg

- Black tea: 14–61 mg

- Decaffeinated black tea: 0–12 mg

- Green tea: 24–40 mg

- Decaffeinated green tea: 0–10 mg

How does green tea help lower blood pressure? First of all, as mentioned in chapter 3 on diet, green tea contains potent polyphenols/antioxidants called catechins, and the most important one is epigallocatechin gallate, or EGCG. EGCG may help lower blood pressure by suppressing the activity of angiotensin-converting enzyme (ACE), a substance that is released by the kidneys. ACE interferes with the flexibility of the arteries, which can cause a significant rise in blood pressure. EGCG helps stop that action. EGCG and other compounds found in green tea may offer other beneficial actions regarding high blood pressure: research continues!

How to Use Green Tea

If you choose to take green tea supplements, look for brands that are standardized to 25 percent or greater polyphenols. You should discuss your use of green tea supplements and any green tea you drink with your health-care provider. A healthy balance of the two—one or two cups of decaffeinated green tea per day plus a moderate dose of caffeine-free green tea extract, 50 milligrams daily or higher—may be a satisfactory way to help manage your blood pressure.

Green tea extracts should be avoided if you are pregnant or breast-feeding, because green tea may interfere with metabolism of iron and result in anemia in nursing infants. Most people do not experience any side effects from using green tea supplements, but in large amounts they may cause heartburn, diarrhea, and a loss of appetite.

COENZYME Q10

Also known as ubiquinone, coenzyme Q10 (CoQ10) is a substance that can be found in every cell in your body, with high concentrations in the heart. Its main job is to regulate energy in muscle tissues. Levels of CoQ10 decline as people age, and low levels are also found in people who have high blood pressure. In addition, if you are taking a statin drug to lower your cholesterol, then you probably have low CoQ10 levels, because these drugs reduce production of CoQ10. Thus it seems natural to believe that taking a CoQ10 supplement may improve blood pressure.

The results of numerous studies support this idea, although the level of benefit from the studies is not all the same. For example, a study published in the *Journal of Human Hypertension* reported on individuals with coronary artery disease who had been taking antihypertensive drugs for about one year. These patients were randomly assigned to take either 60 milligrams of CoQ10 twice a day or a B-complex supplement for eight weeks. Patients in the CoQ10 group experienced an average 16-point decline in systolic and a 9-point decline in diastolic blood pressures as well as an improvement in triglyceride, blood sugar, and insulin levels and an increase in good cholesterol (high-density lipoprotein, HDL) levels. Patients in the placebo group did not enjoy any of these benefits.

In a crossover study, patients with essential hypertension were given either 100 milligrams of CoQ10 or a placebo daily for ten weeks. A crossover study means participants take one of the study supplements, drugs, or placebos for a set period of time, then switch over to the other substance for another period of time. In this study, none of the patients were taking any antihypertension medications during the study period. After all the patients completed the first ten-week portion of the study, they stopped all treatment and placebo for two weeks, then switched to the other therapy for an additional ten weeks.

Each time patients took the CoQ10, there was a significant decrease in both systolic and diastolic pressures. These improvements were noticeable in the third or fourth week of treatment and continued throughout the study. However, the benefits disappeared seven to ten days after patients stopped taking CoQ10. This suggests it's important to continue taking CoQ10 to reap the benefits of lower blood pressure.

How does CoQ10 work in people who may have isolated systolic hypertension? This question was addressed in a study of forty-one men and thirty-five women who had this type of high blood pressure. The participants were randomly assigned to take either 60 milligrams of CoQ10 twice a day along with 150 IUs of vitamin E or a placebo that contained vitamin E only. An additional nine volunteers with normal blood pressure participated as well, and they took the CoQ10 treatment. The entire treatment period lasted twelve weeks.

At the end of the treatment period, systolic blood pressure in the patients with isolated systolic hypertension who took CoQ10 dropped an average of 17.8 mmHg and there was no significant change in diastolic pressure. Overall, 55 percent of patients who took CoQ10 experienced a reduction in systolic pressure of 4 mmHg or greater, while 45 percent did not respond. Although the effect of CoQ10 in this study was not as impressive as seen in other trials, it did show that CoQ10 may be beneficial for some patients who have isolated systolic hypertension and worth discussing with your health-care provider.

How Does CoQ10 Work?

Exactly how does CoQ10 work to lower blood pressure? Experts are not certain, but one theory is that it helps preserve levels of nitric oxide, a substance that relaxes the peripheral arteries, which in turn lowers blood pressure. In some types of high blood pressure, agents called superoxide radicals put nitric oxide out of commission. That's when the potent antioxidant CoQ10 may step in and prevent the damage of superoxide radicals, thus preserving nitric oxide. It's also possible that CoQ10 increases the production of a substance (prostacyclin, or PGI2) that dilates the blood vessels and helps prevent the accumulation of platelets, which can clog up blood flow.

How to Use CoQ10

A typical daily dose of CoQ10 for people who have high blood pressure is 120 to 200 milligrams, taken in two divided doses. To reap the most benefit from CoQ10 supplements, take them along with a (healthy) fatty meal or food, such as salmon (cold-water fatty fish rich in omega-3 fatty acids), nut butters, salad with olive oil dressing, or some low-fat yogurt. Taking CoQ10 in divided doses helps enhance absorption and reduce the chances of experiencing any gastrointestinal discomfort. Also, be sure to take one of your doses of CoQ10 at night, because the nutrient seems to be better utilized by the body late in the day.

There are two main forms of CoQ10 supplements: solubilized and nonsolubilized. The former are better absorbed and used by the body, and so the doses tend to be less than those recommended for nonsolubilized forms. Check with your health-care provider for the proper dose and form for you.

OMEGA-3 FATTY ACIDS

There's something fishy about taking omega-3 fatty acid supplements for high blood pressure, but it's the good kind of fishy. Study after study has shown that omega-3 fatty acids, which are found in abundance in cold-water fatty fish such as salmon, sardines, herring, tuna, mackerel, and others, are beneficial on a number of levels. Not only are omega-3s effective in lowering blood pressure; they also are supportive of the related cardiovascular conditions we've talked about. That means omega-3s can help

- Reduce triglyceride levels

- Lower the risk of developing an abnormal heart rhythm

- Reduce the chances of suffering a stroke or heart attack

- Slow down the accumulation of plaque in the arteries

When I say omega-3s, I am referring primarily to the two main ones, eicosapentanoic acid (EPA) and docohexaenoic acid (DHA), which are found in the fish just mentioned. These omega-3s are a type of polyunsaturated fat, sometimes referred to as a "good fat" or "healthy fat." To get the amount of omega-3 fatty acids you need to benefit your heart and blood vessels, the American Heart Association recommends eating baked, poached, broiled, or steamed fish twice a week, three to four ounces at each meal (see chapter 3).

How to Use Omega-3 Fatty Acid Supplements

If you are rolling your eyes or wrinkling your nose at the thought of eating fish, then taking fish oil supplements may be the alternative for you. The suggested daily dose is three grams unless you use a concentrated ethyl ester form, in which case one gram is usually sufficient. Do not take more than these recommended amounts unless you first consult your doctor. If you do not want to take fish oil supplements for personal or ethical reasons, there are DHA supplements made from algae instead of fish.

Side effects from omega-3 supplements may include diarrhea, belching, and stomach upset. If you are pregnant, talk to your doctor before starting omega-3 supplements. Taking high amounts of omega-3 fatty acids can increase the risk of bleeding. If you are taking blood thinners such as warfarin, you should not take omega-3 supplements without first consulting your health-care provider.

WHAT YOU SHOULD KNOW ABOUT POTASSIUM SUPPLEMENTS

I have already mentioned that potassium is important for managing blood pressure (see chapter 3), so it seems logical for potassium supplements to also be helpful in coping with high blood pressure. Indeed, many people believe they should take potassium supplements for hypertension, but here's what you should know.

Besides being important for healthy function of

all your cells and for heart health, potassium is also an electrolyte, which is a substance that conducts electricity in the body. Other electrolytes are calcium, magnesium (see the connection with potassium?), sodium, and chloride. Sodium and chloride together are salt, so again you can see the intimate relationship between electrolytes and blood pressure.

If you eat a healthy diet, you probably get all the potassium you need. In fact, much of the success of the DASH (Dietary Approaches to Stop Hypertension) diet is due to its focus on foods that are high in potassium, such as fruits and vegetables. Since both vegetarian and vegan diet plans also include lots of potassium-rich foods, these eating programs are effective as well. Meat and some fish (e.g., salmon, flounder, cod) also contain potassium. What you "need" is about 4,700 milligrams daily if you are 19 years or older.

Getting the potassium your body requires to operate optimally isn't the end of the story, however, because your potassium level also depends on how much magnesium and sodium (salt) you take in. If you consume too much salt (and many Americans do), then you need more potassium. Thus it is important to also be aware of your salt intake, especially if you have high blood pressure.

Other things that can cause you to need more potassium are diarrhea, excessive sweating, malnutrition, use of loop diuretics, vomiting, and conditions that affect how well you absorb nutrients, such as Crohn's disease. Drugs that can impact potassium levels include NSAIDs and ACE inhibitors.

So if you have high blood pressure and you think

you need more potassium, should you take a supplement? Although there is some evidence that potassium supplements may reduce blood pressure, other studies have not found this to be true. Potassium may help if you are deficient in potassium, but you don't want to take a potassium supplement arbitrarily and end up with hyperkalemia—too much potassium in the blood. The best way to get potassium is from healthy foods. Be sure to talk to your doctor before taking potassium supplements.

HERBS THAT RAISE BLOOD PRESSURE

Just because something is natural doesn't mean it's healthful, and that applies to herbal remedies that may be suggested to help manage high blood pressure as well as other health issues. In fact, you should be aware that there are a number of herbal remedies that are associated with a rise in blood pressure or can have a negative effect on any medications you are taking to treat hypertension. Be sure to check the labels of any combination supplements to be sure they do not contain any of the following ingredients.

- Arnica (*Arnica montana*)

- Bitter orange (*Citrus aurantium*)

- Ephedra (*ma huang*)

- Ginkgo (*Ginkgo biloba*)

- Ginseng (*Panax quinquefolius, P. ginseng*)

- Guarana (*Paulinia cupana*)

- Licorice (*Glycyrrhiza glabra*)

- St. John's wort (*Hypericum perforatum*)

- Senna (*Cassia senna*)

CHAPTER SEVEN

Manage Stress (Before It Manages You)

If you feel tense and on edge or if you feel "stressed out," then you probably have high blood pressure, right? No, not exactly. Let's clear up this confusion right now: stress does not cause high blood pressure. Yes, it is true that both physical and emotional stress can cause a significant rise in blood pressure. Did you have a fight with your boss? You probably experienced a blood pressure spike. Did you get a flat tire during rush hour? Ditto. Do you have to give a speech for work? Ditto, along with experiencing butterflies in your stomach.

The spike in blood pressure associated with these and similarly stressful situations is natural and typically temporary. Once the stressful situation is over, blood pressure returns to prestress levels. So does that mean stress is not a risk factor for hypertension? Hardly. In fact, stress seems to play an insidious and pervasive role in hypertension for several reasons.

For one thing, stress can exacerbate or has a role in many of the other risk factors for high blood pressure, such as smoking, alcohol use, obesity, and salt consumption. But can chronic stress by itself cause essential hypertension?

That question gets a "yes" response, especially when it concerns job-related stress. According to an important study published in the *Journal of the American Society of Hypertension*, stress related to one's occupation "is considered one of the frequent factors in the etiology of hypertension in modern society."[1] A subsequent study that involved nearly one thousand adults reported there is a significant association between work stress and arterial hypertension, type 2 diabetes, and high lipid levels (cholesterol and triglycerides) in both women and men.

What remains hazy is the exact mechanism behind hypertension related to stress. Forgive me for getting technical for a moment, but one explanation is related to the transient rise in blood pressure that occurs in response to stress. This rise involves something called increased activity of the sympathetic-adrenal medullary that accompanies a heightened level of anxiety and tension. Experts can show evidence of an increased sympathetic tone and that if it persists it may result in high blood pressure. What is unclear is whether anxiety causes the rise in sympathetic tone or it works the other way. Nailing down this distinction is difficult because it relies on personal reports of anxiety, which is subjective.

However, some research has shown that persistent high blood pressure occurs more frequently among people with chronic high anxiety. In a study that involved a nearly twenty-year follow-up period, about 50 percent of the participants eventually developed high blood pressure. Among a subgroup of more than three hundred men, high anxiety was predictive for the development of high blood pressure.

The bottom line is, stress has a significant role in high blood pressure. There is sufficient evidence to support the idea that high levels or long-term chronic stress may increase sympathetic tone enough to result in essential hypertension in some people. At the same time, chronic stress is believed to contribute to hypertension.

And when you add stress to any of the other risk factors for high blood pressure that you may have, the result is not a healthful one for your heart, your cardiovascular system, or your overall health.

Now that I've laid the groundwork for the role of stress in high blood pressure, let's explore some ways to manage stress before it manages you.

ACUPRESSURE

Both acupressure and acupuncture are ancient Chinese medicine techniques that can prove helpful in managing high blood pressure. However, since our focus is on what you can do yourself to cope with hypertension, acupressure fits the bill. However, *do not use acupressure for high blood pressure until you consult with your doctor.* No one with excessively high blood pressure (200/100 mmHg) should ever use acupressure. (If you are interested in learning more about acupuncture and high blood pressure, see "Studies of Acupressure and Hypertension.")

Acupressure is a type of Chinese bodywork therapy in the same category as medical qigong and Tuina. The Japanese also have a form of acupressure called shiatsu. The basic concept of acupressure is that application of pressure to specific points that lie along channels or meridians in the body can relieve blockages that interrupt or disturb the flow of the vital energy or life force called chi or qi. Once the blockage has been removed, balance, health, and harmony can be restored to the body. According to Chinese medicine, there are twelve major meridians and they connect specific organs or groups of organs throughout the body.

You can learn to apply pressure with your fingertips

(practitioners also use their elbows, feet, and palms) to certain points (called acupoints) on your body that correspond to high blood pressure.

In traditional Chinese medicine, hypertension is believed to be closely associated with blockages in the liver meridian. Therefore, the points you apply pressure to correspond to that meridian. Here are several acupressure points you can treat to help in the management of stress and high blood pressure. In each case, once you have located the acupoints apply medium to firm pressure for about sixty seconds and breathe deeply and slowly. Release the pressure slowly. Feel free to practice acupressure several times a day. It's easy to do, and depending on which acupoints you choose to press, you can do acupressure at home, while watching television, at the office, while waiting in line at the bank, or while sitting in a meeting.

Gb20

To find the points, place your thumbs on your earlobes and slide them back toward the center of your neck. Your thumbs should now be about one thumb width above your hairline on your neck and in a slight depression on either side of the vertebra of your neck. You can feel these points more easily if you bend your head slightly forward; the depressions should be obvious. Pressure on these acupoints can help regulate the flow of energy and relieve headaches, neck stiffness, and pain.

Li11 and Ht3

To locate Li11, raise your arm and hold it in front of your chest, as if you were holding a glass in your hand. Li11 is located at the outside end of the crease on your arm, at your elbow joint. Now find Ht3 by holding your palms facing you. Starting at Li11, slide your fingers across the elbow crease until you reach your funny bone (the bony projection in your elbow). Immediately above the bony projection is a natural indentation; this is Ht3. Place your middle finger on Li11 and your thumb on Ht3 and apply equally strong pressure.

St36

To locate St36, place four fingers flat on your leg below the lower edge of your kneecap. You will find St36 one finger width off your shinbone to the outside of your leg. If you flex your foot up and down, you should feel a muscle move under the point. Apply pressure to this point for one minute.

Studies of Acupressure and Hypertension

Despite research (although admittedly limited) showing acupressure can help with relief of stress and help lower blood pressure, some Western practitioners discount the presence of meridians or the concepts behind acupressure. Instead, some say any benefits attributed to acupressure probably are the result of stimulation of the body's natural pain relievers (called endorphins) or that acupressure improves circulation and relieves muscle tension. In fact, acupressure can provide these benefits as well, and if they result in a reduction in high blood pressure so much the better.

The limited amount of scientific evidence to support the use of acupressure in managing high blood pressure is related to the fact that few studies have been undertaken to examine this relationship. Among the studies that have been done, however, evidence suggests a beneficial effect. More convincing are the results of studies using acupuncture for hypertension. For example, a study published in *Acupuncture Today* noted that "acupuncture may offer an alternative antihypertensive therapeutic option" and that "acupuncture effectively lowered systolic and diastolic blood pressures during the treatment period with no or minimal side effects."

The bottom line is that acupressure can be an effective way to help control high blood pressure and you can easily do it on your own without the need for any equipment. Once you have an "all's clear" from your doctor, why not try it?

BIOFEEDBACK

Biofeedback is a technique that can help you control blood pressure and heart rate in the comfort of your own home. When you use biofeedback, you are in charge because you learn from the signals (feedback) from the biofeedback device about your body and how it responds. This knowledge then allows you to make changes that can help lower your blood pressure and stress level and reduce pain.

Using biofeedback to help control high blood pressure has several advantages. One plus is that it doesn't require the use of any medications. While you are learning the technique, you will use a biofeedback machine to help you learn how to control your blood pressure. (I explain how that works under "Trying Biofeedback.") Another advantage of biofeedback is that it can help people who don't want to use or who can't tolerate medications for high blood pressure. Biofeedback may also help you if you have not responded to antihypertensive medications or if high blood pressure is an issue during pregnancy, when it's best to avoid medications if possible.

Although you can practice biofeedback at home, it is recommended you seek some initial help from a professional who can show you how it works. Portable, hand-held biofeedback devices for home use are available and many can be purchased online. Some of these devices hook up to your computer. It is recommended you talk to your doctor about using these devices and also try them on a trial basis before you make your purchase to ensure you know how to use them and that they are beneficial.

Trying Biofeedback

A typical biofeedback session involves having electrical sensors (don't worry, they are painless!) applied to different parts of your body using small adhesive dots or strips. These sensors collect and transmit information to the biofeedback device concerning muscle tension, brain waves, or skin temperature, depending on the type of biofeedback you use.

For example, electromyography (EMG) biofeedback gathers information about your muscle tension so you can learn how to relax. Heart rate variability biofeedback provides information to help you control your heart rate, which in turn can improve your blood pressure and stress level.

Thermal biofeedback uses sensors that attach to your fingers or feet and measures skin temperature. Because body temperature typically declines under stressful conditions, the biofeedback machine will let you know when this occurs, so you can begin to relax. Galvanic skin response devices have sensors that measure the activity of sweat glands, which is an indicator of anxiety.

Biofeedback machines give you feedback in the form of beeps or flashing lights on a small screen to let you know how your body is responding so you can learn how to recognize when your body is responding to stress or your blood pressure may be rising. Once you have that recognition, then you can change your emotions, behavior, or thoughts to eliminate or at least reduce the impact of your response on your blood pressure. For example, visualization and deep breathing are two common techniques people use to lower blood pressure once biofeedback alerts them to their body's response.

If you go to a biofeedback expert at a physical therapy clinic, hospital, or medical center, a session typically lasts thirty to sixty minutes. During that time, you can learn enough about biofeedback so that you can eventually do it yourself at home without the machine, although using a home biofeedback device is also an option. Otherwise, you also can continue to visit a professional biofeedback practitioner and participate in sessions to help reduce hypertension.

Biofeedback Studies

Is biofeedback an effective way to lower blood pressure? Several studies indicate that biofeedback can be a convenient and helpful self-help tool in reducing high blood pressure. For example, an Italian study found that people with prehypertension and hypertension who tried biofeedback experienced a significant reduction in both systolic and diastolic blood pressures after just four sessions while individuals in a control group did not show a reduction in blood pressure. In these cases, guided imagery was used by the participants to help them lower their blood pressure once they got feedback from the machine.

More evidence comes from a meta-analysis, in which researchers evaluated the results of twenty-two controlled studies that included 905 people with essential hypertension. A comparison of self-monitoring of blood pressure or clinical visits with the use of biofeedback showed that the latter resulted in improvements in both systolic and diastolic blood pressures on average of 7.3 mmHg and 5.8 mmHg, respectively.

Finding a Biofeedback Expert

If you would like to find a biofeedback expert, ask your doctor or another health-care professional if he or she can recommend someone. Oftentimes nurses, physical therapists, and other health professionals are also certified in biofeedback. Each state has its own laws regarding certification of biofeedback practitioners, so you should check with your health department.

When looking for biofeedback practitioners, ask if they have experience working with individuals who have high blood pressure, if they are certified or registered, how much training they have had, how many sessions they believe you will need, the cost of their services, and whether they have any references.

BREATHING THERAPY

Breathing therapy is one of the more effective and convenient ways to manage blood pressure. First of all, there's no equipment required (unless you wish to use a device that helps you with breathing therapy, such as RESPeRATE, which is discussed under "Devices to

Help Lower Blood Pressure"). Second, breathing therapy can be done just anywhere and at any time—how much more convenient can you get! So let's discuss how breathing exercises can help you manage your blood pressure.

How to Practice Breathing Exercises

Stressors in life typically cause people to breathe in an unhealthy way—shallow and fast, which only delivers a small amount of essential oxygen to your body, rather than slow and deep, which is energizing. You may never have realized there are many different ways to breathe and some of them are much more healthful and helpful than others. Yogic breathing is called Pranayama, which means "breathing techniques" or "breath control," and it is designed to help keep your body and mind vibrant and healthful.

The two breathing exercises described here are from the yogic tradition, but you don't need to be a practicing yogi to benefit from these exercises! Both breathing exercises can help lower blood pressure and should be practiced daily, several times a day as time permits.

Nadi Shodhana

Nadi shodhana, also known as alternate nostril breathing, is a simple technique that is considered the most important of the breathing exercises (Pranayamas). "Nadi" means "channel" and refers to the energy pathways through which your life force or energy (*prana*) flows. Here's how to do *nadi shodhana:*

- Get into a comfortable seated position and rest your left hand on your left knee.

- Take a slow, deep breath. You can close your eyes or keep them open.

- Use your right thumb to shut your right nostril.

- Exhale slowly through your left nostril.

- While your right thumb is still closing your right nostril, inhale slowly and deeply through your left nostril.

- At the top of your inhale through the left nostril, close your left nostril with the little finger and ring finger of your right hand.

- Exhale through your right nostril.

- Without stopping, inhale through your right nostril while you keep your left nostril closed.

- Then exhale through your left nostril while keeping your right nostril closed.

- You have just completed one cycle of breathing (called *anuloma viloma*). Repeat the entire cycle several times. If possible, practice this breathing exercise several times a day. Bonus: *nadi shodhana* is also good for headaches, asthma, and insomnia.

Bumblebee Breathing

This Pranayama is especially good for high blood pressure, reducing stress and tension, and boosting your energy level. It is called Brahmari, which means "bumblebee" breathing, because you keep your lips together and make a humming bee sound in your throat. When Brahmari is done properly, you can feel vibrations in your face and throat. Children like this breathing exercise, so enlist them to do it with you.

Here's how to do Brahmari. Practice several times a day for the best results. It is recommended you learn Brahmari under the supervision of a trained yoga instructor or consult your health-care provider first:

- Get into a comfortable seated position with your spine and neck straight. Rest your palms on your knees.

- Open your mouth slightly and let your jaw relax.

- Lift your arms so your elbows point to either side and place your thumbs lightly over your ears.

- Place your index fingers above your eyebrows on your forehead and your two middle fingers over your closed eyes

- Place your little fingers against the sides of your nostrils, but do not apply any pressure to your nose.

- Inhale slowly and deeply.

- Exhale slowly through both nostrils and keep your mouth closed.

- As you exhale, make a humming sound in your throat. The goal is to make the sound as loud, continuous, and clear as possible. You should also feel vibrations in your throat and face. This will take some practice, so do not worry if you do not reach this goal for a while.

- Repeat this exercise for two to three minutes per session, preferably several times a day. At the end of your session, release your fingers and open your eyes slowly. Never force your breath when doing this breathing exercise.

Does Breathing Therapy Work? Studies

Studies show that breathing exercises can effectively lower blood pressure after only a few weeks of practice and even immediately in some cases, such as those that involve white coat hypertension. Here's an example.

You may remember the discussion about white-coat hypertension, in which some individuals tend to have an elevated blood pressure associated with being in a doctor's office. In this study, researchers evaluated the impact of a short deep-breathing exercise patients tried after they had their blood pressure taken twice in the doctor's office. Of the seventy-three patients who participated in the study, 62 percent had white-coat hypertension.

The authors asked individuals to practice thirty seconds of deep breathing after they had their blood pressure taken twice in the doctor's office. After the deep breathing, blood pressure was taken immediately and then again two minutes later. The deep-breath test reduced systolic blood pressure by an average of 15 mmHg and diastolic pressure by about 6 mmHg. Although this study was designed to check how a deep-breath test could help detect white-coat hypertension, it also shows that deep breathing has a positive impact on blood pressure levels.

There is more than one way to practice deep breathing and to enjoy the benefits of lower blood pressure. In the *International Journal of Yoga Therapy,* for example, researchers reported on the effects of a yogic deep-breathing technique called *sukha pranayama* on cardiovascular factors in people with high blood pressure. This approach involves a precise breathing method: five minutes of breathing at a rate of six breaths per minute and an equal duration for inhaling and exhaling.

The authors found that adults who participated in the study and practiced *sukha pranayama* for five minutes experienced a highly significant reduction in systolic blood pressure and a significant reduction in heart rate. Although the study did not determine how long such a benefit lasts, it might be assumed that people who practice this technique daily for just five minutes could continue to benefit from the practice.

In another study that included data collected from 21,563 participants, the impact of deep breathing on blood pressure readings taken in a doctor's office was evaluated. The authors reported that deep breathing significantly reduced both systolic and diastolic blood pressures after only thirty seconds.

Daily practice of yogic breathing exercises can have a significant impact on blood pressure. One study involved eight prehypertensive individuals who received weekly training on yogic Pranayama and who practiced the breathing method daily for six weeks. Daily Pranayama practice resulted in an 11-point reduction in systolic and an 8-point reduction in diastolic blood pressure levels. Blood pressure levels remained similar even three weeks after the study ended. Yogic breathing is an easy technique to learn and practice at home on a daily basis, and it's been shown to be effective in lowering blood pressure.

DEVICES TO HELP LOWER BLOOD PRESSURE

Several devices on the market have been shown to help people lower their blood pressure and stress. One such device, approved by the Food and Drug Administration (FDA) for reducing stress and lowering blood pressure, is called RESPeRATE. You don't need a prescription for RESPeRATE, which is available online and from some medical supply facilities.

You can use RESPeRATE in the comfort of your home or office. The portable electronic RESPeRATE device consists of chest sensors, which measure your breathing, and a computerized unit that emits a melody that helps you slow and synchronize your breathing. Numerous scientific studies have shown that RESPeRATE can effectively and safely lower blood pressure without the use of drugs.

For example, one investigative team reported on an evaluation of seven studies that looked at the impact of RESPeRATE on blood pressure. They found that routine use (daily) of the device resulted in significantly lower blood pressure readings both at home and in the doctor's office when used alone, along with lifestyle changes, and along with antihypertensive drugs. The authors concluded that while RESPeRATE is effective, "like all lifestyle modifications, [it] must be practiced consistently to provide benefits."

The similarity between using RESPeRATE and blood-pressure-lowering drugs is that you need to keep using RESPeRATE to keep your blood pressure down. When you quit doing the daily practice—recommended as at least fifteen minutes daily, three to four days a week—then your blood pressure will return to pretreatment levels. However, since there are no side effects associated with using RESPeRATE (and antihypertensive drugs can cause adverse effects; see chapter 8), it seems like a positive treatment option.

Another device that can help lower blood pressure is called Zona Plus. This is a handheld device that involves gripping the instrument with either hand and performing a number of isometric (remember chapter 4 on exercise?) exercises at different levels in response to electronic cues from the device. People who use Zona Plus reportedly experience a decline in blood pressure when they use the device three times a week for twelve minutes per session.

According to the manufacturer, Zona Plus can help lower blood pressure in three ways. One, it helps rebalance your autonomic nervous system, which is known to have a role in high blood pressure when it is overactive. Two, Zona Plus may help improve the health of your arteries by reversing endothelial dysfunction. An improvement in endothelial function is associated with lower occurrences of high blood pressure and various cardiovascular conditions.

Three, the device may help stimulate the production of nitric oxide, which can assist with the dilation of blood vessels, improve blood flow, and maintain normal blood pressure levels.

Naturally, you should consult your health-care provider before you invest in any devices that may help lower blood pressure. If you do decide to try one of these or other products, check with your insurance agent to see if it is covered by your health-care policy.

When using a product to lower your blood pressure, keep a record of your progress. This is important information for your doctor, especially if you are taking blood pressure medication, as use of a device may allow you to reduce or even eliminate your use of drugs.

LAUGHTER

High blood pressure is no laughing matter—except when you use laughter to manage hypertension. A popular saying is that laughter is the best medicine, yet there are always those who say, "Sounds good, but prove it." As it turns out, there are scientific studies showing that humor and laughter can be beneficial when managing a variety of health issues, including high blood pressure. Will you experience dramatic results if you add laughter to your day? Probably not, but the results can be impressive, and can you think of a more enjoyable way to bring your blood pressure levels down?

Some researchers don't think so. A study published in the *Alternative Therapies in Health and Medicine* journal reported on a review of the literature on laughter in medicine. After a comprehensive analysis of the laughter literature, the author concluded: "Laughter has shown physiological, psychological, social, spiritual, and quality of life benefits" and that "there is sufficient evidence to suggest that laughter has some positive, quantifiable effects on certain aspects of health" that would make it "appropriate for laughter to be used as a complementary/alternative medicine in the prevention and treatment of illnesses."

How Laughter Lowers Blood Pressure

How does laughter lower blood pressure? You may be wondering how laughing can lower your blood pressure. Here's one scientific explanation: There are substances called catecholamines that are involved in causing high blood pressure and abnormal heart rhythms. When you block or reduce the effect of catecholamines, you can help your heart. Research has shown that laughter can reduce catecholamine production and thus improve blood pressure and heart health.

Here's an example. In a study from Dillard University in New Orleans, an investigator tested the effect of laughter on catecholamine production. A total of forty-eight people with diabetes who had recently had a heart attack were divided into two groups and followed for one year. One group was asked to watch something humorous for thirty minutes each day along with their standard cardiac therapy while the other group simply followed standard therapy.

The researchers monitored blood pressure and catecholamine levels on a monthly basis in both groups. Overall, patients who used humor on a daily basis had lower blood pressure, fewer episodes of arrhythmia, and lower levels of catecholamines than did participants in the other group. In addition, only two of the twenty-four patients in the humor group experienced another heart attack compared with ten of twenty-four in the control group.

A good laugh also can improve your blood circulation and open up your blood vessels, which in turn helps reduce blood pressure. There are claims by the founder of Laughter Yoga International, Dr. Madan Kataria, that laughter yoga as laughter therapy can help reduce blood pressure and relieve depression and assist with controlling allergies, asthma, arthritis, and more. Laughter yoga is the brainchild of Dr. Kataria, a physician from India, who started the first Laughter Club in 1995, and nearly twenty years later it has grown into more than six thousand clubs around the world.

Laughter yoga is a combination of unconditional laughter (laughing for no particular reason) with yogic breathing (Pranayama; see "Breathing Therapy"), along with chanting and clapping. The concept of Laughter Yoga stems from the fact that the body reaps the same health benefits from real laughter as it does from fake laughter, because the body cannot tell the difference between the two. The important message here is not so much that you should immediately find the closest Laughter Yoga club near you (although you can check the appendix for Web site information) but that this provides further support for the value of laughter in healing. In fact, a scientific study conducted in India found that Laughter Yoga reduced both systolic and diastolic blood pressure levels.

Get Ready to Laugh

Are you ready to write yourself a prescription for a daily dose of laughter? Instead of a prescription pad, however, just turn to a variety of media. For example:

- **TV shows.** Do you have any favorite comedy shows you like to watch? Be sure to tape those you can't catch live and watch them later.

- **DVDs and videos.** Do you have a personal library of movies, comedy shows, or comedians you like to watch? You don't need to purchase them: simply borrow them from your public library.

- **Internet.** The Internet has made laughter therapy so much easier, because you have access to virtually tens of thousands of humorous Web sites and videos, including those on YouTube.

Don't know where to begin? Simply use the search term "laughter web sites" and let the fun begin: you'll find more laughter than you can imagine.

- **Apps.** There's an app for everything, and that includes laughter. Add humorous apps to your iPhone, iPad, or other devices and find humor in life.

- **Plug in.** If you drive to work, take a bus or train, or walk, be plugged into something humorous on your iPod, car DVD player, or radio. Make it a point to start and end each workday with something funny.

MASSAGE

Receiving a massage can be one of the most relaxing experiences of your life, and at the same time it can provide significant health benefits. One of those benefits may be a reduction in blood pressure—but not necessarily. One reason I say this is because research concerning the use of massage for managing high blood pressure has shown some conflicting results, and that may be related to the type of massage a person receives. In fact, there are approximately eighty different types of massage therapy styles and each one is associated with certain pressures, techniques, and movements. Since it's not possible (or necessary) to look at all the different types of massage, let's talk about the few you are most likely to encounter.

Types of Massage

Although there are dozens of different types of massage, all share some common characteristics. Most commonly they all involve manipulating, pressing, or rubbing muscles and other soft tissues using the fingers, hands, or even elbows, feet, or forearms. The most popular and commonly practiced form of massage in the United States is Swedish massage. This also happens to be a form that has shown some benefit among people with high blood pressure.

Swedish massage involves the use of five different types of strokes that can be done with light to firm pressure, usually using the fingers or hands: kneading (petrissage), sliding (effeurage), tapping with cupped hands (tapotement), friction, and vibration. This type of massage involves only the uppermost layers of muscles and tissues, which means it does not (intentionally) include deep or penetrating techniques that can cause discomfort or pain. The goals of Swedish massage are to relieve tension, energize the body, and improve circulation. In the process, it can also help lower blood pressure in people who have prehypertension or hypertension.

Other types of massage, including trigger point, craniosacral, deep tissue, and sports massage, have not been shown to help with blood pressure, however. That's what investigators at National University of Health Sciences in Illinois discovered when they treated 150 adults with a blood pressure lower than 150/95 mmHg using a variety of massage techniques. Swedish massage showed the greatest effect on lowering blood pressure, while trigger point therapy and sports massage increased systolic blood pressure. In fact, all the types of massage except Swedish massage typically involve the use of more pressure and are often administered to treat specific conditions, such as a sports injury, fibromyalgia, headache, or back pain. Therefore, they can be somewhat painful, which is likely at least part of the reason why they cause blood pressure to rise. Also, if people anticipate pain their blood pressure can rise because of the stress they are feeling.

Benefits of Massage: Studies

For some people, a relaxing massage may be just what the doctor ordered (and be sure to check with your doctor first if you have high blood pressure!). Researchers at Isfahan University of Medical Sciences set out to evaluate fifty women with prehypertension who were evenly divided to participate in either ten to fifteen minutes of Swedish massage three times a week for ten sessions or a control group. When the authors tested the blood pressure values of the participants before and after each session, they found that massage significantly lowered both systolic and diastolic blood pressures when compared with controls.

Similar results were seen in another study that included African-American women, who are among those who experience probably the highest prevalence of hypertension of any population. Women in the study who received therapeutic chair massage experienced a significant decrease in both systolic and diastolic blood pressures.

For a chair massage, you sit in a special padded chair and lean forward, placing your head, facedown, in a padded rest. Some massage practitioners use chair massage at trade shows, in clinics, and in business settings because they are a convenient, portable way to give people a massage.

How and Where to Get a Massage

You don't need to pay for a professional massage to reap the blood pressure benefits; a spouse, partner, family member, or friend can learn a few basic techniques of Swedish massage from a class offered by a professional or by watching instructional DVDs or videos, which are available online or for purchase. Many communities offer couples massage sessions where you can learn from a professional the basics of massage you and a spouse or partner can share.

If you want to go to a professional massage therapist, you can ask your health-care provider for a referral or inquire at physical therapy or massage schools in the area. Look for a therapist who is familiar working with people who have high blood pressure. Massage schools often provide services from students (under supervision) for a reduced fee.

MEDITATION

It's free, there are no side effects, you can do it in your pajamas, it requires no special equipment, you don't break a sweat, and did I mention it's free? Meditation is being recommended by conventional doctors everywhere as an effective and safe way to manage many health problems, including high blood pressure. It's been shown to lower blood pressure in teenagers, thirty-somethings, and retirees. For example:

A report from experts at Georgia Health Sciences University noted that the use of Transcendental Meditation was effective in lowering resting and ambulatory blood pressure as well as improving school behavior in adolescents at risk for hypertension. The same technique was helpful in adults as well: those with mild to moderate essential hypertension had a reduction in blood pressure and needed less antihypertensive drugs, and they also experienced reduced symptoms of angina pectoris and atherosclerosis as well as a significant decline in cardiovascular death and symptoms.

In London, 129 adults participated in a group in which 67 practiced Sahaja Yoga meditation daily and 62 served as controls. After just one week, the volunteers in the meditation group experienced significant improvements in blood pressure (especially diastolic blood pressure), anxiety, and quality of life, but these improvements were not seen in the control group. In fact, participants with both high blood pressure and type 2 diabetes showed the best decline in diastolic blood pressure, with an estimated 12 mmHg drop.

At the Medical University of South Carolina, a research team found that breathing awareness meditation for three months was effective in lowering blood pressure in African-American teenagers when compared with a LifeSkills Training program and a health education control group.

Types of Meditation

So far I've mentioned three studies and three different types of meditation, and there are others. Although each study used a different meditation approach, all had the same basic bottom line: meditation helped reduce blood pressure.

Like shoes, not every meditation possibility fits each person the same way. Although there are numerous different ways to meditate, they all share a few basic elements:

- **Quieting the mind.** The intention of meditation is to focus your concentration on one healing element, e.g., your breathing, a candle flame, a sound or phrase.

- **Focus.** When your thoughts begin to wander, slowly and gently bring them back to your focus point. Do not berate yourself for any wandering your mind does: it happens!

- **Ignore distraction.** Try to pay no attention to bodily sensation, irrelevant thoughts, and other distractions while meditating.

How to Use Meditation

Here are four common types of meditation that can be helpful in lowering blood pressure and managing stress. You can get additional information about any of these meditation approaches online and from books, DVDs, and apps (see appendix). You can also enjoy a group experience and learn more about how to meditate by attending meditation programs, which are often offered at community centers, churches, hospitals, health centers, and other facilities in many towns and cities.

Mindfulness Meditation

One of the most commonly practiced types of meditation is called mindfulness meditation, which the Buddhists call insight meditation. This approach involves focusing on what is happening around you and being conscious of your innermost feelings and thoughts. It's critical that you not judge your feelings or thoughts but just allow them to pass through your mind. Mindfulness meditation is often used as a method of self-awakening and can provide a great deal of stress relief.

Breath Meditation

This meditation approach involves focusing on your breathing. It is a good method to try if you have not tried meditation before. To begin, get into a comfortable position, close your eyes, and focus all your attention on your breathing. Breathe in slowly and gently through your nose and feel the air enter your lungs and diaphragm. Focus on your breath as it leaves your body and exits through your nostrils. If your mind wanders—and it probably will—that's okay. Simply refocus on your breathing. Continue for five to ten minutes and try it several times a day if possible. It's a simple and effective way to relax and relieve stress.

Walking Meditation

This meditation technique allows you to walk and meditate at the same time. Instead of focusing on your breath or a specific sound or thought, you target your attention on the way your body moves and the sensations associated with walking. For example, concentrate on the way each foot feels when it makes contact with the floor or the ground, how your foot rolls into the movement. Focus on how the breeze feels against your arms, face, and body as you walk. If your mind wanders, refocus on your body. Of course, you need to pay enough attention to where you are walking so you are safe. In fact, focusing on the ground beneath your feet and the area you are walking in is part of your walking meditation. If you jog or run, you can also use this idea as basis for a jogging or running meditation.

Transcendental Meditation

If your idea of meditation has always included chanting a mantra, then you may have been thinking about Transcendental Meditation. This form of meditation has been the subject of more than 350 studies and is a meditation tradition practiced since ancient Vedic times. However, it became more recognized and popular in the middle of the last century when the Maharishi introduced Transcendental Meditation to the Western world.

Transcendental Meditation involves use of a mantra—a sound, word, or phrase that one repeats—and is practiced twice a day for twenty minutes while sitting comfortably. It is not a lifestyle, religion, or philosophy but simply a path to self-awareness and development. Many people find Transcendental Meditation to be helpful because repeating a mantra helps prevent the mind from wandering and also helps achieve a relaxed, dream-like state.

OTHER WAYS TO MANAGE
STRESS AND HYPERTENSION

Here are some other suggestions for how to manage stress before it manages you and, in the process, help lower your blood pressure:

- **Get creative.** Unrealized, bottled-up desires to create or to produce something beautiful or of value can fuel slow-burning stress and frustration, which can support high blood pressure. Allow yourself to take some time each day, or perhaps a few times a week, to be creative or play. That may mean doing watercolors, planting flowers, learning an instrument, carving something out of wood, making puzzles, or creating a patchwork quilt. The important thing is that it's something just for you that relieves stress and nurtures your creative spirit. In fact, a German study found that among people with essential hypertension who were being treated with medication, those who had a more positive attitude toward creativity and life were able to reduce their medication use.

• **Spend time with animals.** If you have a pet, share some quality time with the animal. Although research results are inconclusive, some studies show that people who have a dog have lower blood pressure and are less sedentary than people without dogs. A State University of New York at Buffalo study looked at 240 married couples, half of whom had a pet. Individuals with pets had significantly lower blood pressure, experienced less of an increase during stress, and recovered faster than did people without a pet. These benefits were especially evident when the pets were present.

• **Listen to music.** Listening to slower music tends to help lower blood pressure while faster music seems to increase blood pressure. Write yourself a prescription to listen to stress-reducing music every day. You can plug into your iPod or turn into your stereo system. Scientists have even developed an MP3 player that detects a person's blood pressure and then selects certain types of music to help relieve hypertension of patients. Dozens of apps related to music therapy for hypertension are available online.

CHAPTER EIGHT

Consider Medications

Although high blood pressure is largely a disease associated with lifestyle, sometimes making changes in routine habits and altering lifestyle does not provide all the help you need to effectively manage and lower your blood pressure. Sometimes the use of one or more medications is necessary for a short or longer period of time to help bring blood pressure under safe control. After all, high blood pressure doesn't develop overnight and so it may take some time for your body to adjust as you make changes to bring it under control. I want to emphasize that you should never stop taking medications that have been prescribed without first consulting with your healthcare provider.

The good news is that the lifestyle changes discussed throughout this book work in synch with medications. Therefore, if you and your doctor do decide you should start a medication program—or continue medications that you were previously taking—you can still explore the natural approaches discussed in this book. Oftentimes people find they are able to significantly reduce or eventually eliminate use of prescription medications for high blood pressure and continue with lifestyle modifications as their means of hypertension control.

That said, it's important for you to understand the

different types of medications your doctor may recommend and prescribe for high blood pressure. This chapter introduces you to those drugs, their benefits and side effects, other warnings about their use, and how they may interact with other medications or supplements.

DO YOU NEED MEDICATION?

The first question many patients with high blood pressure ask is do they really need antihypertensive medications? This is a question all individuals with high blood pressure are encouraged to ask their health-care providers, and the answer should be fully explained, including a discussion of how natural treatment options can be included in a treatment program should medication be chosen.

Research indicates that the chances of experiencing serious health problems (e.g., heart attack, kidney disease, stroke, and early death) increase twofold for every 20-point increase in your systolic pressure or 10-point increase in diastolic pressure from a starting point of 115/75 mmHg. Yes, even though the accepted "normal" blood pressure is 120/80 mmHg, trouble can begin brewing even at that level.

The answer to the question "Do you need medication?" is highly individual. If you have mild hypertension and are not overweight, have no history of heart problems, and have recently stopped smoking, you and your doctor may decide to forego medication as your body adjusts to your recent smoking cessation and you gradually increase your exercise level and practice stress reduction.

If, however, you have mild hypertension, are overweight, have type 2 diabetes, and your attempts at weight loss have not (yet) been successful, then your doctor may prescribe medication for your blood pressure. Once you are able to lose weight and have success using other natural ways to lower your blood pressure, you may eventually eliminate your need for the drugs.

Generally, doctors prescribe medications for patients who have a blood pressure of 140/90 to 159/99 mmHg or higher. Patients who also have diabetes, kidney disease, or heart problems are often handed a prescription if their blood pressure is as low as 130/80 mmHg.

The fact is, most people who have high blood pressure are prescribed medications, and not just one (see "Combining Medications"). That doesn't mean everyone with a prescription needs the medication. It also doesn't mean that the patients are actually taking the medication as prescribed. Indeed, patient compliance is low: 50 percent of patients stop taking their medications within the first year of treatment, and many patients take only half of their prescribed doses. Neither of these actions is recommended. If you want to stop taking your prescription or are unable to continue for any reason, you should contact your doctor immediately and discuss an alternative plan, such as making significant lifestyle changes. But stopping your medication or taking it only some of the time can be dangerous.

The bottom line when it comes to using medications for high blood pressure is that each individual case is different. Therefore, you should be prepared to discuss the pros and cons of taking antihypertensive drugs with your health-care provider. Also, discuss the lifestyle changes you are willing to make and any you are already doing to lower your blood pressure so you and your doctor are on the same page regarding your treatment.

DRUGS TO TREAT HYPERTENSION

Doctors typically prescribe medication to treat high blood pressure for anyone who has a sustained systolic pressure greater than 160 mmHg or a diastolic pressure greater than 100 mmHg. A wide variety of drugs are available from several different categories, as explained here. While some people with high blood pressure take only one drug, about 10 percent of patients may need up to three medications to control their blood pressure. It's important to remember that lifestyle changes can and should be used along with any medications prescribed by your doctor, because those modifications can not only reduce or even eliminate your need for drugs, but they also can help improve cardiovascular health and quality of life on many levels.

Now let's discuss the most commonly prescribed medications for high blood pressure and what you might expect if you take them. A few words of caution: never stop taking any prescribed drug without first consulting your doctor. Suddenly stopping a medication can result in serious side effects.

DIURETICS

Diuretics, often referred to as water pills, help the kidneys eliminate water, sodium, and other substances from the body in urine. Removal of excess fluid and salt from the body lowers blood volume, which in turn helps make it easier for the heart to pump blood and thus lowers blood pressure. Doctors typically prescribe diuretics not only for high blood pressure but also for heart failure, glaucoma (because of elevated pressure in the eye), and various liver and kidney conditions.

Diuretics can be helpful for people who are salt sensitive, blacks, and anyone who tends to consume too much salt. For help reducing your salt intake, see chapter 3.

Types of Diuretics

There are three types of diuretics: loop, thiazide, and potassium sparing. Your doctor may prescribe one or more of these drugs at the same time.

- Loop diuretics (e.g., bumetanide [Bumex], furosemide [Lasix], torsemide [Demadex]) do not have a significant impact on blood pressure, but they are often prescribed for people who have symptoms of congestive heart failure. Therefore, if you have congestive heart failure and high blood pressure your doctor may give you a prescription for a loop diuretic as well as other medication to help lower your blood pressure. Along with water and sodium, loop diuretics cause the body to lose potassium, which means you will need to be sure to eat more foods rich in potassium and/or take potassium supplements if you take these medications.

- Thiazide diuretics (e.g., chlorothiazide [Diuril], chlorthalidone [generic], hydrocholorothiazide [Esidrix, Microzide], indapamide [Lozol]) are prescribed for hypertension and for edema associated with heart failure. These diuretics also may reduce potassium levels. A side effect of thiazide diuretics is an increase in blood sugar and cholesterol levels, so you will need to keep a close eye on these factors if you take a thiazide diuretic.

• Potassium-sparing diuretics (amiloride [Midamor], spironolactone [Aldactone], triamterene [Maxzidel]) have an obvious advantage over the other two types of diuretics because of their ability to preserve potassium levels. However, because they do not significantly reduce blood pressure levels they are often prescribed along with one or two other diuretics.

Side Effects of Diuretics

Generally, diuretics are associated with weakness, dizziness, nausea, leg cramps, fatigue, gout, an increase in blood sugar levels (be especially careful if you have diabetes), reduction of sex drive, and impotence. Some people find the need to use the bathroom more frequently annoying or disruptive. If you already experience urinary urgency or some urinary incontinence (e.g., urine leakage when you sneeze or cough), you may want to ask your doctor about taking something other than diuretics.

BETA-BLOCKERS

The beta-adrenergic blockers, or beta-blockers for short, have been prescribed for high blood pressure and heart disease since the 1960s. Beta-blockers work by stopping or blocking neurotransmitters from attaching themselves to beta-receptors, which are found on cells. This action prevents the neurotransmitters from stimulating the heart and blood vessels and in turn slows the heart rate and how much blood the heart pumps, which lowers blood pressure. If you have suffered a heart attack or you have the heartbeat abnormalities known as arrhythmias, you may be prescribed beta-blockers as well.

For high blood pressure, doctors typically prescribe beta-blockers along with other anti-hypertensive medications. Beta-blockers are not effective when used alone in African Americans but produce better results when taken with a thiazide diuretic.

As an interesting aside, many sports organizations, including the Olympics, the PGA, the United States Anti-Doping Agency, and the World Anti-Doping Agency, have or plan to add beta-blockers to their banned substance lists for athletes. Why? Because beta-blockers are also effective at calming nerves in stressful situations, such as athletic competition.

Examples of Beta-Blockers

The beta-blockers available for treatment of high blood pressure include the following:

- Atenolol (Tenormin)

- Bisoprolol (Zebeta)

- Carvedilol (Coreg)

- Labetalol (Trandate)

- Metoprolol (Lopressor, Toprol XL)

- Nadolol (Corgard)

- Nebivolol (Bystolic)

- Pindolol (Visken)

- Propranolol (Inderal)

- Sotalol (Betapace)

- Timolol (Blocadren)

Side Effects of Beta-Blockers

If you have a chronic lung condition such as asthma, use of beta-blockers can make it worse. Ironically, beta-blockers can also increase the risk of heart failure in some people but improve it in others. Research also suggests that taking some of the older beta-blockers (e.g., atenolol, metoprolol, propranolol) may increase a person's risk of type 2 diabetes by more than 25 percent. The most common side effects include depression, erectile dysfunction, fatigue, insomnia, shortness of breath, and reduced exercise tolerance.

ALPHA-2 AGONISTS

The drugs in the alpha-2 agonist category, also called centrally acting alpha agents, differ from other antihypertensive drugs because they act in the brain by turning off activity that causes the arteries to constrict. Several drugs in this category are used for women with high blood pressure who are pregnant (see "Treating Hypertension with Drugs During Pregnancy").

Examples of Alpha-2 Agonists

Here are some of the alpha-2 agonists your doctor may

prescribe. Note in the section "Side Effects of Alpha-2 Agonists" that the adverse reactions to these drugs differ among them.

- Alpha-methyldopa (Aldomet)

- Clonidine (Catapres)

- Guanabenz (Wytensin)

- Guanfacine (Tenex)

Side Effects of Alpha-2 Agonists

All four of the alpha-2 agonists listed are associated with the common side effects of sexual dysfunction and sleepiness. In addition, alpha-methyldopa may cause your blood pressure to decline significantly when you walk or stand. Methyldopa is also associated with dry mouth, fever, anemia, and sluggishness. The latter three drugs are more likely to cause severe dry mouth, constipation, or drowsiness.

ANGIOTENSIN-CONVERTING ENZYME (ACE) INHIBITORS

The ACE inhibitors get their name from the fact that they prevent the kidneys from retaining water and salt by inhibiting the activity of angiotensin-converting enzyme. This enzyme changes inactive angiotensin I to active angiotensin II, a substance that causes blood pressure to rise. ACE inhibitors tend to be effective in most people who have high blood pressure, while causing fewer side effects. Another positive trait of ACE inhibitors is that they protect the hearts of people who have congestive heart failure, and they are also protective of the kidneys of people who have kidney problems or diabetes.

A downside of ACE inhibitors is that they are less effective in African Americans when used alone, but they do lead to better results when taken with a thiazide diuretic.

Examples of ACE Inhibitors

Your doctor may prescribe one of the following ACE inhibitors:

- Benazepril (Lotensin)

- Captopril (Capoten)

- Enalapril (Vasotec)

- Fosinopril (Monopril)

- Lisinopril (Prinivil, Zestril)

- Quinapril (Accupril)

- Ramipril (Altace)

- Trandolapril (Mavik)

Side Effects of ACE Inhibitors

The most common side effects of ACE inhibitors are dry cough and a reduced sense of taste. ACE inhibitors may also cause you to retain potassium, so if you have kidney problems you should use them with caution.

CALCIUM CHANNEL BLOCKERS

Calcium channel blockers address the problem of high blood pressure by interfering with the entry of calcium into heart muscle cells and arteries. This action in turn reduces the strength of the heart's contractions and increases the dilation of the blood vessels, which improves blood flow and lowers blood pressure.

Examples of Calcium Channel Blockers

Here is a list of some of the calcium channel blockers your doctor may prescribe.

- Amlodipine (Norvasc)

- Bepridil (Vascor)

- Diltiazem (Cardizem)

- Felodipine (Plendil)

- Isradipine (DynaCirc)

- Nicardipine (Cardene)

- Nifedipine (Adalat, Procardia)

- Nimodipine (Nimotop)

- Nitrendipine (Cardif, Nitrepin)

- Pranidipine (Acalas)

- Verapamil (Calan, Isoptin)

Side Effects of Calcium Channel Blockers

You may experience any of the following side effects if you take calcium channel blockers: constipation, gum problems, headache, heartburn, nausea, slowed heart rate (bradycardia), and water retention (edema). Avoid drinking grapefruit juice or eating grapefruit if you are taking calcium channel blockers.

ANGIOTENSIN II RECEPTOR BLOCKERS (ARBS)

Among the more recent additions to the treatment options for high blood pressure are angiotensin II receptor blockers, which help stop the effects of a chemical called angiotensin. Interference with this chemical helps lower blood pressure. Your doctor may prescribe ARBs if you are not able to take ACE inhibitors.

Examples of ARBs

Here are some of the ARBs your doctor may prescribe:

- Candesartan (Atacand)

- Eprosartan (Tevetan)

- Irbesartan (Avapro)

- Losartan (Cozaar)

- Olmesartan (Benicar)

- Telmisartan (Mycardis)

- Valsartan (Diovan)

Side Effects of ARBs

If your doctor prescribes ARBs, you may experience any of these side effects: back or leg pain, confusion (contact your doctor immediately), diarrhea, dizziness, fainting (strongest after the first dose), insomnia, irregular heartbeat, muscle cramps, sinusitis, and upper respiratory infection.

COMBINING MEDICATIONS

Many clinicians prescribe more than one antihypertensive medication for their patients who have high blood pressure. As mentioned earlier, people who have resistant hypertension are routinely prescribed three or more different drugs in an attempt to manage their blood pressure.

The usual course of treatment for individuals with stage 1 hypertension is to prescribe one drug at the lowest possible dose and to gradually increase it with the goal of reaching a healthier range, which is typically less than 140/90 mmHg or less than 130/80 mmHg if they have diabetes or kidney disease. If blood pressure does not decline, then a second medication may be prescribed. While taking antihypertensive medications you should always also be following lifestyle changes.

In addition to the single-ingredient drugs already discussed, drug companies also market combination prescription medications that consist of two drugs from different categories. In this way, patients can take one drug instead of two, but the two drugs in one combination medication can work in two ways to help lower blood pressure. At the same time, a single combination medication may treat both hypertension and other medi-cal problems, especially heart disease. Patients are more likely to take one drug rather than two, so compliance may be better.

Here is a sample of some of the combination antihy-pertensive drugs on the market. The most commonly combined drugs for high blood pressure are two differ-ent types of diuretics, or hydrochlorothiazide plus a beta-blocker, an ACE inhibitor, or an ARB, but there are others, as the following list demonstrates:

- Amiloride plus hydrochlorothiazide: Moduretic

- Triamterene plus hydrochlorothiazide: Dyazide

- Prazosin plus polythiazide: Minizide

- Atenolol plus chlorthalidone: Tenoretic

- Metoprolol plus hydrochlorothiazide: Lopressor HCT

- Enalapril plus hydrochlorothiazide: Vaseretic

- Captopril plus hydrochlorothiazide: Capozide

- Candesartan plus hydrochlorothiazide: Atacand HCT

- Losartan plus hydrochlorothiazide: Hyzaar

- Valsartan plus hydrochlorothiazide: Diovan HCT

- Amlodipine plus benazepril: Lotrel

- Diltiazem plus enalapril: Teczem

- Methyldopa plus hydrochlorothiazide: Aldoril

- Amlodipine plus valsartan: Exforge

- Amlodipine plus olmesartan: Azor

Side effects of combination medications typically include the adverse reactions from both of the drugs in the mixture. The side effects associated with each of the ingredients in the combination medications are mentioned earlier in the chapter.

TREATING HYPERTENSION WITH DRUGS DURING PREGNANCY

Hypertension in pregnancy is defined as systolic blood pressure of 140 mmHg or higher and/or a diastolic blood pressure of 90 mmHg or higher. If you are pregnant or have plans to get pregnant and you have high blood pressure, you and your health-care provider should discuss ways to manage your blood pressure without the use of medications. However, in some cases the use of antihypertensive medications is necessary.

A small percentage of women (about 5 to 8 percent) develop preeclampsia during pregnancy, a condition characterized by a spike in blood pressure and the presence of protein in the urine, typically appearing around week 20. Treatment of preeclampsia is especially critical to protect the health of the mother and baby. Women with preeclampsia may be administered intravenous magnesium sulfate or prescription antihypertensive drugs. In addition, women who have or develop high blood pressure during pregnancy (called gestational hypertension) also may need medication.

Therefore, if your doctor has recommended prescription drugs you should know there are several that researchers have identified as being safe to take during pregnancy. You will recognize these drugs as those discussed earlier in the chapter:

- **Methyldopa.** This drug is typically prescribed as the first choice in the United States and the United Kingdom because it has not been shown to affect the mother's heart or blood flow to the uterus or kidneys.

- **Labetalol.** Similar to methyldopa, labetalol does not seem to have a negative impact on blood flow to the uterus. If you have asthma, chronic obstructive pulmonary disease, a heart condition, liver disease, kidney disease, or diabetes, you may need to consider other medication to manage hypertension. Labetalol may be taken orally or intravenously.

- **Nifedipine.** The long-acting form of this drug is usually prescribed during pregnancy. However, nifedipine is used less often than are methyldopa or labetalol. Nifedipine should not be used along with magnesium sulfate because it can cause the mother's blood pressure to drop to dangerously low levels.

- **Atenolol (Tenormin) and clonidine (Catapres).** These two drugs are not among the more commonly prescribed medications, but they are still regarded as safe

- **Hydralazine (Apresoline).** This drug is used mainly intravenously and for women with preeclampsia. If you have coronary artery disease, rheumatic heart disease, kidney disease, or a history of stroke, your doctor may need to prescribe another medication for preeclampsia.

Drugs in the ACE inhibitor and angiotensin receptor blocker categories should be avoided.

MEDICATIONS THAT CAN RAISE BLOOD PRESSURE

Did you know that an over-the-counter drug you take to relieve your headache or help you cope with cold or flu symptoms can raise your blood pressure? Many common OTC medications can cause your blood pressure to rise, and if you take them for a prolonged time their use can be especially detrimental if you have high blood pressure. Here are some of the drugs you should be aware of, but be sure to talk to your health-care provider about any medications you are taking.

Cold Medications (Decongestants)

If you have high blood pressure and you catch a cold or the flu, stop and think before you take a decongestant. These over-the-counter medications can cause your blood vessels to constrict, which interferes with blood circulation and thus boosts your blood pressure. Decongestants are available as nasal sprays as well as tablets, capsules, and liquid. Also be aware that some OTC cold and flu medications contain a combination of ingredients, one of which may be a decongestant. Ask your doctor or pharmacist which OTC products for cold and flu are safe if you have hypertension. Look for these decongestants when shopping so you know what to avoid:

- Phenylephrine (e.g., Neo-Synephrine)

- Phenylpropanolamine (e.g., Accutrim, Propan)

- Pseudoephedrine (e.g., Sudafed)

Immunosuppressants

Generally, immunosuppressants are drugs used to suppress the immune system. They are usually prescribed for individuals who have undergone an organ transplant, in which case they help prevent the body from rejecting the new organ. They are also prescribed to treat some autoimmune diseases and similar conditions, such as psoriasis, rheumatoid arthritis, Crohn's disease, and alopecia areata (hair loss).

If you have been prescribed immunosuppressants and you have high blood pressure, you should check your blood pressure regularly and talk to your doctor about alternatives to these medications, especially if you have difficulty managing your hypertension. Instituting lifestyle changes as suggested throughout this book may help reduce or eliminate your need for hypertension drugs while allowing you to continue with any immunosuppressants that are necessary. Examples of immunosuppressants that may raise blood pressure include:

- Cyclosporine (e.g., Neoral, Sandimmune)

- Tacrolimus (e.g., Prograf)

Nonsteroidal Anti-inflammatory Drugs (NSAIDs)

This is a popular category of OTC drugs often used to treat headache, muscle aches and pains, arthritis, and general pain. However, these drugs also can cause you to retain fluids, which can result in a rise in blood pressure. Talk to your doctor about the use of NSAIDs and consider finding alternative means to address pain (e.g., herbal remedies, massage, heat therapy, among others). NSAIDs that may increase blood pressure include the following:

- Ibuprofen (e.g., Advil, Motrin)

- Meloxicam (e.g., Mobic)

- Naproxen (e.g., Naprosyn)

- Naproxen sodium (e.g., Aleve)

Other Drugs

Some other drugs that can elevate your blood pressure include stimulants, such as methylphenidate (Ritalin), which also boosts your heart rate along with your blood pressure. Use of illicit drugs such as amphetamines (e.g., methamphetamine), anabolic steroids, cocaine, Ecstasy, and phencyclidine (PCP) is extremely dangerous for the heart and blood pressure.

ANTIHYPERTENSIVE DRUGS, SUPPLEMENTS, AND FOOD INTERACTIONS

In addition to the side effects associated with antihypertensive medications, there is also a risk of experiencing adverse reactions if you combine some antihypertensive drugs with natural supplements or foods. Here are a few interactions of which you should be aware:

- **Thiazides.** If you take large amounts (1,500 mg or more) of calcium along with thiazide diuretics, a serious condition called milk-alkali syndrome may result. This syndrome occurs if you ingest too much calcium along with taking thiazides, resulting in abnormally high calcium levels, or hypercalcemia, and possibly leads to kidney failure. Talk to your doctor before taking calcium supplements if you are also taking a thiazide.

- **Calcium channel blockers.** If you are taking calcium intravenously, it may reduce the effects of any calcium channel blockers you are taking. Use of oral calcium supplements, however, does not appear to interfere with calcium channel blockers.

- **Grapefruit.** You should avoid eating grapefruit or drinking grapefruit juice when taking antihypertensive medications. This fruit can interfere with the absorption and stabilizing effects of the drugs.

APPENDIX

SUGGESTED READINGS

Allen, Marc. *How to Quiet Your Mind: Relax and Silence the Voice of Your Mind Today.* CreateSpace Independent Publishing Platform, November 2012.

Barnard, Neal D. *Dr. Neal Barnard's Program for Reversing Diabetes: The Scientifically Proven System for Reversing Diabetes Without Drugs.* Emmaus, PA: Rodale Books, 2008.

Brill, Janet Bond, PhD, RD. *Blood Pressure Down: The 10-Step Plan to Lower Your Blood Pressure in 4 Weeks—Without Prescription Drugs.* New York: Three Rivers Press, 2013.

Casey, Aggie, and Herbert Benson, MD. *Harvard Medical School Guide to Lowering Your Blood Pressure.* New York: McGraw Hill, 2006.

Cohen, Jay S. *The Magnesium Solution for High Blood Pressure: How to Use Magnesium to Help Prevent & Relieve Hypertension Naturally.* Garden City Park, NY: Square One, 2004.

Frank, Rachel. *Stress the Silent Killer: Stress Management Techniques for Fighting Back*. Columbia, SC: Happy Health, 2013. Kindle edition.

Froberg, Stig, and Stefan Frobert. *Decrease Hypertension and Cholesterol Naturally*. Vol. 1. CreateSpace Independent Publishing Platform, July 16, 2012.

Kornfield, Jack. *Meditation for Beginners*. Pap/Com ed. Louisville, CO: Sounds True, 2008.

Kowalski, R. E. *The Blood Pressure Cure: 8 Weeks to Lower Blood Pressure Without Prescription Drugs*. Hoboken, NJ: John Wiley & Sons, 2007.

LaGrande, Jack. *High Blood Pressure: Experience the Health Benefits and Healing Power of Fruits and Vegetables*. Amazon Digital Services. Kindle Edition.

Lidell, Lucinda, with Sara Thomas, Carola Beresford Cooke and Anthony Porter. *The Book of Massage: The Complete Step-by-Step Guide to Eastern and Western Technique*. 2nd ed. Greenwich, CT: Touchstone, 2001.

Mann, Samuel J. *Hypertension and You: Old Drugs, New Drugs, and the Right Drugs for Your High Blood Pressure*. Lanham, MD: Rowman & Littlefield, 2012.

Physicians Committee for Responsible Medicine. *Healthy Eating for Life for Children*. New York: John Wiley & Sons, 2002.

Snyder, Dr. Mariza, Dr. Lauren Clum and Anna V. Zulaica. *The DASH Diet Cookbook: Quick and*

Delicious Recipes for Losing Weight, Preventing Diabetes, and Lowering Blood Pressure. Berkeley, CA: Ulysses Press, 2012.

Sparrow, Sarah. *High Blood Pressure.* Amazon Digital Services. Kindle edition.

Townsend, Raymond R., MD. *100 Questions & Answers About High Blood Pressure.* Sudbury, MA: Jones and Bartlett, 2008.

RESOURCES

Apps

There are apps for everything, including ones that will help you monitor your blood pressure, meditate, sleep well, manage stress, eat healthy (DASH diet), and more. Several Web sites offer scores of apps for these purposes. Since it's not possible to list them all, feel free to visit the main Web sites and search for appropriate apps. Here are a few to get you started:

- Blood Pressure Monitor, by Family Lite, offered by iTunes

- Blood Pressure Companion Free, by Maxwell Software, offered by iTunes

- BloodPressure Pro, by RumbleApps, offered by iTunes

- iBP Blood Pressure app, by Leading Edge Apps, offered by iMedicalApps

- The Mindfulness App, by MindApps, offered by iTunes

• Buddhify, by 21 awake Ltd, offered by iTunes

• DASH Diet Pro—Prevent and Lower High Blood
  Pressure, by FitKit, LLC, offered by iTunes

Acupressure.com
Information about acupressure, including charts of acupoints, articles, and more
http://www.acupressure.com/

American Heart Association
Information on high blood pressure, including an online
risk calculator
http://www.heart.org/HEARTORG/Conditions/High
BloodPressure/High-Blood-Pressure_UCM_002020
_SubHomePage.jsp

Centers for Disease Control and Prevention
Comprehensive information on high blood pressure, including lots of links to fact sheets and information on
self-monitoring of blood pressure
http://www.cdc.gov/bloodpressure/

DASH Diet Eating Plan
Lots of information on the DASH diet to get you started
http://dashdiet.org/

Laughter Yoga International
Everything you'd ever want to know about laughter yoga,
including how to find a group near you
http://www.laughteryoga.org/

National Heart, Lung, and Blood Institute
Information on high blood pressure
http://www.nhlbi.nih.gov/health/health-topics/topics/hbp/

National High Blood Pressure Education Program
Information on everything from prevention to medications
http://www.nhlbi.nih.gov/hbp/

National Institute of Diabetes and Digestive and Kidney Diseases
Provides information on high blood pressure and your kidneys
http://kidney.niddk.nih.gov/

National STROKE Association
Nonprofit offering information on stroke prevention, treatment, and rehabilitation
http://www.stroke.org/

RESPeRATE
Web site for RESPeRATE, a device that can help lower blood pressure when used regularly
http://www.resperate.com/us/welcome/index.aspx

Tai Chi
Information on the National Center for Complementary and Alternative Medicine Web site regarding tai chi
http://nccam.nih.gov/health/taichi/introduction.htm

Transcendental Meditation
The official Web site for Transcendental Meditation, which has been shown to significantly reduce stress and help lower blood pressure
http://www.tm.org/

WebMD Alternative Treatments for High Cholesterol
Nondrug approaches to treatment of high cholesterol
http://www.webmd.com/cholesterol-management/guide/high_cholesterol_alternative-therapies

VEGETARIAN AND VEGAN FOOD MANUFACTURERS

Note: This is only a representative list . . . there are many more! This list in no way endorses any of these products, nor does the absence of any other manufacturers suggest they are any less desirable.

Amy's Kitchen
Annie's Naturals
Barbara's Bakery
Bob's Red Mill Natural Foods
Boca Food Company
Cascadian Farms
Celentano
Chocolate Decadence
Dr. McDougall's Right Foods
Eden Foods
ENER-G Foods
Essential Living Foods
Fantastic Foods
Foods Alive
Gardenburger
Genisoy

Gluten-Free Pantry

Go Veggie!

Hain Celestial Group (includes but not limited to Alba Botanica, Arrowhead Mills, Casbah, Celestial Seasonings, Estee, Garden of Eatin', Hain Pure Foods, Weight Watchers, Westbrae Natural, Yves Veggie Cuisine)

Kashi

LightLife Foods

Lumen Soy Foods

Muir Glen Organic Tomatoes

Pacific Foods

Rella Good Cheese Company

ShariAnn's Organics

Tofutti Brands

Tree of Life

Vitasoy

WhiteWave Foods

Worthington Foods, which includes MorningStar Farms, Natural Touch, and Loma Linda

NOTES

PART I. INTRODUCING HIGH BLOOD PRESSURE

Chapter 1. High Blood Pressure Basics

1. X. Urrutia-Rojas et al., "High Blood Pressure in School Children: Prevalence and Risk Factors," *BMC Pediatrics* 6 (Nov. 16, 2006): 32.

2. American Heart Association, "Energy Drinks May Increase Blood Pressure, Disturb Heart Rhythm," *ScienceDaily* March 21, 2013, retrieved March 22, 2013, from http://www.sciencedaily.com-/releases/2013/03/130321205524.htm.

3. D. A. Calhoun et al., "Resistant Hypertension: Diagnosis, Evaluation, and Treatment: Scientific Statement from the American Heart Association Professional Education Committee of the Council for High Blood Pressure Research," *Circulation* 117 (2008): e510–e526.

Chapter 2. High Blood Pressure and Your Body

1. R. J. Glynn, et al., "Development of Predictive Models for Long-Term Cardiovascular Risk Associated with Systolic and Diastolic Blood Pressure," *Hypertension* 39, no. 1 (Jan. 2002): 105–10.

2. Y. Zhang et al., "Prehypertension, Diabetes, and Cardiovascular Disease Risk in a Population-Based Sample: The Strong Heart Study," *Hypertension* 2006 47, no. 3 (March 2006): 410–14.

3. Karen M. Rodrigue, "Risk Factors for B-Amyloid Deposition in Healthy Aging: Vascular and Genetic Effects, *JAMA Neurology* 18 (2013): 1–7.

4. P. A. Newman-Casey et al., "The Relationship Between Components of Metabolic Syndrome and Open-Angle Glaucoma," *Ophthalmology,* 2011.

PART II. HOW TO PREVENT AND TREAT HIGH BLOOD PRESSURE

Chapter 3. Eat Your Way to a Healthy Blood Pressure

1. W. J. Craig et al., "Position of the American Dietetic Association: Vegetarian Diets," *Journal of the American Dietetic Association* 109, no. 7 (July 2009): 1266–82.

2. G. E. Fraser, "Vegetarian Diets: What Do We Know of Their Effects on Common Chronic Diseases?," *American Journal of Clinical Nutrition* 89, no. 5 (May 2009): 1607–12S.

N. Brathwaite et al., "Obesity, Diabetes, Hypertension, and Vegetarian Status Among Seventh-Day Adventists in Barbados: Preliminary Results," *Ethnicity and Disease* 13, no. 1 (Winter 2003): 34–39.

L. T. Coles, and P. M. Clifton, "Effect of Beetroot Juice on Lowering Blood Pressure in Free-Living, Disease-Free Adults: A Randomized, Placebo-Controlled Trial," *Nutrition Journal* 11 (December 2012): 106.

J. A. Conquer, "Supplementation with an Algae Source of Docosahexaenoic Acid Increases (N-3) Fatty Acid Status and Alters Selected Risk Factor for Heart Disease in Vegetarian Subjects," *Journal of Nutrition* 126, no. 12 (1996): 3032–39.

S. C. Couch et al., "The Efficacy of a Clinic-Based Behavioral Nutrition Intervention Emphasizing a DASH-Type Diet for Adolescents with Elevated Blood Pressure," *Journal of Pediatrics* 152, no. 4 (April 2008): 494–501.

M. Galleano et al., "Hypertension, Nitric Oxide, Oxidants, and Dietary Plant Polyphenols, *Current Pharmaceutical Biotechnology* 11, no. 8 (December 2010): 837–48.

S. M. Ghosh et al., "Enhanced Vasodilator Activity of Nitrite in Hypertension," *Hypertension,* April 15, 2013.

Diana I. Jalal, Gerard Smits, Richard J. Johnson, and Michel Chonchol, "Increased Fructose Associates with Elevated Blood Pressure," *Journal of the American Society of Nephrology* 21, no. 9 (Sept. 2010): 1543–49.

L. L. Moore et al., "Intake of Fruits, Vegetables, and Dairy Products in Early Childhood and Subsequent Blood Pressure change," *Epidemiology* 16, no. 1 (Jan. 2005): 4–11.

J. S. White, "Challenging the Fructose Hypothesis: New Perspectives on Fructose Consumption and Metabolism," *Advances in Nutrition* 4, no. 2 (March 1, 2013): 246–56.

Chapter 4. Be on the Move

R. D. Brook et al., "Beyond Medications and Diet: Alternative Approaches to Lowering Blood Pressure: A Scientific Statement from the American Heart Association," *Hypertension*, April 22, 2013, Epub before print.

V. A. Cornelissen and N. A. Smart, "Exercise Training for Blood Pressure: A Systematic Review and Meta-analysis," *Journal of the American Heart Association* 2013 2, no. 1 (Feb. 1 2013): e004473.

R. M. Cunha and P. C. Jardim, "Subacute Blood Pressure Behavior in Elderly Hypertensive Women After Resistance Exercise Session," *Journal of Sports Medicine and Physical Fitness* 52, no. 2 (April 2012): 175–80.

F. Dimeo et al., "Aerobic Exercise Reduces Blood Pressure in Resistant Hypertension. *Hypertension* 60, no. 3 (Sept. 2012): 653–58.

G. A. Kelley and K. S. Kelley, "Isometric Handgrip Exercise and Resting Blood Pressure: A Meta-analysis of

Randomized Controlled Trials," *Journal of Hypertension* 28, no. 3 (March 2010): 411–18.

C. L. Lin et al., "The Effect of Tai Chi for Blood Pressure, Blood Sugar, Blood Lipid Control for Patients with Chronic Disease: A Systematic Review," *Hi Li Za Zhi* 60, no. 1 (Feb. 2013): 69–77.

H. M. Lo et al., "A Tai Chi Exercise Programme Improved Exercise Behavior and Reduced Blood Pressure in Outpatients with Hypertension," *International Journal of Nursing Practice* 18, no. 6 (Dec. 2012): 545–51.

P. J. Millar et al., "Isometric Handgrip Effects on Hypertension," *Current Hypertension Reviews* 5 (2009): 54–60.

N. Sousa et al., "Long-Term Effects of Aerobic Training Versus Combined Aerobic and Resistance Training in Modifying Cardiovascular Disease Risk Factors in Healthy Elderly Men," *Geriatric Gerontology International*, Feb. 26, 2013.

R. E. Taylor-Piliae and E. S. Froelicher, "Measurement Properties of Tai Chi Exercise Self-Efficacy Among Ethnic Chinese with Coronary Heart Disease Risk Factors: A Pilot Study," *European Journal of Cardiovascular Nursing* 3, no. 4 (Dec. 2004): 287–94.

Chapter 5. Lose Weight, Sleep Better, and Other Lifestyle Matters

P. Bogdanski et al., "Green Tea Extract Reduces Blood Pressure, Inflammatory Biomarkers, and Oxidative Stress and Improves Parameters Associated with Insulin

Resistance in Obese, Hypertensive Patients," *Nutrition Research* 32, no. 6 (June 2012): 421–27.

M. A. Denke, "Nutritional and Health Benefits of Beer," *American Journal of the Medical Sciences* 320, no. 5 (Nov. 2000): 320–26.

K. Kozuma et al., "Antihypertensive Effect of Green Coffee Bean Extract on Mildly Hypertensive Subjects," *Hypertension Research* 28, no. 9 (Sept. 2005): 711–18.

M. G. Jensen et al., "Effect of Alginate Supplementation on Weight Loss in Obese Subjects Completing a 12-Wk Energy-Restricted Diet: A Randomized Controlled Trial," *American Journal of Clinical Nutrition* July 2012, ajcn.025312.

H. Maeda et al., "Effect of Medium-Chain Triacylglycerols on Anti-obesity Effect of Fucoxanthin," *Journal of Oleo Science* 56, no. 12 (2007): 615–21.

H. Maeda et al., "Fucoxanthin from Edible Seaweed, Undaria Pinnatifida, Shows Antiobesity Effect Through UCP1 Expression in White Adipose Tissues," *Biochemical and Biophysical Research Communications* 332.2 (2005): 392–97.

MedicineNet.com, "Black Pepper May Help Fight Fat. MedicineNet, accessed April 15, 2013, http://www.medicinenet.com/script/main/art.asp?articlekey=157866.

A. E. Mesas et al., "The Effect of Coffee on Blood Pressure and Cardiovascular Disease in Hypertensive Individuals: A Systematic Review and Meta-analysis,"

American Journal of Clinical Nutrition 94, no. 4 (Oct. 2011): 1113–26.

R. Ochiai et al., "Green Coffee Bean Extract Improves Human Vasoreactivity," *Hypertension Research* 27, no. 10 (Oct. 2004): 731–37.

Y. Okumura et al., "Adiposity Suppression Effect in Mice Due to Black Pepper and Its Main Pungent Component, Piperine," *Bioscience, Biotechnology, and Biochemistry* 74, no. 8 (2010): 1545–49.

U. H. Park et al., "Piperine, a Component of Black Pepper Inhibits Adipogenesis by Antagonizing PPARy Activity in 3T3-L1 Cells," *Journal of Agricultural and Food Chemistry* 60, no. 15 (April 18, 2012): 3853–60.

H. D. Sesso et al., "Alcohol Consumption and the Risk of Hypertension in Women and Men," *Hypertension* 51, no. 4 (April 2008): 1080–87.

J. D. Shlisky et al., "Partial Sleep Deprivation and Energy Balance in Adults: An Emerging Issue for Consideration by Dietetics Practitioners," *Journal of the Academy of Nutrition and Dietetics* 112, no. 11 (Nov. 2012): 1785–97.

J. A. Vinson et al., "Randomized, Double-Blind, Placebo-Controlled, Linear Dose, Crossover Study to Evaluate the Efficacy and Safety of a Green Coffee Bean Extract in Overweight Subjects," *Diabetes, Metabolic Syndrome and Obesity* 5 (2012): 21–27.

B. Wansink and K. van Ittersum, "Portion Size Me: Downsizing Our Consumption Norms," *Journal of the*

American Dietary Association 107, no. 7 (July 2007): 1103–6.

T. Watanabe et al., "The Blood Pressure-Lowering Effect and Safety of Chlorogenic Acid from Green Coffee Bean Extract in Essential Hypertension," *Clinical and Experimental Hypertension* 28, no. 5 (July 2006): 439–49.

W. C. Winkelmayer et al., "Habitual Caffeine Intake and the Risk of Hypertension in Women," *JAMA* 294, no. 18 (Nov. 9, 2005): 2339–35.

W. Zhu et al., "Calcium plus Vitamin D3 Supplementation Facilitated Fat Loss in Overweight and Obese College Students with Very-Low Calcium Consumption: A Randomized Controlled Trial," *Nutrition Journal* 12 (2013): 8.

Chapter 6. Try Nutritional and Herbal Remedies

G. A. Benavides et al., "Hydrogen Sulfide Mediates the Vasoactivity of Garlic," *Proceedings of the National Academy of Sciences USA* 104, no. 46 (Nov. 13, 2007): 17977–82.

A. M. Bernstein et al., "A Meta-Analysis Shows That Docosahexaenoic Acid from Algal Oil Reduces Serum Triglycerides and Increases HDL-Cholesterol and LDL-Cholesterol in Persons Without Coronary Heart Disease," *Journal of Nutrition* 142, no. 1 (Jan. 2012): 99–104.

F. R. Beyer et al., "Combined Calcium, Magnesium and Potassium Supplementation for the Management of Primary Hypertension in Adults," *Cochrane Database Systematic Reviews* 3 (July 19, 2006): CD004805.

G. Block, "Ascorbic Acid, Blood Pressure, and the American Diet," *Annals of NY Academy of Sciences* 959 (2002): 180–87.

P. Bogdanski et al., "Green Tea Extract Reduces Blood Pressure, Inflammatory Biomarkers, and Oxidative Stress and Improves Parameters Associated with Insulin Resistance in Obese, Hypertensive Patients," *Nutrition Research* 32, no. 6 (June 2012): 421–27.

S. Brankovic et al., "Comparison of the Hypotensive and Bradycardic Activity of Ginkgo, Garlic, and Onion Extracts," *Clinical Experimental Hypertension* 33, no. 2 (2011): 95–99.

T. E. Brinkley et al., "Effect of Ginkgo Biloba on Blood Pressure and Incidence of Hypertension in Elderly Men and Women," *American Journal of Hypertension* 23, no. 5 (May 2010): 528–33.

R. M. Bruno et al., "Effect of Acute Administration of Vitamin C on Muscle Sympathetic Activity, Cardiac Sympathovagal Balance, and Baroreflex Sensitivity in Hypertensive Patients," *American Journal of Clinical Nutrition* 96, no. 2 (Aug. 2012): 302–8.

B. E. Burke et al., "Randomized, Double-Blind, Placebo-Controlled Trial of Coenzyme Q10 in Isolated Systolic Hypertension," *Southern Medicine* 94 (2001):1112–17.

M. R. Cesarone et al., "Kidney Flow and Function in Hypertension: Protective Effects of Pycnogenol in Hypertensive Participants—a Controlled Study," *Journal of Cardiovascular Pharmacology and Therapy* 15, no. 1 (March 2010): 41–46.

J. Chen et al., "Serum Antioxidant Vitamins and Blood Pressure in the United States Population," *Hypertension* 40 (2002): 810–16.

H. O. Dickinson et al., "Potassium Supplementation for the Management of Primary Hypertension in Adults," *Cochrane Database of Systematic Reviews* 3 (July 19, 2006): CD004641.

J. P. Forman et al., "Effect of Vitamin D Supplementation on Blood Pressure in Blacks," *Hypertension* 61 (2013): 779–85.

F. C. Griffin et al., "Vitamin D and Subsequent Systolic Hypertension Among Women," *American Journal of Hypertension* 24, no. 3 (March 2011): 316–21.

I. M. Hajjar et al., "A Randomized, Double–Blind, Controlled Trial of Vitamin C in the Management of Hypertension and Lipids," *American Journal of Therapy* 9 (2002): 289–93.

M. C. Houston and K. J. Harper, "Potassium, Magnesium, and Calcium: Their Role in Both the Cause and Treatment of Hypertension," *Journal of Clinical Hypertension* 10(7 Suppl. 2) (July 2008): 3–11.

S. H. Ihm et al., "Decaffeinated Green Tea Extract Improves Hypertension and Insulin Resistance in a Rat Model of Metabolic Syndrome," *Atherosclerosis* 224, no. 2 (Oct. 2012): 377–83.

S. P. Juraschek et al., "Effects of Vitamin C Supplementation on Blood Pressure: A Meta-analysis of Randomized Controlled Trials," *American Journal of Clinical Nutrition* 95, no. 5 (May 2012): 1079–88.

Chris Kilham, "The Healing Power of Olive Leaf," accessed March 11, 2013, http://www.foxnews.com/health/2013/01/23/healing-power-olive-leaf/.

X. Liu et al., "Pycnogenol, French Maritime Pine Bark Extract, Improves Endothelial Function of Hypertensive Patients," *Life Science* 74, no. 7 (Jan. 2, 2004): 855–62.

P. R. Miller, in "Extra Vitamin C May Help Lower Blood Pressure," WebMD, accessed March 24, 2013, http://www.webmd.com/hypertension-high-blood-pressure/news/20120420/extra-vitamin-c-may-help-lower-blood-pressure.

P. K. Myint et al., "Association Between Plasma Vitamin C Concentrations and Blood Pressure in the European Prospective Investigation into Cancer—Norfolk Population-Based Study," *Hypertension* 58, no. 3 (Sept. 2011): 372–79.

Y. Nakasone et al., "Effect of a Traditional Japanese Garlic Preparation on Blood Pressure in Prehypertensive and Mildly Hypertensive Adults," *Experimental and Therapeutic Medicine* 5, no. 2 (Feb. 2013): 399–405.

T. Perrinjaquet-Moccetti et al., "Food Supplementation with an Olive (*Olea* Europaea L.) Leaf Extract Reduces Blood Pressure in Borderline Hypertensive Monozygotic Twins," *Phytotherapy Research* 22, no. 9 (Sept. 2008): 1239–42.

C. B. Rasmussen et al., "Dietary Supplements and Hypertension: Potential Benefits and Precautions," *Journal of Clinical Hypertension* 14, no. 7 (July 2012): 467–71.

K. Ried et al., "Aged Garlic Extract Reduces Blood Pressure in Hypertensives: A Dose-Response Trial," *European Journal of Clinical Nutrition* 67, no. 1 (Jan. 2013): 64–70.

R. B. Singh et al., "Effect of Hydrosoluble Coenzyme Q10 on Blood Pressures and Insulin Resistance in Hypertensive Patients with Coronary Artery Disease," *Journal of Human Hypertension* 13 (1999): 203–8.

E. Susalit et al., "Olive (Olea Europaea) Leaf Extract Effective in Patients with Stage-1 Hypertension: Comparison with Captopril," *Phytomedicine* 18, no. 4 (2010): 251–58.

H. Tamez and R. I. Thadhani, "Vitamin D and Hypertension: An Update and Review," *Current Opinion in Nephrology and Hypertension* 21, no. 5 (Sept. 2012): 492–99.

University of Maryland Medical Center, Hawthorn, accessed March 12, 2013, http://www.umm.edu/altmed/articles/hawthorn-000256.htm.

Vitamin D Council, accessed April 14, 2013, http://www.vitamindcouncil.org/.

A. F. Walker et al., "Hypotensive Effects of Hawthorn for Patients with Diabetes Taking Prescription Drugs: A

Randomized Controlled Trial," *British Journal of General Practice* 56, no. 527 (June 2006): 437–43.

Andrew Weil, "Vitamin C," accessed March 26, 2013, http://www.drweil.com/drw/u/ART02811/facts-on-vitamin-c.

G. Wu et al., "Potassium Magnesium Supplementation for Four Weeks Improves Small Distal Artery Compliance and Reduces Blood Pressure in Patients with Essential Hypertension," *Clinical Experimental Hypertension* 28, no. 5 (July 2006): 489–97.

M. Wyman, "Coenzyme Q10: A Therapy for Hypertension and Statin-Induced Myalgia?," *Cleveland Clinic Journal of Medicine* 77, no. 7 (2010): 435–42.

Chapter 7. Manage Stress (Before It Manages You)

1. T. Rosenthal and A. Alter, "Occupational Stress and Hypertension," *Journal of the American Society of Hypertension* 6, no. 1 (Jan.–Feb. 2012): 2–22.

K. Allen et al., "Cardiovascular Reactivity and the Presence of Pets, Friends, and Spouses: The Truth About Cats and Dogs," *Psychosomatic Medicine* 64, no. 5 (Sept.–Oct. 2002): 727–39.

K. Arhant-Sudhir et al., "Pet Ownership and Cardiovascular Risk Reduction: Supporting Evidence, Conflicting Data and Underlying Mechanisms," *Clinical and Experimental Pharmacology and Physiology* 38, no. 11 (Nov. 2011): 734–38.

V. A. Barnes and D. W. Orme-Johnson, "Prevention and Treatment of Cardiovascular Disease in Adolescents and Adults Through the Transcendental Meditation Program: A Research Review Update," *Current Hypertension Review* 8, no. 3 (Aug. 2012): 227–42.

A. B. Bhavanani et al., "Immediate Effect of Sukha Pranayama on Cardiovascular Variables in Patients with Hypertension," *International Journal of Yoga Therapy* 21 (2011): 73–76.

J. A. Cambron et al., "Changes in Blood Pressure After Various Forms of Therapeutic Massage: A Preliminary Study," *Journal of Alternative & Complementary Medicine* 12, no. 1 (Jan.–Feb. 2006): 65–70.

S. C. Chung et al., "Effect of Sahaja Yoga Meditation on Quality of Life, Anxiety, and Blood Pressure Control," *Journal of Alternative and Complementary Medicine* 18, no. 6 (June 2012): 589–96.

N. Djindjic et al., "Associations Between the Occupational Stress Index and Hypertension, Type 2 Diabetes Mellitus, and Lipid Disorders in Middle-Aged Men and Women," *Annals of Occupational Hygiene* 56, no. 9 (Nov. 2012): 1051–62.

W. J. Elliott and J. L. Izzo Jr., "Device-Guided Breathing to Lower Blood Pressure: Case Report and Clinical Overview," *MedGenMed* 8, no. 3 (Aug. 1, 2006): 23.

M. J. Gregoski et al., "Breathing Awareness Meditation and LifeSkills Training Programs Influence upon Ambulatory Blood Pressure and Sodium Excretion Among

African American Adolescents," *Journal of Adolescent Health* 48, no. 1 (Jan. 2011): 59–64.

L. L. Jefferson, "Exploring Effects of Therapeutic Massage and Patient Teaching in the Practice of Diaphragmatic Breathing on Blood Pressure, Stress, and Anxiety in Hypertensive African-American Women: An Interventions Study," *Journal of the National Black Nurses Association* 21, no. 1 (July 2010): 17–24.

H. A. Kahn et al., "The Incidence of Hypertension and Associated Factors: The Israeli Ischemic Heart Disease Study," *American Heart Journal* 84 (1972):1721.

J. A. McElroy et al., "Take a Deep Breath: A Pilot Study Demonstrating a Significant Reduction in Blood Pressure with 15 Minute Daily Pranayama Breathing," *Annals of Behavioral Science and Medical Education* 18, no. 2 (2012): 15–18.

M. Mocini et al., "The Effect of Massage Therapy on Blood Pressure of Women with Pre-Hypertension," *Iran Journal of Nursing and Midwifery Research* 16, no. 1 (Winter 2011): 61–70.

R. Mora-Ripoll, "The Therapeutic Value of Laughter in Medicine," *Alternative Therapies in Health and Medicine* 16, no. 6 (Nov.–Dec. 2010): 56–64.

H. Mori et al., "How Does Deep Breathing Affect Office Blood Pressure and Pulse Rate?," *Hypertension Research* 28, no. 6 (June 2005): 499–504.

M. Nakao et al., "Blood Pressure-Lowering Effects of Biofeedback Treatment in Hypertension: A Meta-analysis of Randomized Controlled Trials," *Hypertension Research* 26, no. 1 (Jan. 2003): 37–46.

D. Palomba et al., "Biofeedback-Assisted Cardiovascular Control in Hypertensives Exposed to Emotional Stress: A Pilot Study," *Applied Psychophysiology and Biofeedback* 36, no. 3 (Sept. 2011): 185–92.

H. Potz et al., "Influence of Out-Patient Training on Locus of Control and Health-Relevant Attitudes in Hypertensive Patients," *Psychotherapie Psychosomatik Medizinische Psychologie* 52, nos. 9–10 (Sept.–Oct. 2002): 417–24.

M. Sharma et al., "RESPeRATE: Nonpharmacological Treatment of Hypertension," *Cardiology Review* 19, no. 2 (March–April 2011): 47–51.

S. A. Tan et al., "Humor, as an Adjunct Therapy in Cardiac Rehabilitation, Attenuates Catecholamines and Myocardial Infarction Recurrence," *Advances in Mind and Body Medicine* 22, nos. 3–4 (Winter 2007): 8–12.

M. Shahidi et al., "Laughter Yoga Versus Group Exercise Program in Elderly Depressed Women: A Randomized Controlled Trial," *International Journal of Geriatric Psychiatry* 26, no. 3 (March 2011): 322–27.

J. Y. Yu et al., "Implementation of MP3 Player for Music Therapy on Hypertension," *Conference Proceedings: Annual Conference of the IEEE Engineering in Medicine and Biology Society,* 2009, 6444–47.

P. Yu et al., "Treatment of Essential Hypertension with Auriculoacupressure," *Journal of Traditional Chinese Medicine* 11, no. 1 (March 1991): 17–21.

W. Zhou and J. C. Longhurst, "Review of Trials Examining the Use of Acupuncture to Treat Hypertension,"
Future of Cardiology 2, no. 3 (May 2006): 287–92.

Chapter 8. Consider Medications

R. R. Baliga et al., "B-blockers in Heart Failure: Breaking Tradition to Avoid Diabetes?," *Heart Failure Clinics* 8, no. 4 (Oct. 2012): xiii–xvi.

Harvard Medical School, accessed April 24, 2013,
http://www.health.harvard.edu/newsletters/Harvard
_Womens_Health_Watch/2009/August/Medications
-for-treating-hypertension.

B. Pennington, "Heart Medications May Also Calm
Nerves, Keeping Them Banned," *New York Times*. Nov.
14, 2012, accessed April 12, 2013, http://www.nytimes
.com/2012/11/15/sports/golf/heart-medications-may
-also-calm-nerves-keeping-them-banned.html?_r=0.

T. Podymow and P. August, "Antihypertensive Drugs
in Pregnancy," *Seminars in Nephrology* 31, no. 1 (Jan.
2011): 70–85.

A. R. Vest and L. S. Cho, "Hypertension in Pregnancy,
Cardiology Clinics 30, no. 3 (Aug. 2012): 407–23.

CONTENTS

In
Herschel's
Wake

A MEMOIR

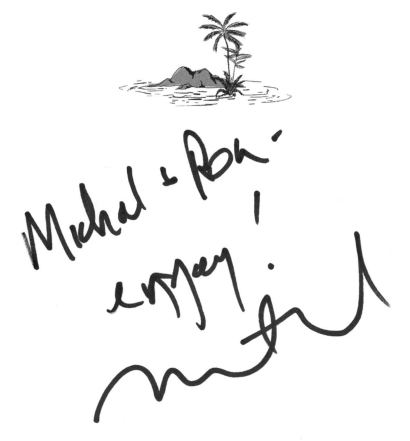

In Herschel's Wake

A Memoir

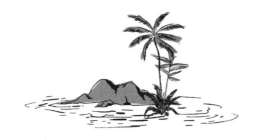

Michael Wohl

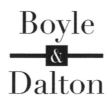

Boyle
&
Dalton

Book design & production:
Boyle & Dalton
www.BoyleandDalton.com

Paperback ISBN: 978-1-63337-627-4
E-book ISBN: 978-1-63337-628-1

Printed in the United States of America
1 3 5 7 9 10 8 6 4 2

DEDICATED TO:

My children,
my siblings,
my incredible wife,
and to my father . . .
who would have probably hated it.

AUTHOR'S NOTE:

THE FOLLOWING STORY IS TRUE. Mostly. In an effort to present an emotionally honest and resonant version of this story (and to provide a certain degree of anonymity for the people mentioned), I have simplified, reordered, combined, complexified, or otherwise fictionalized certain details, names, and events; I have recreated dialogue from memory or conjecture; and in more than one instance I have assumed I knew what was going on inside another person's head. I may have been wrong. As a questionably wise man once told me (or I think he told me), "Fiction can often be more honest and truthful than nonfiction." Please consult local traffic and weather conditions before utilizing this material as a guide.

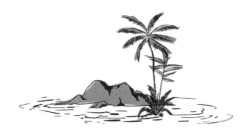

PROLOGUE
1984

IT WAS UNSETTLING to see my father in a suit. His beard was unusually kempt and trimmed, his bouncy Jew-fro surprisingly tame and adorned with a white silk yarmulke bobby-pinned a little off-center. He was wearing a loud, wide '70s necktie, no longer remotely in style now that it was 1984. He opened his face into a big dopey grin, his yellow smoker's teeth glowing in the dim light of the synagogue antechamber where I stood waiting by myself.

"Hey kiddo."

"Look at you," I whispered. "All dressed up." My freshly tightened braces caused my words to slur a bit.

He nodded and gave an amused shrug as he looked around. "I feel like I'm in the other team's locker room." He wiggled his shoulders in an exaggerated shudder. We could hear the rabbi talking to the congregation on the other side of the curtain beside us.

"You still have time to change your mind, you know. Jilt God at the altar and keep your integrity."

I

"You had a bar mitzvah," I shot back. "You survived."

He rocked his head back and forth: perhaps.

"I am kinda nervous," I confessed. "I'll be glad when the reading is over."

He put his hand on my shoulder. "Relax. Have fun. Remember: religion's nothing more than a human construct. Plus, from here on in you get to make your own rules."

I smiled back at him and nodded, not really following.

He continued, "That's at least a little consolation. For, you know, being *a man* now." He winked. Then, looking around to ensure we were alone, he slipped a small, fat envelope into my hand. "And of course, this'll help too."

I looked down and spread the top of the envelope open with my thumb and finger. Inside were three chubby marijuana joints. They smelled glorious.

"Happy birthday, buddy."

I grinned, covering for the guilt of holding the contraband right there in the synagogue. He turned to leave.

"Don't uh . . . you know, just keep it from your sister."

"Of course," I said, playing it cool, tickled to share a secret with him, already trying on the posture of what I thought adulthood required. He nodded and headed back out, disappearing just as the cantor appeared waving at me to step onto the stage.

"Come on. It's time!"

I stuffed the envelope into my inside suit pocket, took a breath, and tried to steady myself, but the grin kept fighting its way back to my face. The cantor led me through the curtain, and I stepped up to the bimah, where an ornate Torah was splayed out. We had rehearsed all of this, but still, I started to sweat. I thrust my hand into my pocket and made a fist.

The rabbi laid his heavy hand on my shoulder. "Bar mitzvah is both blessing and obligation. I was overjoyed when young Michael here came to us, determined to find his own way, to mark his passage into adulthood with me and with all of you."

I looked out at the audience, at my friends all sitting politely and patiently, at my eighteen-year-old sister, Anais, with her over-earnest, overencouraging smile, and at my mom beside her in the front row, gritting her teeth with anxiety on my behalf and probably focused most on how her rich, successful brother and his perfect family were judging our *ungapatchke* attempt to pretend we were normal.

My mom was ambivalent about her Judaism. As a toddler during the Holocaust, safely growing up in Queens, she remained blissfully unaware of the horrors being committed, least of all her own family's connection to it. Her parents never spoke of their religion, until at thirteen she came upon her father crying after a meeting with a doctor who "knew people from the old country." Only then was she forced to absorb the reality of why she had no relatives on her father's side.

For me, Judaism was a part of my identity that I understood to be a bit unfortunate—like a cleft palate or being short. Something that made me different, but that I could compensate for with wit or mathematical acumen. I didn't know anything about bar mitzvahs until my friends started having these elaborate parties and getting showered with gifts and savings bonds. Best of all, a bar mitzvah was an excuse to invite all the girls from school to a party where I'd be the center of attention. I wanted in.

Dad slipped into the sanctuary through a side door and managed to trip over and knock down a stack of collapsed folding chairs lined up along the side aisle, creating a cascading eruption

of noise and garnering the attention of everyone in the room. He flashed a smile and a quick wave to the congregation, and, making no effort to clean up the mess, he scanned the seats for a place to sit.

The rabbi continued, trying to overcome the distraction. " . . . and so it's quite fortuitous that today's passage is one about self-determination above all things. And about duty to oneself, to one's family, and to God."

He nodded grandly at me, a cue for me to begin, but I just stood there frozen. He moved his hand from my shoulder to the small of my back and forcibly pulled me forward a step.

"Begin whenever you're ready," he grunted.

I watched my dad make his way to a seat in the third row, forcing a few of my classmates to get up to let him pass.

He was smugly oblivious to my struggle to muster the courage to speak, to proceed with this thing, this commitment I had made—perhaps to spite him, though my teenage emotions were hardly coherent enough for me to consciously recognize that.

He finally sat down, of all places, right next to my goy crush, Mary Ann O'Malley.

I cleared my throat and began my memorized Hebrew. The rabbi stuffed the *yad* into my hand, and then, with his hand on top of mine, roughly dragged the pointer along the hand-drawn glyphs on the scroll. As I spoke, he unconsciously mouthed the reading along with me, occasionally vocalizing that plosive "kh" sound that is so common in Hebrew.

When I next looked up, my eyes went straight to that third pew, four seats in, and I watched as my dad leaned over and whispered something in Mary Ann's ear, making her blush. She covered her face with her hand as she tried to stifle a laugh. I darted

my eyes back down to the scroll, then closed them as I struggled through the last few stanzas.

God, please make him die, I thought.

CHAPTER 1

THE ODYSSEY

TWENTY-FOUR YEARS LATER, it was 2008, April. George W. Bush was president. Barack Obama was just an idealistic senator from Illinois. Facebook didn't even have a "like" button yet. Apple's iPhone was brand new, and it would be months before anyone even uttered the term "app." And the world was flush with easy subprime credit. Few people had any idea of the string of catastrophes that were imminent, least of all me. I was on an airplane, in a window seat, at night. Leaning my body against the curved fuselage wall and crowding against the stiff armrest, trying to will myself to sleep. I was wrapped in the cheap airline-supplied blanket. I'd left in such a hurry that I didn't think to bring a sweatshirt for the flight. The seats rattled as the airplane bounced and shook as we passed through the cold air pockets over the Rockies. A sharp dip forced my stomach to leap to my throat.

My mind turned to probabilities. Calculating. Forecasting. Pondering the likelihood of dying in a plane crash. Of course, it was statistically minuscule, but nonetheless it was possible. It

did happen. Even if it was one in a million, there's still that one. And how many people fly every day? Ten thousand? That would mean at least one person every hundred days was destined to die in a fiery crash. Had there been a crash in a hundred days? I located a crumpled receipt in my pants pocket and smoothed it out on the plastic table. I did some quick math. It was hard to keep the pen steady with all the bouncing around, but I did my best. *If there are five thousand flights every day, and they hold an average of two hundred people per flight, that's a million right there. One in a million means one passenger flying right now.*

I looked at the people around me as the plane shook. The guy next to me was sound asleep, but the guy in the aisle seat was visibly anxious. The seats clattered and shook. *How old is this plane anyway?* Some middle-seat shithead in the row in front of me decided it was a good time to go to the bathroom and forced the woman in the aisle seat to stand up so he could get out. I shook my head in disgust and tried to make eye contact with the woman to give her a sympathetic smile, to show her my solidarity against assholes everywhere, but she never looked over.

I looked out the window. There was nothing out there. Just darkness. No lights below, no moon or stars above. The plane stopped shaking and was eerily still and quiet. For a moment, I couldn't tell if we were flying or falling. I listened to the hum of the engine and tried to find some comfort in its constancy. I loosened my grip on the seat cushion and felt my fingers pulse and tingle from holding them so tightly.

I realized my whole body was tensed up, and I tried to relax each set of muscles, systematically, using the Buddhist meditation method my dad taught me when I was a teenager. I inhaled and held the air in for a moment. As I breathed out, I wiggled my toes

and then my ankles. Tensing each set of muscles and then releasing them. I took another breath in and repeated the process with my calves, my thighs, the muscles in my ass. I progressed through my whole body, breathing in and breathing out until I felt a deep calm. The warm air in the dark plane began to feel safe and even comfortable. I sighed a little smile.

And then the plane started shaking all over again.

I was flying from Los Angeles to Miami, and then on to San Juan, Puerto Rico. From there I was to go on to Sint Maarten in the Lesser Antilles, which was way farther out in the middle of the Atlantic Ocean than I could have imagined before I'd consulted a map. From Sint Maarten, I had to figure out how to get to an even more remote island: Sint Eustatius in the Netherlands Antilles. Which was where my father had been living for the past few years.

Only he wasn't living there anymore. He was dead.

CHAPTER 2

THE STRANGER

EARLY THAT MORNING, lying in bed in my Los Angeles apartment with my cat, Butterscotch (a long-haired, lawnmower-loud vestige of a recent failed relationship), I read the email from some woman named Natasha, who was, I guessed, a student of my father.

I regret to inform you that Herschel Wohl has died . . .

He was seventy years old. He had gotten some kind of infection, and two weeks later it was over. The date was April 20. Universal pot-smoking day, Hitler's birthday, and from that moment on, also the day my dad died.

I hadn't been in contact with him in almost a year, and that was on email. I couldn't remember the last time we spoke. There was a brief Skype around my birthday. I'd turned thirty-nine. He'd remarked that he had a friend who'd died of a heart attack at thirty-nine, then bragged that if he hadn't dropped out and dedicated his life to his art, he was sure he'd have been dead by forty himself.

I wasn't so worried about a heart attack. I had taken a different route. While I acceded his guidance and found an artistic outlet for myself as a filmmaker, I had coupled that with a lucrative day job in software, one that many others would have comfortably considered a career. Balancing the job and my creative aspirations kept me from fully investing in either, but for the most part I found a balance, supporting myself well enough to produce a string of creative works without having to live on ramen and Pepsi.

When I was offered the full-time tech gig, Dad scolded me for selling out at the first possible opportunity. He mocked me as "making great strides toward my executive vice-presidency." While some might consider that a legitimate goal, to him it was nothing short of betrayal. I took the job but couldn't shake that specter of doubt: Had I made a catastrophic mistake?

Natasha's message was brief, and in fact, the news was secondhand. She had been contacted by the couple who ran the inn where my dad had been living on Sint Eustatius (or *Statia* as the locals call it). She had visited him a few months before, so they had her contact info, and I guess they didn't have any of ours. I wondered if the people living on this island with him even knew he had children. He had changed his name when he got there. Who knows what other aspects of his story he had reinvented.

Natasha herself only knew how to contact us because there had been a spam email a few weeks earlier from my dad that went to everyone in his address book. Some fountain of youth supplements scam. She remembered it, she said, because it was so amusing to get such a brazenly commercial email from the most anti-capitalist person she'd ever met. When she got this bad news, she scoured the email addresses in the spam message to find all of us, his next of kin.

My phone rang shortly after I read the email: it was Anais, my sister, in Austin, Texas. She just sobbed for the first couple minutes of the call. We shared our confusion and shock.

"I just don't understand. Did you know he was sick?" Anais asked.

I didn't. "Who's Natasha?" I asked.

"Must have been a girlfriend," she said.

"He ever mention her to you?"

"No, but that doesn't mean anything. She said she was a student of his."

"Of course she was," I said. "What are we going to do?"

"Someone's got to go down there," she said.

"Well . . ." I hesitated, fantasizing for a moment that there was some way we could get out of the giant hassle that had landed like a dead rat on our doorstep, Dad's Cheshire smile still glimmering nearby as the rest of him slipped away.

"Max! There is a dead body just lying there on that island. Jews have three days to bury their dead. We're not permitted to leave the body unattended. Somebody must make a proper funeral."

"Or else what?" I couldn't resist taunting her.

And she couldn't resist taking the bait. "Do you have any idea how shallow and callous you sound?"

"Do you have any idea how cloying and melodramatic you sound?"

She sighed. Then I did. Neither of us had the energy for a real fight.

She changed tack. "Did you see Tobias was on the email too?"

At that point, I hadn't bothered to look at who else received

the message. Hearing that name was both shocking and familiar. Tobias was our twenty-five-year-old half-brother, whom I hadn't spoken to . . . ever. I'd last seen him when he was a toddler. When Margo (Dad's second wife) finally sued Herschel for divorce and spirited Tobias away to New Jersey. While there had been a letter or two in the intervening decades, we were effectively cut off from one another. Until now.

Holy shit! I have a brother! I thought.

"We've got to call him," she said.

I agreed, but neither of us had his—or even his mom's—number. I crafted a brief email to his address from the spam list and fired it off into the void.

Soon after, my phone rang.

CHAPTER 3

THE IMPORTANCE OF BEING EARNEST

IT WAS THE FIRST TIME Tobias and I had ever spoken to one another. He was a total stranger, yet we shared the most personal, the most intimate aspect of our identities: we shared a father.

"He's dead?" Tobias asked.

"I know. When was the last time you talked to him?"

It suddenly occurred to me that I had no idea if Tobias had a better, more connected relationship with Dad than I did. He was younger, and maybe they were in regular touch. Just because I had grown to resent and reject my father as I grew into an adult, that didn't mean Tobias had the same experience.

"Shit, I don't even remember." He laughed. "He met me and Julie on Saint Martin when we took a cruise a couple years ago, but since then . . . I don't even know."

Question answered.

In between the calls with Anais and Tobias, I had emailed the couple on the island that ran the inn to see if they could provide any more information about what happened. The reply came

in while I was talking to Tobias. I read it aloud for him: "*We're very sorry to have to share this sad news with you. He had been sick for a few weeks, and we had been looking after him now and then to make sure he was all right. A couple weeks ago he had come by to borrow the mop, and I hadn't given it much thought, but when I went to call on him on Friday, I understood why he had borrowed it. He was too sick to get out of bed, so I had to clean up for him. He had been vomiting blood all over the apartment.*"

"Jesus!" Tobias said.

"*Every Thursday we have a community dinner, and he came out last week and was in good spirits, but he didn't eat anything. Then on Friday he was stuck in bed. I called for his friend Ralph, who brought him some medicine. But on Saturday he was even worse. He started talking about 'If I die—' and I kept saying, 'Nonsense. You're not going to die.' But he went on and told me that he wanted to be buried here on the island, and that he wanted a proper Jewish burial.*" I stopped, a little shocked. "A proper Jewish burial? For him?"

Tobias was still stuck on the vomiting blood part.

"*He asked that you bring a white burial shirt.*" I stopped reading. "This is all so weird. Are we sure this is the right guy?" I asked.

"Maybe he just means that we shouldn't wear black," Tobias reasoned. "That it should be casual. He couldn't possibly want us to wear a tie."

"Yeah, you must be right," I said. "So are you going to come?"

"Can I?" he said.

"He's your dad just as much as mine. Do you want to?"

"I don't know. I've got finals this week. I'm, uh . . . finishing up my engineering degree."

I was reminded that I knew absolutely nothing about my brother—what he was studying, where he was in school, if he was

married, or even if he had other siblings. I opted not to inquire. Not now. "Of course. It's totally up to you." I punted.

"The white burial shirt is for him. Not you." I was back on the phone with Anais. "It's called *tachrichit*. In the traditional Jewish ceremony, the body is wrapped in a simple white sheet, a burial shroud. And interred in a simple unadorned pine box." She had inherited Dad's facility to pontificate on any subject matter at hand.

"It's really kind of beautiful . . ." I could hear her choking up a little. "The idea is that we shed all our worldly possessions, that we don't need anything for this journey, least of all a fancy ornate casket. In Israel, they don't even use caskets at all—"

I interrupted. "Did you hear from your synagogue?"

"Not yet. But if you go to any synagogue near you, I'm sure they'll be happy to give you a tachrichit for free. Is Tobias going to come?"

"I don't know. I think he might. It'll be so weird to see him."

"I know I can't really afford it, but I want to come," she said.

"Then you should. We'll find a way to make it work," I said, trying to sound sincere.

• • •

Anais was perpetually broke. I found that hard to understand given her Ivy League honors bachelor's degree and a master's from Harvard. She was currently working at a big grocery store chain, dishing out food samples to the impatient, irritable shoppers. She said she enjoyed it, but it was a minimum wage job, and she had been doing it for five years and counting. Even if she was satisfied, it was hard for me to accept that this was where she had wound up. I imagined her giving ten-minute lectures to each customer on

the biochemical qualities of the frozen beef Stroganoff entrée, a fascinated crowd gathering around her sample station. Maybe she was good at it, but still—I wanted more for her.

Of course, it was no mystery where her rejection of traditional success originated, but she was working full-time hours, on her feet, and she couldn't scrape up five hundred dollars to go to her father's funeral. Not even on a credit card.

It wasn't always that way. At twenty-two she married Mitchell, a successful stockbroker, whom Herschel constantly mocked for being a symbol of everything wrong with the world. While Dad did show up for their wedding (tuxedo and all), when Mitchell was promoted to vice president at the investment bank, Dad refused to even come to the celebratory dinner.

After earning a master's at the University of Texas, Anais enrolled at Harvard for a PhD in educational psychology. Unfortunately, she was never politic enough to navigate the minefield of academic egos, and early on, she alienated one of the esteemed faculty by disagreeing with her scholarship. Knowing Anais, her critique was probably supportable, but it was a miscalculation to prioritize accuracy over authority and she made few friends.

Undeterred, she embarked on a massive, multiyear research project about teenage girls and disillusionment—hoping to prove that romance novels created dangerous and unrealistic expectations that were ultimately a danger to their target audience. I always remembered her as reading heavier fare than romance, but I guess her early teens were full of the stuff, and the world wasn't quite turning out as those books had promised.

She and Mitchell settled in New Jersey, Anais sitting down at the computer long into every night to bang away at her dissertation, while Mitchell took the train to Wall Street early every morning to

support the two of them. Not surprisingly, their relationship grew strained. Then, one day, Mitchell was nearly killed in a car accident. His recovery was slow, and he was left with severe chronic pain. After, they attempted to resume their lives, but it was impossible to just pick up where they had left off. A near-death experience like that gives you permission to rethink everything, and soon after Mitchell asked for a divorce.

Unable to complete her ever-expanding dissertation, Anais reluctantly accepted Harvard's gracious offer of a master's degree instead of the doctorate she was unable to complete after ten years. Adrift, she wandered back to Austin and struggled to gain any professional traction. The only job she could hold was the minimum wage supermarket gig.

• • •

"My synagogue says that they can come up with the money for me to come, but not until after the first of the month. If you buy my ticket, they'll reimburse you." It was a question disguised as a statement, a rhetorical trick of hers that I was familiar with.

Despite the fact that she was four years my senior, I was used to playing the role of the older sibling—or at least the more responsible one. I agreed to front the money for her ticket, but that wasn't the whole story. Her passport was expired, and this was an international flight. So, she had to drive three hours to Houston to the passport office to get a waiver or a temporary travel document or something. Oh, and she wanted her new husband to join her, but he didn't have a passport at all, so she needed to find out if the passport office could provide him some kind of similar temporary travel document.

I don't know why that all pissed me off. They weren't doing a lot of international travel, but to me, keeping your passport current was just a basic civic responsibility. I mean what if the government started rounding up Jews? It felt to me like just another example of her general negligence and flakiness. At the very least I felt like she always managed to make things far more difficult than they needed to be.

The husband, Stan, a butcher at her grocery store, could not have presented a more extreme contrast to Anais; she was a garrulous, overeducated, overearnest Jewish intellectual from New York, and he was a taciturn, small-town, small-minded Christian Texan with nary a high school diploma and two teenage kids from a previous marriage. He was also a recovering alcoholic. Oh, and he was almost sixty. The whole thing was odd if not downright creepy. They had married unceremoniously without any family in attendance. I just assumed she had gotten pregnant, but no baby ever materialized.

"Of course, I'll buy the ticket," I capitulated. "Just send me the details."

CHAPTER 4

THE SOUND
& THE FURY

THERE WAS ANOTHER PERSON on the email from Natasha: Marcy, Dad's third serious long-term relationship. Though they never married and their relationship was turbulent, Marcy was a major part of his life for well over a decade. They met when he was fifty-six and she was twenty-four—two years younger than I was at the time. To his credit, Dad seemed to recognize that Marcy was a bit too young for him to date, so he first tried to set her up with me. "She's exotic and sexy and incredibly smart!" He was sure we would hit it off.

On my next visit to New York from California, he arranged for the three of us to go out. We sat at a little table in the back room of Kiev on Second Avenue. Marcy dominated the conversation, earnestly complaining about how gentrification was ruining her local bodega. Breadlines and riots were imminent, and really it was all for the best, as civilization as we knew it was irreparably broken, and Mother Nature should probably just kill us all and start over.

Dad just nodded and egged her on as he slurped his borscht, its bloody red color clouded by the sour cream he stirred in. I was offended that he had even imagined she would be someone I was attracted to, but in retrospect it was easy enough to see what was going on.

Marcy had visited him several times since he moved to the Caribbean—in one instance staying for three months, which explained her friendship with Luuk and Belinda, the couple who ran the inn. She knew far more than any of us what was going on in Dad's life. Marcy was also partially responsible for why he was living there in the first place, in precarious exile from the United States. I was the only one who knew the truth about that, and sharing this secret bonded Marcy and me (in a twisted way). So, in the emotional upheaval and confusion regarding the news of his death, I took some comfort when she called that morning. There were very few people with whom I could share my grief, and she was one of them.

"It's so deeply unfair," she moaned.

"Do you know what happened?" I interrupted. "I got this email from Natasha saying he was vomiting blood and was bed-ridden. I didn't even know he was sick."

Marcy had spoken to them before calling me, and now I received even more unpleasant details. "Ralph was his best friend there," she explained. "They taught at the school together. Ralph brought him some antibiotics, but it must have been too little, too late."

Butterscotch began rubbing his face against mine, purring aggressively and competing with the sound of Marcy's voice through the phone. "They found him in the bathroom, crumpled on the floor. He had probably died in the middle of the night before."

I stopped breathing. The cat stopped purring and looked up at me. Then he crawled into the half-packed suitcase on my bed and curled up inside.

It's customary for people to say that they hope the deceased didn't suffer. I'm pretty sure my dad suffered. I'm pretty sure that he was in excruciating agony for a number of days, if not weeks. Sitting there, I tried my best not to picture him struggling to get out of bed that last time, weakened by fever and agony. I tried not to envision him stumbling to the bathroom, breath labored, trying to reach the toilet to literally puke his guts out. And I tried not to visualize him finally succumbing to death, there on the cold tile floor. Alone, covered with blood and bile. I pushed the images away, but they kept oozing back into my mind, each time with more gruesome detail.

"You must find the manuscript." Marcy's impatient voice pierced the nightmare I was indulging.

"What manuscript?" I asked.

"He was working on his book. It was pretty close to being done. I've already talked to Rupert, his editor, who had an incomplete draft from about a month ago. Whatever more he was able to get done, we need to make sure it's safe. If you can get me the manuscript, I'll pass it on to Rupert. Please!"

It was a little hard to take her request seriously, given my complex relationship with his so-called manuscript. That was the thing that always came before me. Before us. Before everyone. His *work* was all that mattered. But the thing was, he never finished it.

· · ·

17

Years ago—just a few months after he castigated me for taking that software job—I confronted him about his manuscript, and we got in a fight. He had recently asked to borrow five thousand dollars. I gave him the money, and at the very least, I felt like that bought me the right to speak my truth. When I next visited him in New York, he was lamenting that another publisher had rejected his manuscript.

We were in Tompkins Square Park. It was snowing, and he was having trouble lighting his cigarette. I impatiently walked a few steps ahead, eager to get out of the cold.

"How many publishers have rejected you at this point?" I probed.

He managed to get his Marlboro burning but refused to walk any faster. "Why does it matter to you if I get published?"

I swung around. "Because it would mean someone else thinks it's good. Thinks it's worthwhile."

"You think some NYU grad intern at Random House is the arbiter of great art?" he scoffed. "You live in a fantasyland."

"You don't get to explain away all your bad parenting decisions by hiding behind some supposedly great piece of art if it's never realized."

"It's not about me! My mistakes. It's about the work. Who cares what kind of father I am? What kind of man I am? We're all fucked, we're all shitty. But if my art reaches even two or three people, and inspires or enlightens or even just entertains them, then maybe my time here was worth it." He gestured a grandiose wave, a mix of gallantry and genuflection.

"Wait, I was wrong," I mocked. "You are a master storyteller after all—if you can convince yourself of that." I scoffed and walked ahead.

18

He caught up to me and lowered his voice to a less confrontational tone. "I can't say whether or not I'll be recognized, or *when* I'll be recognized. Van Gogh wasn't regarded till years after his death—"

"Look," I interrupted, "I can accept the logic that, objectively, a great piece of art could be measured to be of more benefit to society than the cost to the people who suffered the asshole artist who created it. Jackson Pollack, Miles Davis, Hemingway—their contributions *might* justify the havoc they wreaked on the people in their lives. I couldn't believe how much I sounded like him when I was angry. "But if you never publish the fucking book," I snarled, "it doesn't matter, because no one will ever benefit at all. And all that's left in the balance are your selfish decisions to prioritize your own 'pursuit of truth' over the well-being and happiness of everyone around you."

"Fuck you," he bristled. "I never denied you well-being or happiness. *You* have to decide to be happy. Not glom onto my ankles hoping I'll drag you there."

His cigarette had been put out by the falling snow. He threw it to the ground and stopped again to light a new one, and I just walked away. We didn't talk for about a year after that.

• • •

"Sure. If I find the manuscript, I'll make sure it's safe," I told Marcy and hung up the phone.

CHAPTER 5

THE AGE OF INNOCENCE

TOBIAS WAS BORN when I was fifteen. That was an era when I spent a lot of time with Herschel. It was when we were at our closest. Anais was four years older, so she'd gone off to college, which meant I had him all to myself.

I don't think my parents had a formal custody arrangement, but in those years I eagerly spent every possible weekend moment with him in his East Village railroad apartment. It was impressive that my mom allowed him access to my sister and me at all, given that he neglected to pay several years' worth of child support. But to her credit, I guess Mom figured it was better that we know our father—even if he wasn't living up to his paternal responsibilities. Or maybe she just desperately needed a break from parenting, whether or not it was in our best interests. She suffered from clinical depression throughout our childhood. It's hard to gauge who was the more pernicious caregiver.

• • •

When we were younger, at the end of our visits, Dad would accompany us to Port Authority Bus Terminal to catch the bus back to New Jersey. Most of the time we'd hike three blocks to Broadway and 8th and hop the RR train up to midtown, but if it was raining or really cold, he'd splurge and hire a taxi.

Walking through the streets of New York with him was always a little harrowing. He seemed to believe that the faster you walked, the more authentic a New Yorker you were. And until I was eleven or twelve, I would often have to switch to a trot if not a full-blown sprint to keep up. He was also an enthusiastic jaywalker, and he would frequently dart out into the street without warning, never looking back to make sure we were keeping up. More than once I found myself stuck in the middle of Second Avenue—a wall of yellow taxis careening toward me on their way downtown—scrambling to make my way across the five wide lanes while Dad hurried ahead onto the far sidewalk, oblivious to my harrowing experience.

At the bus terminal, he'd usually wait with us at the gate until the bus was ready to board. He'd read a book while Anais and I played. We liked to stand behind the stone statues of queuing passengers or sneak away to one of the cigarette kiosks that sold candy and pornographic magazines, hoping to steal a glance of the latter or a handful of the former. If the proprietor yelled at us, we'd race back through the crowds, collapsing onto the pale orange plastic chairs beside our inert, unmindful guardian.

One time he didn't have the few dollars required to pay for the bus tickets, and my sister had to pull out the emergency ten-dollar bill from her little girl purse, where our mom had stashed it.

"You may not be able to count on me for money, but you can always count on me for love," he explained in the tone of a grand scientific theory.

The arrangement seemed reasonable enough to my child's mind, though I could tell something was off as he hugged us a little too quickly and disappeared as soon as our bus arrived at the platform. Anais at eleven could be moody and mean, but she was especially kind to me that night, letting me have the window seat, which she usually hoarded. As we rode back through the Lincoln Tunnel in silence, I watched for the place in the middle of the underground channel where the border between states is highlighted with a colorful tile display: the words *New York* on one side and *New Jersey* on the other. We tried to hold our breath upon entering the tunnel, only letting it out once we passed that threshold—from dirty, unsafe New York to the relative comfort and banal familiarity of New Jersey.

• • •

Years later, as a teenager, I'd count the hours each week until Friday afternoon when I got to hop the Community Coach bus going the other direction into the city for the weekend. Those years, I'd hold my breath on the way in; taking a deep, eager breath once we'd escaped miserable, conformist suburbia and crossed the border into the city, where real life happened.

As soon as the bus pulled into the gate on the top floor of the bus station, I'd put on my city face and fast-walk through the terminal, expertly navigating my way through the maze of tunnels, four levels beneath the midtown streets, to find the subway that would take me down to the Village and to my dad's apartment on East 6th Street.

That two-bedroom railroad apartment was sacred space, and most sacrosanct of all was his writing desk. It was the center of

the universe. Three-feet deep and six-feet wide, this was no modern, assemble-at-home computer stand. It must have weighed three hundred pounds. It commanded a prominent position in that apartment, filling the nook at one end of the living room and splitting the space into two areas. I could only imagine the effort it must have required to transport it up the five flights of narrow stairs. Given that it was the first thing you saw when you entered the apartment, his priority of workspace over living space was very apparent. The surface of the wood divulged a lifetime's worth of scars and bruises—a story each, and a custom cut slab of quarter-inch-thick, green-edged glass covered its uneven surface, turning the gouged and dented antique into a perfectly smooth writing surface.

The upper right drawer held the *medicine*, and it was always equipped with all the essential accoutrements: rolling papers, a cardboard box for cleaning and de-seeding, an ashtray of roaches, and a hemostat or two stolen from the medical research company where he worked before he dropped out. (He pompously claimed the hemostat—created for clamping veins during surgery—was the perfect roach clip.)

He smoked constantly, both tobacco and pot. The connoisseur-quality joints were just cycled in with the Marlboro reds, and those days there was always one or the other lit, thin blue or brown smoke gently dissipating into the subtle layer of perpetual smog that was slowly turning the ceiling sepia.

He was never shy about it; even when we were very young, he brazenly smoked joints in front of my sister and me. In some ways, I appreciated how ordinary he made it. Just like the way he and his second wife decided to be nudists one year and shamelessly wandered through the apartment baring all right in front of

us. As a teenager, I found the normalness of it a refreshing relief to the pretense of propriety that the rest of the world seemed obsessed with maintaining.

He was who he was, unabashedly.

He preached, above all else, the importance of art, most specifically the art of *writing* (a word always pronounced with a certain reverence). His apartment was lined floor to ceiling with bookcases, in some places stuffed two books deep. And not just in one or two rooms, but everywhere. And his books were arranged not by topic or alphabetically, but mapped to his own internal understandings and interconnections: Heinlein, Huxley, and Hawking were all grouped together, but not because of the letter H.

His taste was eclectic, and he read everything, from trashy sci-fi to the Russian classics.

In what I could only assume was a practical joke, I was named for Miguel de Cervantes—sentencing me to a life of windmill-tilting. (Thankfully, at least my mother put her foot down and anglicized it—lest I suffer a lifetime of apologizing for appropriating a Spanish name.) But his favorites were his sex-obsessed contemporaries: Philip Roth, Henry Miller, and John Updike. Their works were always within arm's reach of his primary workspace, a massive wooden writing desk topped with a big beige IBM Selectric typewriter and several neat stacks of scribble-full yellow legal pads.

He had an encyclopedic knowledge of his library. In the midst of a conversation about tropical birds, he'd rush straight over to the stack near the stereo by the kitchen and pull out his dog-eared copy of Michael Herr's Vietnam journo-memoir *Dispatches*. He'd flip right to a section describing the Khe Sanh

jungle in its terrifying lushness, just to find one glorious sentence about a red-headed trogon flying away like a phoenix through the smoke as the *rolling thunder* of napalm decimated a forest. He was like Google—decades before it existed—only with a penchant for anything dirty or psychedelic.

He constantly pushed books on me, and not the same ones being assigned in school. I wrote a book report on *Rabbit, Run* in seventh grade, which impressed my English teacher enough to recommend me for the AP class the following year. He served up Kerouac and Vonnegut, Rilke and Ginsburg, Ram Dass and Kahlil Gibran. By fifteen, I could recite most of *Howl*, and glibly wax on about Hemingway's lesser-known, posthumous *A Moveable Feast*, cherishing its portrayal of the 1920's expat scene in Paris—obviously a high point for literature. At his urging, I shared *Portnoy's Complaint* with each of my teenage girlfriends under the pretense of serious intellectual study, though it was really just a poorly disguised attempt to gauge their comfort discussing sex. At the time, I didn't think to question his insistence on a full report afterward.

One night I watched as he prepared for his nightly ritual of getting stoned and going to work for several hours at the typewriter. I had started getting high already, but I was still young enough that I wasn't sure if he would share with me, and I was too shy to ask. But on that night, he nonchalantly passed me the joint, and we fell into some conversation or another, and before I knew it, he had pulled out *Finnegans Wake* and began reciting Joyce's spectacular, rich, poetic gibberish, stopping occasionally to explain a reference or to take a hit off the joint.

It was transformative. Magical. It left me gleeful and ecstatic. I couldn't believe that it could be real. He went on for an hour, skipping around to share his favorite passages and puns, pointing

out each sentence's (or each word's) double, triple, or sometimes quadruple meanings, providing the context of Joyce's life in Dublin as well as explaining Joyce's references to Irish history, to classic literature, and to the events of the time it was written.

I had been invited into the highest secret elite level of the cult of language. He had skipped right past *Ulysses* and taken me right to the mother lode: *Finnegans Wake*, and he could read it as if it were normal English.

"It might seem ironic, but fiction is the secret to understanding what's real. Nonfiction may convey facts, but you can only see what's real when you squint. And nothing is more important than seeing the world for what it really is. Unflinchingly." He put his hands on my shoulders and looked me right in the eye. "That's where the magic is."

I nodded solemnly. I guess it's normal for a son to worship his father, at least for a moment in time.

And all the while throughout these years, he was hard at work writing his own great American novel. And so, every night, after the rest of us went to sleep, he would sit up and bang away at the loud electric typewriter, stopping only occasionally to light a cigarette or to cough loudly after a long pull on a joint. I would lie there awake (the pull-out couch was only a few feet from the noisy machine), but I understood that nothing was more important than his writing—than the creation of his art.

CHAPTER 6
ON THE ROAD

I DROPPED OFF THE CAT at my ex-girlfriend's apartment and took a taxi to the airport. It was easy enough to get time off from my technical writing day job, but I had been working for months on this elaborate virtual-reality film project about a bunch of squatters who manage to secure a subprime mortgage on a Beverly Hills mansion. I had a meeting with a potential investor scheduled for the following day, and honestly, I was a little relieved to have an excuse to postpone it. In the taxi I called my coproducer and rescheduled for three days later. This couldn't possibly take longer than a day or two, right?

Surviving what the pilot called "moderate chop," I arrived in Miami at 11:25 p.m., and my flight to San Juan wasn't until 6:45 a.m. With seven hours to kill, I wasn't sure what to do with myself. My plan had been to sleep for a few hours there in the terminal, but the airport turned out to have been specifically configured to prevent people from sleeping. All the rows of seats were interrupted by armrests so you couldn't possibly lie down,

and the ground was only carpeted on the walkways that led from the gates to the baggage claim. I spotted a few other people who shared my predicament. One guy was just sprawled out on the hard cold floor next to a bank of windows, and another couple was huddled around a laptop watching a movie. I wandered the terminal looking for a store that was open so I could get something to eat, but I couldn't find one.

I called my mom. I had left her a message with the news before I left, but I wasn't able to reach her. This was the first time we'd had a chance to talk.

"I'm sorry for your loss, kiddo. I know you had a complicated relationship, but he was still your father."

"Your loss too, I guess. In some way," I offered, trying to be kind and avoid exploring my feelings.

"Oh, I mourned his departure a long time ago," she started. "It is weird, though, to think he's actually gone-gone. Hate to say it, but it kinda feels like a burden lifted." She laughed gently. I nodded silently in agreement.

• • •

Much of my mom's adult life had been hampered by depression and anxiety. I'll never know how much was purely chemical and how much was the result of the existential disappointment driven by divorce and the challenge of being cajoled into the workforce, largely against her wishes. Like countless women of the 1970s, she was robbed of the predictable lifestyle of comfort that she was raised to expect. Despite being trained in suburban housewifery, she was thrust into single-parenthood with insufficient resources. And if just managing that struggle wasn't enough, timing and

circumstances (and a few of her hippie friends) demanded she publicly celebrate her liberation and revel in her independence. She attended ERA marches and wore a NOW button, but I think she was happiest when quietly wrapping an elaborate pile of Hanukkah gifts, each in its own perfect color scheme, or putting on a kid's birthday party, or teaching me at ten to iron and fold laundry—something I needed to learn, since my eventual wife would likely be too freethinking to do it for me.

Add to that the insult that she had put her husband through medical school on his way to that pharmacology degree, and just a few years later, he had discarded a lucrative career (and the support she was counting on) in exchange for a younger girlfriend and a bohemian fantasy. Her entire life became about keeping her kids clothed and fed. She was forced to trade the upscale midcentury house, where she'd imagined gracefully fledging her children, for a compact two-bedroom apartment in a town with a questionable school district.

Intrepid or just resigned, she took night classes and earned a master's in education and social work at a community college. That lead to her teaching "assertiveness training" seminars to other divorced women. Knowing now how desperate and frightened she was, I can only imagine what that was like. I can also only imagine how little income it generated at a time when inflation was raging and food staples were becoming increasingly unaffordable. When we got down to skipping meals, her parents stepped in and enrolled her in a computer trade school where she learned COBOL to program the mainframe computers that were already running corporate America. During those years, she accepted whatever part-time work she could while she took her courses at night. At one point, she did a stint at a cafeteria in a

hospital, wearing a hairnet and dishing out single serving bowls of Jell-O.

Whatever shame or embarrassment I felt at the time dissolved, as I grew up, into downright admiration. She was determined to do whatever was necessary to keep us fed and safe—her own well-being be damned.

Eventually she developed a stable career. But along the way, she was largely emotionally (and often physically) absent as my sister and I grew up. When she was around, she would spend a lot of time screaming at us, then disappearing to cry in her bedroom. I took to appeasing her, using humor to de-escalate conflict. But my sister went the other direction, and the two of them engaged in routine screaming matches. One night at ten years old, trying to sleep, I threw myself out of my bed just to create a distraction (my child's brain somehow thinking it was plausible that I might accidentally fall out of bed). It paused their fight for the evening, though my sprained wrist lasted for weeks. I still freeze up in panic when I hear voices raised in anger, or any loud noises really.

Their rancor has faded over the decades, but their relationship remains strained.

• • •

"Listen, Anais missed her flight," Mom informed me.

Of course she did, I thought. "What happened?"

"Well, apparently, Stan had some delinquent child support payments, and they wouldn't grant him a passport. So he can't come at all."

"That seems somehow ironic."

"I suppose. Anyway," she continued, "I wired her some money so they could spend the night in Houston, and she's getting on the next flight tomorrow morning and is supposed to arrive in Sint Maarten around ten p.m."

"That's after the last flight to Statia," I sighed.

"I'm only the messenger."

"I know. Was there a warrant out for Stan?"

My first thought was that this was yet another indicator of Anais's bad judgment. Marrying a guy who was late on his child support to his first wife? Really? Did she not recognize that as repeating the past? Marrying the worst traits of her own father?

Back in 1980, at a time when we were particularly broke, my mom had a warrant put out for my dad to collect some child support. The warrant was only active in New Jersey, so as long as he didn't enter the state, he didn't have to face the charges. However, that spring, I played the Artful Dodger in our sixth-grade production of *Oliver!* I had a big role, and I begged him to come. When he arrived at the bus stop near the elementary school, a cabal of cops was waiting for him. He never made it to the play, to my great disappointment.

Later he talked about his brief jail experience with a bit of bravado, and how it was such great fodder for his writing, though I'm sure it was at least a tad harrowing. My mom described it as the unfortunate outcome of his own actions. It was only a few years later that I realized she must have tipped off the cops.

• • •

"Did Dad ever get square on the money he owed you?" I asked her on the phone. "Maybe if there's anything in his bank account—"

33

She cut me off. "I don't need his money now. If there's anything there, it should go to you kids. It's the least he could do for you."

THE HEART IS A LONELY HUNTER

I WANDERED AROUND the empty Miami terminal, feeling melancholy and lost. There's something so disconnecting and isolating about airports. They all look the same and smell the same and have the same view of planes and runways out the window. And there's no sense of time—it could be 6:00 a.m. or 6:00 p.m., and somewhere in the world it was both. The rules of real life cease to apply. I could have been anywhere, and I was almost able to forget the reason I was travelling in the first place. I let myself indulge in that odd out-of-life, out-of-time feeling.

I eventually left the secure area and wandered outside. The humidity was literally breathtaking. The air was so thick I felt like I was walking through gel. Like if I lifted my arms, they wouldn't fall back down on their own, defying gravity. With three hours left to kill, I walked a full transit around the perimeter of the airport. Dawn was still hours off, and there was no one else around. A few times I got a chill of fear, though I'm not sure if I was more afraid of some crazy person with a

machete or an errant alligator. But mostly, I felt protected. Like I was in some kind of bubble.

At one point I heard the familiar, plaintive whistle of a killdeer. I couldn't see her in the darkness, but I imagined her protecting her fledglings against a hungry gator. In my head, I listened to Dad explaining the curious behavior to me. "The killdeer pretends it's injured and leads the predator away from the nest," he'd narrate. "The female's wings are specially designed to be folded in a way to look broken, and she puts on a whole show, crying and limping and looking all vulnerable, and then as soon as she lures the predator sufficiently far away from the nest, she drops the charade and flies away."

He seemed delighted in the profound truth that deceit was not an exclusively human trait.

Back inside the airport, I watched out the window as the first glow of the morning light emerged through the trees on the far side of the runway. First, just a faint purple bulge at the bottom of the sky, but soon there was a thin red corona leaching through. And over what seemed like just a few minutes, the sky woke from slumber. The red rolled up from the horizon, opening into an orange that almost immediately yawned into yellow, and then the pale blue of day crept up and eagerly swallowed the whole of the sky.

On the television in the waiting area, they were showing a video of a Brazilian priest who had tied himself to a giant bunch of balloons as a publicity stunt to support a labor strike. Evidently, his gimmick worked too well, and he floated away and no one could find him.

Despite my brief second wind, I fell asleep almost instantly once I got to my seat on the plane, and I didn't wake up until we touched down in Puerto Rico two and a half hours later. I had a

short connection, and the San Juan airport was surprisingly big. So I jogged through the corridors in a bit of a daze, never fully waking up. I arrived at the connecting gate as they were already boarding. The flight attendant checking passengers in was strikingly beautiful, with sexy Latin features and bouncy auburn hair, all of which was undermined by her impossibly warm corporate-sponsored smile.

"Have a wonderful vacation in Sint Maarten, *Señor*." She must have assumed that everyone going on that flight was there to frolic on the beach. I considered telling her I was going to a funeral, to dampen her animatronic enthusiasm, but decided it wasn't my business to puncture her veil.

"Thanks. You too," I muttered.

There was no Jetway here. I walked through a glass door and straight out onto the tarmac and into the hot sun. A mustachioed young man in a well-pressed blue uniform guided me to the airstairs, beckoning me in Spanish. "*Vamos, por favor. Aquí.*"

"*Gracias*," I blurted, embarrassed by my poor accent. I lifted my roller bag in front of me and climbed the short, steep stairs to board the plane.

The guy at the top of the stairs greeted me in English. This plane was a lot smaller than the one from Miami. It was an old turboprop with a narrow aisle and only fifteen rows. As I made my way to 7B, I noticed that nearly everyone else on the plane was Black, and the majority of them were overweight, middle-aged women. They chattered gregariously in the chirpy island patois that I remembered from the one time I had visited my dad several years before.

Oh. The woman at the gate didn't wish everyone a happy vacation, just the pasty white guy from the mainland.

It was only two hundred miles, so we never climbed up to a regular cruising altitude, and we experienced full-on roller-coaster ups and downs as we careened through the clouds. The local women who dominated the cabin were not shy with their reactions either. Every time we hit a bump or a dip, the whole plane erupted with a chorus of full-voice hoots, whoops, and gasps. Like they were all singing along with the movement of the plane in a bizarre symphony of human agony. It was almost too funny for me to feel scared. Almost.

The flight was about an hour long. I spent the first half wishing it was over and the second half wishing it would never end as I considered what was waiting for me at my destination. It dawned on me that any panic about the plane crashing was just an attempt to protect myself from the more serious fear of what lay ahead for me. Not just in the sadness and unpleasantness of the funeral, but beyond that: what life would be like without my father in the world.

This part of my voyage—being by myself in the unreal world of airplanes and airports, deprived of sleep and proper hydration—had been a purgatory, a time-out between the shock of learning the news and the reality of having to deal with it. As we careened awkwardly toward a tiny landing strip on the edge of a splinter of land, surrounded by so much ocean, I lamented that this leg of the journey was finally coming to its end.

CHAPTER 8
GREAT EXPECTATIONS

I HAD NO IDEA what Tobias looked like. That fact was going to make it hard to find him in the airport, but it also made me feel ashamed, like I had been such a shitty brother all those years. We weren't even linked on Myspace. I didn't remember his birthday. Why hadn't I been sending him birthday presents for the last twenty years? Not even a card. What kind of an asshole was I? I was repeating my dad's own legacy of abandoning his family. He was a kid. How much comfort might I have been able to offer as an older brother, during whatever trials and troubles he'd suffered through?

I didn't even know what he looked like. I waited in the Sint Maarten Immigration line and looked beyond the security kiosks, scanning for someone who looked vaguely familiar. I inched my way forward as the security officers stamped the visitors' passports and ushered them into this supposed island paradise. Finally, I reached the desk.

"What's your name?"

"Michael Wohl."

"Where are you coming from?"

"California."

He gave me a look.

"Oh, Sorry. San Juan. It was a connecting flight."

He nodded.

"Purpose of your visit?"

"Uh, funeral. My dad died. On Statia, er, Sint Eustatius. He'd been living—"

He cut me off, forcefully stamping my passport and holding it out to me. "Enjoy your visit. Next!"

The terminal was busy with impoverished families and single travelers lugging giant overstuffed luggage or pushing carts stacked high with cardboard boxes labeled in marker and secured with duct tape. These were people moving their lives or going on big trips, not coming down to the islands for a quick getaway. I guess I had been expecting Maui. I was wrong.

I suddenly wondered if I'd packed properly. I'd been so distracted that I'd just thrown a handful of t-shirts and underwear into my bag, plus my favorite "nice-casual" outfit for the funeral. I did not bring a tie.

As I approached a bank of payphones, I noticed a guy leaning on a nearby wall, facing away. There was something about his posture that grabbed my attention. Something about his silhouette, the way his leg was bent, the way his head was slightly slouched, it didn't just look familiar—he looked exactly like me. It was uncanny. I called out to him.

"Tobias?"

He turned around and saw me, and he smiled. "It's Toby," he said. "Michael?"

"I usually go by Max."

Glimpsing his face, I didn't recognize him so much. He was way too good looking. He had a chiseled chin and a stylish short haircut. His biceps bulged under his T-shirt. I was oddly jealous; I could have looked like that had I just made different choices. We hugged warmly and then pushed each other to arm's distance to examine each other's faces.

"Wow," I said aloud. "So crazy to see you."

"You too," he said, still smiling. "Bro!" he said. Trying it on maybe.

"Yup," I nodded. Still admiring him, a little incredulous at the whole thing. "You're fucking built. Jesus."

He shrugged.

"Can you believe this? What the hell are we doing here?" I asked. "Have you tried the payphones?"

"Yeah, but they're pretty lame. You have to put in a credit card number, but half the time it just hangs up after you dial."

"Perfect. How about tickets to the other island?"

"Yeah. We're kinda screwed," he said. "There's only one outfit that flies there, Winair. And there were three seats on the afternoon flight today, but tomorrow everything's sold out. It's Carnival."

"Carnival? Are you kidding me? Jesus fucking Christ." I kept smiling. Just looking at him.

"What?"

I shook my head, but he knew what I was smiling about, at least I hoped he did. I noticed he was wearing a big fancy wrist-watch. It was impressive looking, like everything about Tobias, but I was reminded that watches were on Dad's no-go list, like television and owning a car. "Why would you want to live by someone else's clock?" he'd prodded me when, at age sixteen,

I had shown up in New York for the weekend with a new rub-ber-banded Swatch. "The only reason to wear a watch is to keep up with someone else's schedule. And if you live your life prop-erly, you should let other people keep up with you. A watch is a symbol of conformity. Of capitulation. Plus it's capitalist, made-in-China crap," he ranted. I never wore a watch again.

. . .

I wanted to try to reach Luuk on the phone to tell him we were late. Our cell phones had no service, and the payphones weren't much better, so Tobias and I stood at adjacent payphone booths and alternated our dialing efforts. We tried nine or ten times. Sometimes it rang, but no one ever picked up. Sometimes we got an error message in English saying the call couldn't go through. Sometimes there was an error recording in Dutch, and we had no idea what it said. And sometimes it just never connected. The variety of failure types would have been amusing if it hadn't been so infuriating.

Eventually we gave up. We had to move on to the next task: securing us a hotel for the night. Working together was surpris-ingly easy. I felt like I could cut through the bullshit politeness that I might afford a stranger, and we were just instantly in a groove. In seconds, I'd worked up a whole story in my head. I got a flush of warm excitement, fantasizing about what it would be like to have grown up with a brother—an intrinsic ally and con-fidante. This was what I had been missing my whole life! Then I remembered what it was like to "work together" with Anais. My warm feeling subsided. He was just being polite and deferential. Nothing is easy. Nothing is free.

CHAPTER 9
CRIME &
PUNISHMENT

THE TERMINAL WAS one grand hall. The interior wall was lined with ticket counters, and on the windowed side, near the road, was a row of booths offering tourist services: car rentals, hotel bookings, scuba boat adventures, and other activities. Strangely, the booths were all empty. It was the middle of the afternoon, so we wondered if it was siesta or a lunch break or . . .

"Maybe..." Toby suggested, "it's just self-service."

I was skeptical but followed him over to a booth advertising hotels. There was an old-fashioned desk telephone on a table and a list of hotels posted on the wall nearby, each with a phone number. We slipped into an instant organic flow—he read the numbers, I dialed. We had no idea where the hotels were or what they might cost for the night, but we picked one at random and gave it a try. It was booked solid. "It's Carnival," they explained. We called the next one on the list. Booked. And so on.

Suddenly a slight man with close-cropped white hair and coffee-dark skin came running over, straight toward us. He was

tucking his shirt into his pants as he ran, as if he had just come out of the bathroom, and he was yelling. "Hey-ya! Hey-ya! Watcha doin', mon?" in a funny island accent. Turned out the booths were not self-service after all, and the guy was furious that we had been charging all these calls on his telephone line. He scolded us, explaining impatiently that there were no hotels with space anywhere near the airport, but then softened and told us he might have a friend who could put us up. We were dubious about it, but it appeared we had little choice.

Around that time, a few of the taxi drivers who had been parked outside the terminal had caught a whiff of possible tourists in need and headed over to tout their services. They were mostly young men in their twenties, all local, which meant they had a particular dark caramel skin, curly hair, and spoke with the same accent. "Tek-see fer you, sir?" they asked as they approached. "You need tek-see? You need hoh-tel?" There was a slightly desperate, aggressive air to their competitive offers. I looked to Toby and took some comfort in his youthful, brawny virility. If I appeared middle aged, soft around the middle, easy prey, Toby most certainly did not. I wondered if he knew martial arts.

• • •

When I was eleven, Dad was studying Aikido. I was going to have to learn, he explained, that there were dangerous people out there who might want to cause me harm. Like it or not, I was responsible for my own safety. He proudly demonstrated the *taki-waza* pose, the ultimate defensive position. "If I hold my body in this particular posture"—he crouched slightly and arranged his feet to point in opposing directions—"it's physically impossible

to knock me over, no matter if you come at me from the front, the back, the right, or the left," he said. "I'm invincible!" He told me to come at him and he would prove it. I ran at him and gave him a shove, completely knocking him off his balance and to the ground. I'm sure he had some verbal explanation for his physical blunder, though the message was loud and clear, and suitably unsettling: there was, in fact, no posture that could not be upset. There was no safe place to hide. At least not with him in charge.

A couple years later, on my thirteenth birthday, I was mugged. Right on Washington Place at 6th Avenue, in broad daylight, in what I thought was my safe backyard. I had fifty dollars in cash in my pocket—a birthday gift from my maternal grandmother—and I was eager to spend it at one of the used record shops on West 8th Street.

It was a beautiful day, so I walked through Washington Square Park and passed two guys sitting on a stoop, who offered to sell me a watch. I got a sketchy vibe and laughed them off as I told them I couldn't afford to buy anything, feeling clever that I had subtly communicated that I didn't have any money worth stealing. But a moment later they flanked me. One put me in a headlock and yanked me down to the ground. The other held a rusty bowie knife against my neck and yelled at me to empty my pockets. Just before they ran away, one of them punched me in the face. It wasn't all that hard of a punch, but it was startling enough and frightening enough to do just what was necessary, keep me from following or yelling for help while they ran away toward the park.

I took a minute there on the ground, and then stood up, brushed myself off, and made my way back to East 6th Street. I burst into the apartment and relayed what had happened. And then the tears finally came.

I guess I expected that Dad might go back out there and find them and get me some justice. Instead, he brought me some ice for my face. He told me I had passed an unfortunate rite of passage: my first mugging. As if it was an inevitability, like getting pimples or jury duty. He offered to take me out to Gem-Spa for a chocolate malt, but I didn't want to go back outside. Instead, Margo made me a warm milk with orgeat syrup and I nursed my sorrows in its thick, sweet whiteness.

■　●　●

No one would mess with Toby. How different our upbringings must have been that he had been encouraged to take care of his body while I was allowed to grow lazy and fat. Had Dad taught him that? Did Toby know Aikido? Maybe my mugging was the inspiration for them to bond about martial arts—or more likely, that was the most ridiculous thought I'd ever had. After thirty-two hours of travel, I clearly needed a real night's sleep. I needed a hotel room.

One of the taxi drivers offered to take us to a hotel that he thought might have a room, but another guy was absolutely sure he had a place for us, and then the two of them started fighting about it. Tout One told us that Tout Two was a liar, and Tout Two told us that Tout One was just trying to steal our money. We skittered away from them both, still without a plan.

A third, younger guy then began following us. He spoke clearer English, and he told us we had to go to the French side of the island, which was farther away from the airport but would likely have space. Except he couldn't take us there himself for some reason.

The two guys who were fighting reappeared, now suspiciously friends. Tout Two seemed to have won, and Tout One smiled far too broadly and gave us his blessing. Clearly, they had decided to join forces to maximize the advantage they planned to take of us.

We reluctantly followed our soon-to-be murderer outside. His car wasn't marked in any way as a taxi. The dashboard was covered in brightly colored beads and religious figurines, a diorama like some kind of sci-fi fever-dream where Jesus and Mary have arrived on a remote planet swarming with multicolored ping-pong balls. He drove us from the airport toward Phillipsburg, the urban center of the Dutch side. On one side of the road there was lush forest, and on the other side was a shantytown that stretched on for several miles, full of impromptu structures, debris and trash everywhere. It was close to dusk. People wandered on and off the highway, oblivious to the cars. I hadn't realized until that moment how undeveloped the island really was. The driver asked us what we were doing there, and I had the opportunity to say, "We're brothers." Which felt really weird, but nice too.

Eventually he turned off the road and into a residential area. Toby and I looked to each other, still not entirely convinced that we weren't getting robbed or worse, but after a few minutes, the driver pulled into the curved driveway of what looked like a luxury hotel.

We made our way into the lobby, and it was no Four Seasons, but it was no motel either. It was called Pleasure Island—which I recalled was where Pinocchio was tricked into going and turned into a donkey as punishment for being lazy and self-indulgent—but I guess the proprietors just thought it was a nice-sounding name. The design was a ludicrous aquatic theme: aqua blue

47

wallpaper covered with large framed pictures of starfish and seahorses. An enormous fishing net was elaborately draped over the front desk as if it was frozen in time the moment before seizing everyone in the entire reception area like so many tuna. Yet, the traditional brown leather furniture and green banker's lamps expressed a far more conservative affect. Still, there was that giant tarnished brass captain's wheel that I had to reach over in order to hand the receptionist our passports.

All the women working at the desk took their job far more seriously than I expected (and they were all women). Again I was reminded that I was in an undeveloped country—one where a desk job at a hotel was a coveted opportunity. The woman helping us somberly explained that all they had were their luxury suites because everything else was sold out. "It's Carnival," she explained.

It was four hundred dollars, but we figured a bird in the hand kept us from having to trust the taxi driver to find us another option, so we agreed. When we got to our room, we laughed out loud at how magnificent it was: a two-room suite with a patio door that opened out directly onto a gorgeous (if a bit pebbly) beach with calm, turquoise waves lapping less than twenty feet from our window.

There was also internet access. Finally. Being disconnected from the outside world for over twenty-four hours had been excruciating. Both of us whipped out our laptops and disappeared into the familiarity of our email accounts. There was still no word from the investor for my project. Oh joy.

CHAPTER 10
STRANGER IN A STRANGE LAND

TOBY AND I TOOK a couple beers from the mini-fridge and went outside to check out our own private beach. Waves gently lapped with a creamy foam on top, illuminated yellow by the faux-candle sconces on either side of our living room's sliding glass door. Taking in the cool night air, we reclined on chaise lounge chairs and sipped our beers. Familiar strangers, strange familia.

Our conversation started slowly. Toby seemed a bit shy, or at least quiet. And I didn't want to interrogate him about his life, especially since I felt so much guilt that I hadn't been in touch all along. After a while, we took off our shoes and rolled up our pants and waded into the water to feel how warm it was. And it was warm indeed. Toby joked about skipping the funeral and camping out there for a few days instead. I was half serious when I told him what a good idea that sounded like. Neither of us could possibly have imagined at the time how prophetic that sentiment would prove to be.

We decided to go into "town" to get something to eat. A five-minute cab ride took us to the waterfront in downtown Phillipsburg, which was lined with bars and restaurants, all with open-air seating along the water. And there, finally, were the tourists that I had expected to see at the airport: mostly twenty-something Americans and slightly older Europeans, all in couples or boisterous groups. I was taken with a weird feeling of incongruity from being in such a beautiful place, surrounded by all these happy people on vacation, when we were supposed to be there for this solemn and sad occasion.

We wandered into a bar and grill and ordered burgers and more beers. Finally, I got to hear some of Toby's story. He was living in New Jersey, earning a mechanical engineering master's at a school in Hoboken, with a year left. And he'd been dating a girl named Julie for five years. I asked if he planned to marry her.

"I guess so," he said.

"That's not a very convincing answer. Are you happy?" I asked.

"Yeah. You know. Sure. Enough. Or maybe not enough. I don't know. Getting married's what you do, right?"

"I haven't. At least not yet," I said. "And I don't see any good options on the horizon."

"We'll see," he said. "She's great. She is. But, you know . . ."

He trailed off. I was a little concerned by his ambivalence, but we were new friends so I bit my tongue. What did I know of the details? Who was I to judge or give advice? I told him about the woman I had recently hooked up with who turned out to be a porn star.

"Are you kidding me?!" He jabbed me in the ribs.

"It sounds a lot better than the truth of it. She's more than a little bit crazy," I said.

"Crazy hot! You're the man."

I suddenly felt old. I rattled off the highlights of my romantic history. Hearing myself tell it to him, I realized I was a long way from finding someone to settle down with—that my story was the painful cliché of the forty-year-old child of divorce, terrified of commitment but still endlessly pursuing it.

"What about kids?" Toby asked.

"I don't know. Dad sure made it look pretty unappealing," I said. "How 'bout you?"

Toby shrugged. "Maybe if Julie wanted to, I guess."

I shook my head, seeing too much of myself in him, knowing that we were both cursed with the affliction of this father of ours and the terrible legacy he left. Would either of us ever find someone we could trust? Could we even trust each other?

After a few more beers, we decided to walk back to the hotel. We weren't sure of the way, but there seemed to be a lot of people out and about so we figured we could probably ask for help if we got lost. We headed down the main street. When we found the street where we thought we should turn into a dark, residential neighborhood, a car pulled up and the driver asked if we needed a taxi. Now knowing that "cabs" were unmarked and unregulated, this didn't seem all that strange.

We told the guy we were fine, that we were going to Pleasure Island and asked if this was the right place to turn. He started laughing and told us we couldn't walk there. We were both confused, as it was only a five-minute taxi ride on the way over.

"Not safe, mon." He dragged an imaginary knife across his throat, though his smile never dipped.

Toby figured it was a ploy to get us to pay him for a ride. "Nice try, buddy," he said.

"We're fine to walk."

The driver turned serious. "No, please. Let me drive you, mon. No charge. This is not a safe area for you. Believe me, mon."

This was a little disconcerting, and after conferring for a moment, we got into the car. He drove us through the streets which did seem especially dark and ominous. At one point we heard a quick barrage of gunfire, and the driver shot us an I-told-you-so smile. I thought about how tourists killed in a plane crash would at least make the news back home, but a pair of Americans murdered during a mugging on a Sint Maarten back street wouldn't generate any notice whatsoever. We arrived back at the hotel, and I thanked the driver with a twenty-dollar bill.

CHAPTER 11
A PORTRAIT OF THE ARTIST AS A YOUNG MAN

AS MY DAD GREW DISILLUSIONED with his predetermined, by-the-numbers life with two kids and two cats and three bedrooms in the 07006, he fell depressed. Toby's mother, Margo, was my dad's secretary during this time, when he was a drug researcher for Schering-Plough in the early seventies. Margo was young and beautiful, and I can imagine she was adoring of his intellect and charisma. Working a job he didn't believe in and with nothing to give his life meaning, it was only natural that my dad took up with Margo—family commitments be damned. (There are obviously different, less generous versions of this story.)

Around that time, he started working on the novel that would become his primary preoccupation for the rest of his life, and that was also when he first discovered psychedelic drugs. He may have been a few years late to the party, but once he dropped out, tuned in, and turned on, he could never go back. He took over the basement of our suburban house and began the ritual of spending hours every night at the typewriter in a cloud of pot smoke.

At some point my mom found out about Margo, and shortly thereafter I was woken up late one night to the sounds of furious screaming. A few days later, my sister and I were marched to the end of the bedroom hallway near the front door, and my mom did all the talking as she explained that Dad would be moving out. I had just turned four.

"You'll still see him on the weekends, but he's going to live in another house." She repeatedly smoothed the creases from her high-waisted polyester pants as if wiping away invisible crumbs that just wouldn't go.

Dad muttered an awkward apology and slipped out the front door. Anais cried openly, and Mom tried to comfort her. I just stood there, staring blankly at the three small vertical windows in the door and the blackness beyond them. My mom sat between the two of us on the two-step stairway between the foyer and the bedroom hallway. She looked dazed, with a hint of smeared mascara from tears we hadn't seen fall. Anais settled down, and I just stared straight ahead. Mom took off the cat-eye glasses she was too old to be wearing and crumpled them in her hand.

"I'm going to need both of you to help me through this. Okay?" She put her arm around me and pulled me to her. "Mikey, you're the man of the house now."

I nodded, furrowing my tiny brow in an effort to appear serious and mannish. She smiled softly and let out a long slow whistle of a sigh, collapsing against me, unwittingly bestowing an unsupportable responsibility upon me even though I barely came up to her hip.

Dad moved in with Margo. Soon thereafter, he quit his "straight" job and dedicated his life to the pursuit of his art while she paid the rent. It was 1973. Everyone was a hippie, or wished

they were. He and Margo were idealistic and carefree. Sure, they were broke, but they had each other, and her secretarial job could support them until his novel hit. He wrote and she danced ballet, and eventually they moved into that fifth-floor walk-up with a cockroach problem and the occasional rat. At that time, the East Village was where the artists congregated, which is another way of saying it was cheap and charmless.

Over the next decade, Margo matured and, as one does, grew tired of living in poverty. Like any self-respecting young adult of the seventies, she rejected security and comfort in exchange for freedom and independence, but as she reached her mid-thirties and the crow's feet began to pull at the outer corners of her eyes, the cost of those decisions became increasingly irrefutable. Plus, her time was running out to have a child of her own. She presented Herschel with an ultimatum, and given that she was supporting them both, he didn't have a lot of options so he married her. By 1983 she was pregnant with Tobias.

• • •

I looked over at Toby, sleeping soundly on the bed beside me as I lay awake, listening to the waves and the cicadas. I was desperately wishing I was unconscious. I tried to time my breathing to the rhythm of his. Okay. I have a brother. I wondered what other surprises awaited me.

CHAPTER 12
OUR LADY OF THE FLOWERS

WE WERE THERE at the gate as Anais's plane arrived the next morning. I calculated that it had been well over a year since I had seen her. And more than twenty since she and Toby had been in the same room. She was lugging a giant carry-on, but as soon as she saw us she dropped it. Her face split open into a wide smile, and she broke into a near run. I was reminded of just how intensely she felt every emotion. This was going to be unbearable.

She wore a flowy, flowery floor-length dress, which fluttered dramatically as she whisked toward us, ahead of the other deplaners. A dried-flower broach on her breast skewed the ensemble from hippie to hick. Despite myself, I recognized the flowers as sage and statice, and I was reminded of her insufferable herbalism.

I got a perfunctory hug and then she was on to Toby. "Oh my God! Look at you." She regarded him voraciously, undeterred by his growing expression of concern. "Would you look at him, Max?" She looked at me, somehow actually expecting some sort of response to her clearly rhetorical question.

I nodded, trying to keep things moving along. "Yes. It's quite the reunion."

She grabbed him and held him tightly for an interminable minute, her face moving from delight, to sadness, to grief, and then to relief. I could see Toby's face too, and he gave me a half-smile as he waited for her to release him from her grasp. I found myself taking a surprising amount of pleasure in his awkward reaction. For the first time in my life, I wasn't the only one who was Anais's brother.

"The last time I saw you, you were like four years old. Running around naked. And now . . . you're a fully grown young man. And so handsome!"

Suddenly our whole tone shifted. Whereas Toby and I could keep things at a politely casual level, Anais lived at such a deep emotional place all the time. And now, especially in the context of why we were all there, I feared we were going to be faced with indulging every feeling that might find its way into our brains. She was going to make sure of it.

She launched into the story of her ordeal. First with the passport office, and then the cancelled flight, the inevitable delay, and on and on. Toby listened good-naturedly, but I had less patience.

"We've got to go right away to the ticket counter to see about getting on the flight to Statia," I said, grabbing her carry-on roller and heading off without waiting for a response.

"Wait! I've still got to get my bag. I had to check my other bag," she yelled after me.

How many days are you planning to be here? I thought. *Did you really need to pack two suitcases?* But I didn't speak.

Toby was more patient. "No problem. The luggage comes in over there." He pointed in the opposite direction of the Winair ticket booth. I groaned.

We all went over to the luggage carousel while Anais inter-rogated Toby about his life. She seemed to have none of the guilt or shame that throttled my own stream of questions, or at least she wasn't letting it get in the way of pulling his story out of him. As the two of them talked, I became less and less present, as if I was disappearing into the humid island air. I had barely said two sentences since Anais arrived, and she hadn't stopped talking. She was all raw nerve. Her feelings came fast and fully formed, and she was never quiet about them. So, while she talked about what was going on for her, I withdrew to a familiar, quiet numbness—disconnected from the world and from myself.

"I was crying on and off throughout the plane ride, just reminiscing about stories and moments we had shared," she explained. "Like the time we painted his car. Do you remember that, Max? It was before you were born, Tobias."

I did remember, and it was a fond memory. In the year after he had moved out when I was five and Anais was nine, Dad had bought a used red VW Beetle. And at some point, out of activity ideas for his visitation days, he came up with the idea to paint the car like a ladybug. He drove us all out to a big empty field for the occasion and handed out cans of spray paint.

I didn't know that he was on the verge of selling the car, as he and Margo were soon to move into the city. The idea of hand-painting a car to look like an insect right before selling it seems like a questionable marketing tactic, but at the time I thought it was genius. And Anais and I had a grand time playing with the spray cans, adding black circles to the body and roof of the car, and drawing a little face and antennae onto the hood and front grill.

But as the day went on, we got caught in a storm. And not just any storm. There was a hurricane passing over New Jersey,

and for some reason we were out driving in it. The rain was so heavy and intense that it overpowered the car's weak windshield wipers, and visibility was reduced to zero. I sat in the front seat and looked out the windshield. It was like opening your eyes underwater without goggles. There was a solid wall of water all around us.

At one point, I decided that I had to see and touch this unreal experience, so I rolled down the window. Water began pouring into the car, and Anais screamed from the backseat, but Dad just laughed, and after a minute, he joined in, rolling his window down in solidarity. In moments we were completely drenched. Finally, accepting that it was impossible to drive, Dad pulled over onto the shoulder, and we sat there listening to the torrents beat down on us. We waited, hoping the storm would ease up.

Without warning, the water rushing down the side of the road turned into a spontaneous river, and our little insect of a car got swept up by the flow and carried backward, keeling a bit to the side. At that point, even Dad got a bit flustered, grabbing the window and the roof to brace himself. After a few seconds we were deposited back on the ground, albeit tilted heavily to the left and with the leeward wheels dug deeply into the mud.

A few hours later, Anais and I sat squeezed between Dad and an auto mechanic in the bench seat of a tow truck's cab, the driver's grease-stained towel wrapped around both Anais's and my wet heads and shivering shoulders.

The rain had stopped and Dad, never one to miss an opportunity to share the wonders of the natural world, excitedly pointed out the window at how the storm was surrounding us on all sides, but there was clear blue sky right above us. We were right in the eye of the storm. And sure enough, as we kept driving toward

the wall of gray clouds ahead of us, soon we were back in the pounding rain.

I didn't remember the episode as scary or unpleasant, but I did recall how furious and terrified Mom was when the tow truck dropped us off at her apartment, ending our weekend with Dad prematurely.

"I could kill you," she said coldly to him, as she ushered us into the house.

CHAPTER 13
PRIDE & PREJUDICE

"YOU'RE WELCOME to wait at the gate and try to fly standby," the young Winair ticket counter clerk explained kindly, "but the plane to Statia only holds eleven passengers, so finding three seats is unlikely."

I kept quiet, but I was steaming under the surface. I blamed Anais for the whole predicament, even though I knew it wasn't really her fault. Still, nothing made me more furious than logistical incompetence, making life more complicated and frustrating by getting tripped up by simple problems that could be avoided through smart planning and efficient execution. This sort of "smart living" was what I excelled at, and what Anais appeared to be incapable of. And sure, there may have been no reason she needed to have her passport ready for last-minute travel, and she couldn't have known that Stan's past would rear up and thwart his attempt to leave the country. And I suppose it was hard to pin on her the weather that delayed her second flight. But still, why did she even have to come? If I had been there alone, I could've

taken care of the whole thing quickly and efficiently. I'd get in, make the arrangements with the funeral home, settle whatever outstanding financial complications he'd left behind, clean out his apartment, send his stupid manuscript to Marcy, and be back in California in a day or two to return to real life.

Then it struck me. What were we going to do with his belongings? What were we going to do with the fucking books? He'd fled New York in a panic six years earlier, but had somehow managed to pack all 9,526 of his books into boxes and secured them in a storage unit. At the time, I suggested that perhaps it was time to let the books go. He wouldn't lose the knowledge within them, and what with Google and the internet, he could probably find any passage or detail that he wanted from the palm of his hand. "Imagine how much lighter you'd feel if you shed the weight of all those dead trees?" I was trying to be helpful.

That was the second time he told me to fuck off. He was totally broke and needed to leave the country (for reasons I'll get to soon), but he was determined to take care of his books and get them all safely squared away, no matter the cost—care he never thought to dispense on Anais or me.

• • •

We waited in the gate area, and after an hour the first flight began to load up. It turned out there was, in fact, one seat available. Naturally, of the three of us, I was the logical choice to be the first one to go. I don't really know why this was, but the decision was unanimous, and as always, I complied.

Since I was flying standby, I boarded the plane last, through the door at the rear. This was a seriously tiny plane: five rows,

with one seat on each side, except for the last row where there were three seats together. I spotted the one empty spot in the first row on the left behind the cockpit—which was separated from the cabin only by a tatty mauve curtain.

I made my way up the aisle and sat down, then I fished around for the seat belt. I found one half, but the other side was missing the clasp. I looked around nervously and observed that no one else seemed to have a seat belt on, so I just sat there, holding the unlatched belt in my hand.

The pilot, a young local guy in his twenties with his uniform shirt unbuttoned a little too far, arrived and shut the passenger door from the outside. Then he went around and climbed into the cockpit through a separate door. He settled in quickly, revved the engines loudly, and the plane jerked into motion. No announcements, no illuminated seat belt sign, nothing.

After a short bit of high-speed taxiing, the pilot opened the throttle and we accelerated quickly. In a moment we were off, into the air, wobbly accelerating through the thermals rising over the warm Caribbean. I grabbed the seat firmly with both hands and looked out the window as we soared up over the crystal-blue water. We banked hard to the left, and I watched the tiny strip of beach on Sint Maarten disappear below us. I closed my eyes and fought to keep my stomach below my throat.

The pilot swiveled around in his chair and yelled to us over the considerable noise of the plane. "We git some wither now. No worries. Jus-ta li'l bumpy-bumpy. We be safe on da ground een fifteen minutes." He seemed to recognize the woman sitting behind me, and he winked at her with a smile.

Almost immediately, the plane began quivering and jerking in an unnatural horizontal motion. I looked out the window at the

endless blue of the ocean and the continuous hue of the sky, and I searched for the line where they met out at the distant horizon. A few thunderheads were visible ahead of us. I wondered how close we were to the Bermuda Triangle.

Still, despite the bumpiness, a strange calm overtook me. If this little plane, with its broken seat belts and distracted pilot, did me in, no one could fault me. At that moment I wasn't living on my own behalf. I was taking care of a duty so much older and bigger than me. I was honoring my father—honoring an ancient tradition, older than God, one as old as humankind itself. No matter what happened, I felt clean, justified, worthy.

Just then we hit an air pocket and seemed to fall a hundred feet in an instant. I blurted out a loud "Whoa!" with all the gusto of the Caribbean women on my flight from Puerto Rico. The rest of the passengers remained silent. I smiled to myself. Maybe it was all going to be okay.

And in a few minutes, we swooped down hard, banked left and then right, and I saw we were heading directly toward a volcano sticking out of the ocean, Sint Eustatius. The pilot maneuvered deftly, cutting the engines to a quiet hum a moment before we gently touched down onto the tiny runway. Once we were on the ground, he turned around to the cabin and smiled and winked again at the one woman sitting behind me.

"We at Statia now," he said. "May you all have a meaningful stay."

CHAPTER 14
LORD OF THE FLIES

WHEN I WAS FIFTEEN, I spent a few weeks of my summer break with Margo and Herschel in the Florida Keys. I looked forward to the trip for months. They had rented a houseboat. For them, it was a vacation to precede the difficult first months (or years) of having a new baby, but also it was a place where Dad could escape and really focus on his writing.

He had warned me as the trip approached that he would be busy and I'd have to entertain myself sometimes. I thought that sounded great; I was old enough to want to be on my own anyway, and doing it in Florida with them meant no authority figure to answer to. I was giddy with anticipation. Plus, I got to travel all by myself.

When the day finally arrived, my mom walked me onto the plane in Newark and helped me get my bags secured in the overhead compartment. After a brief kiss, she whispered something to one of the flight attendants and slipped off the plane. Once she was gone, the stewardess (as they were called at the time) gave

me a big wink. I felt small and alone, but I steeled myself and returned the wink, pretending we were flirting.

My father's parents had immigrated with a caravan of Jews from the Caucasus after Lenin established the Soviet Union and decided that Jews were no longer welcome. They settled in Long Island where they raised my dad and his younger brother. Ever the assimilators, they joined the sunbird movement upon retirement and moved to Hollywood, Florida, where they bought a condo and promptly sheathed their floral-patterned furniture with thick plastic covers.

Having only seen them a handful of times during my childhood, I felt little kinship or connection to them, and evidently, that feeling was mutual. They picked me up at the Fort Lauderdale airport, and as we drove to their apartment, they argued about whether I would prefer to eat lunch before or after going swimming in the pool, referring to me in the third person, even though I was sitting right there in the backseat.

I slept that night on an unopened sofa bed in the living room. I awoke at 2:00 a.m., soaking wet from the sweat that had pooled beneath me in the plastic-covered indentations of the couch pillows. I lay there quietly, awake and wet, listening to my grandfather's snoring until the dawn finally broke. After an awkward breakfast, Dad showed up in a rental car and drove me the hour and a half down to Conch Key, a crumb of an island about midway down the archipelago on the way to Key West.

As excited as I was to get away and to have some time on my own, it turned out there was very little with which to entertain myself; it was just me and my sneakers in the heat and humidity. For fun, I'd walk down to the footbridge near the entry road to the complex of houseboats. An old stingray lived in the lagoon

under the bridge, and I found his huge, undulating shape end-lessly fascinating. There was also a family of nurse sharks. I was fearful at first but soon learned that nurse sharks were harmless, and once I even reached into the water to pet the big eight-foot momma that would frequently ascend to the surface.

In the evenings I'd go out and look for fireflies. I developed a game where I'd hold my breath and count how many flashes I could see before having to release the air in my lungs. I'd make a wish, and if I saw ten lightning bug flashes before breathing out, the wish would come true. At first it was challenging, but after I while I observed their behavior and learned how to rig the game. To avoid challenging my belief in magic, I was careful to choose wishes whose outcome would be far off or somehow controlla-ble—I'd wish that I'd someday buy a camper van and escape to California, or that Dad would publish his book before he died.

Always the naturalist, Dad joked that I'd better stay away from the lightning bugs. He explained how some of the females mimicked the flickering-light mating patterns of a similar species. When the unsuspecting males approached, all fired up for light-ing bug sex, the females would kill and eat them. Dad thought it was hilarious, and he teased Margo that this was a common trait of females of all species. The image stayed with me. At fifteen, looking for attractive females took up an outsized percentage of my time and attention, and I found it especially creepy that just innocently looking for love could, in fact, prove to be deadly.

While Dad originally seemed excited about having me join them in Florida, once I arrived, he was constantly trying to get rid of me. One morning, returning after a long solitary walk and eager to get out of the heat of the midday sun, I found the house-boat locked. I banged on the door, and Dad and Margo yelled out

in unison, "Go away!" I didn't have anywhere to go, so at first I just sat in the folding chair on the dock beside their boat. But after a moment or two, I realized the sounds I was hearing were of them having sex. (Wasn't she pregnant already?) I wandered back off, careful not to come back until sundown.

Another time, Dad and I rode rented bicycles through Marathon Key to the Seven Mile Bridge to go fishing. The plan was to catch some red snapper for dinner. We got some minnows for bait, and he showed me how to affix them to the fishhook. His intention was to leave me there alone fishing for an hour or two, but my beginner's luck spoiled his plan. He mounted his bike and began to ride off, but almost instantly I got a strong nibble and yelled to him to come back for help. Despite his skepticism, I wasn't bluffing. And he helped me reel in a nice foot-long snapper. We put the catch into a bucket and I dropped my line in the water again. He tried again to ride off, but a few seconds later I got another bite. This went on two more times, until we had more than enough fish to eat for dinner and our fishing expedition was abruptly over. I was proud of having such success catching the fish so quickly, but he was visibly annoyed and frustrated that he had to come up with yet another activity to keep me busy.

At the end of my stay, we all flew back to New York together. While we sat in the Miami airport terminal and waited for the flight, Margo was upset for some reason about whether people could tell that she was pregnant. Dad pointed out (rather gleefully) that indeed everyone there could tell that she was knocked up, and not only that, he relayed with a twinkle in his eye just for me, "They all knew exactly what we did to put you in that state!" Margo was not amused.

She had grown up, but my dad never matured. He remained emotionally stunted. He used to brag that if you woke him up in the middle of the night and asked him how old he was, he would blurt out "Nineteen." He was still saying that into his sixties. He thought this was funny or charming, but clearly Margo ceased to think so, especially now that they would soon have a baby to care for.

And despite the thousands of typewritten pages he churned out, there was still no coherent novel and certainly no prospects for financial return from his efforts. Later, with Margo's earning capacity extirpated while she stayed home with the new baby, he was forced to take on a variety of jobs, some more well-suited to him than others. He taught writing classes at NYU; he worked as a prep cook in a greasy spoon; he answered phones in a real estate office; he worked as a handyman for his landlord; and he later claimed that he even did a stint as a roustabout at a carnival somewhere. But nothing lasted very long, and none of it was enough to support them.

Eventually, as things got tighter and tighter financially, Margo gave up and took Toby with her back to New Jersey and to the support of her parents. Dad had become a burden, and she needed a fresh start to figure out how she was going to survive and raise this child.

"Just get a job so you can keep the apartment. So you have a place to write. So there's a place I can come see you," I urged him. "Is that such a sacrifice? Such a violation of your principals?"

"I was put here to do something important. So what if I have to starve along the way?" His defiance was wrapped up in a pride I couldn't fathom.

"You have to live in the real world, Dad. People have responsibilities."

"You're an imbecile," He snorted. "It's okay. I was an imbecile at your age too. But let me tell you something: At some point you gotta choose what's important. We don't live forever."

CHAPTER 15

BEING THERE

THE STATIA AIRPORT was a tiny building at the end of a single landing strip. Inside, there were only two "gates" and a tiny waiting area between them. The whole place was only big enough to hold twenty or thirty people standing. A frosted plexiglass security wall separated departures and arrivals, but it appeared more for show (and to comply with international regulations) than to actually provide any security.

As I approached the immigration desk, the clerk, a big, cocoa-skinned woman with frizzy black hair, pointed at me and gasped. "Look at that!" she shrieked. "Alesha! Come look!"

I worried about what she must have seen. I tried to stay cool as I looked down to make sure there wasn't some giant tropical spider climbing up my shirt. But when her friend approached in her polyester Winair vest, my apprehension waned. Alesha was also oversized, with a beautiful Caribbean complexion and big brown eyes. She came right up to me with a look of great sympathy on her face, her arms open, compelling me toward her for a hug.

"Ah! You must be Joe's son!" she sang.

When my dad moved away from New York, he adopted his middle name, Joe. It was obvious enough to me why he dropped the less common—and therefore more easily traceable—Herschel. But without knowing Dad's secret, Anais was left to make her own sense of it. She said she figured it was because he wanted to reinvent himself as more of "an average Joe." I kept my mouth shut, no matter how absurd that idea seemed to me.

"Sweet Jesus. Ya look just like 'im!" Alesha continued. She appeared torn between the comicality of my resemblance to my dad and the solemnity of the occasion. She wrapped her arms around me tightly. I didn't have much choice but to accept her affection.

Eventually she released me. She clicked her tongue. "We all so sorry about Doctor Joe," she said with requisite sadness, but then she smiled, scrunching her nose and shaking her head again at me. "Incredible."

I shrugged and smiled gently, not sure what to say. The woman at the immigration desk called me back over. She made a spitting motion toward the ground, though I didn't see any fluid leave her mouth. "Keep them spirits away." Then, she shook her head sadly. "Ah, we're so glad you've come. What a terrible shame about your papa." She took my passport and studied the picture, a big smile creeping slowly across her face.

"Lookit!" She held the picture up to show the bored-looking young man standing nearby in loose-fitting fatigues and an automatic rifle on his shoulder. The soldier nodded and then looked to me, silently touching his forehead and bowing his head in some sort of act of piety. I nodded to him in appreciation, although I was a bit unnerved by the way everyone seemed to recognize me. I was also aware of (and starting to feel guilty

about) the three other passengers who got stuck in line behind me. I tried to apologize with a polite smile, but they seem wholly unbothered. Finally, the clerk stamped my passport and handed it back to me.

She called out again to her friend. "Alesha, wontcha go an call Mr. Luuk? Tell 'im Joe's son has finally arrived."

I gestured to my cell phone, to show her that I could call myself, but she shook her head.

"That won't likely do you much good around here." She pointed to the waiting area by the outgoing gates. "You go in wait there, and we'll have Mr. Luuk come and fetch ya. He been coming around every hour or so since Monday to check if you done come in yet. But . . ." She trailed off and got a funny look on her face, like she was withholding a secret. Then, she came around from behind the desk and squeezed me to her chest before bowing her head. "We're so very sorry for you. You come and let us know when the funeral be. Okay?"

I nodded. "Sure. Of course. We're hoping it'll be . . . well, hopefully tomorrow."

One of the rules of a Jewish funeral is that the family is required to bury the body within three days of death. Despite my dad's lifelong repudiation of organized faith, he had specifically requested a proper Jewish funeral, and despite my own disdain for such things—not to mention my ambivalence about him— that instruction had been driving my urgency to get the whole thing taken care of promptly and efficiently. It was already day three. He had died on Sunday, we didn't find out until Monday, and it had taken two more days to finally arrive at the island. I knew it was futile and absurd, but until that moment, I'd been holding onto the possibility that we could get it done under that

seemingly arbitrary deadline. But I finally accepted that, like it or not, we were going to have to be a day late—or so I thought.

CHAPTER 16
A MAN WITHOUT A COUNTRY

I SAT IN THE WAITING AREA as the rest of the passengers left on foot or got picked up by loved ones. The little plane reloaded and took off again, leaving a disquieting silence in its wake. With only me and the few airport employees remaining, the place felt desolate. While Sint Maarten was at least part beach resort with the obligatory tourist services, Statia had none of that. It was just a bleak rock tossed in the middle of the Atlantic. The airport didn't even have so much as a vending machine. And I was getting hungry.

• • •

It wasn't that much of a surprise to anyone when Dad announced he had decided to leave New York, despite his impassioned identity as a New Yorker. The city itself had changed. As the Village gentrified, he moved to the Lower East Side. And when that neighborhood began to improve, he moved deeper into Alphabet

City. He had long boasted that he'd get a nosebleed if he had to go north of 14th Street, and when he had finally succumbed to the rent pressure and found another hole in the wall at 13th and A, it was clear he was running out of room to run.

Of course, I knew the true story of why he was absconding, and it was awkward when I had to lie about it to Anais and my mom by going along with the absurd alternative story he had cooked up.

The irony was that he enjoyed his life in this forsaken part of the globe. He thrived in a way that he never had before. First of all, there was work. It turns out that throughout the Caribbean, there are dozens of little medical schools. They're generally second-rate colleges for wealthy European and Asian students who can't get into Johns Hopkins or other major American universities. These schools have a hard time attracting top teaching talent. So, when an American with a pharmacology doctorate came a-calling, they were thrilled to have him. Never mind that he hadn't thought about the subject in twenty years and that the drug industry had expanded from five thousand to over a hundred thousand products in the intervening time. He was articulate and charismatic, and he got himself hired.

And though they did require him to have proper paperwork, they were willing to let him work while he waited for his "lost" passport to arrive—and he was able to stretch that out for a good long time. He didn't make great money, but his expenses were low, and his local credit was good. And what's more, he turned out to be a terrific teacher. He had a way with his students and quickly grew to be one of the more popular professors at the school.

He also finally found a way to publish his book. By then, he had decided that his novel was actually six books: a triptych

where each third was further split into two four-hundred-page tomes. (You have to at least admire his hubris.) And while he had been submitting samples to publishers for many years, no one had been willing to take a risk on him. But technology had caught up, and he was now able to afford a vanity press who would print copies of his books on-demand as orders came in from Amazon. His friend Rupert had a light enough touch that his edits didn't destroy the brittle integrity of Dad's vision. And lo and behold, one day I got a package in the mail, and in it was a novel with my dad's name on it.

Far too little, far too late. Though I can't deny feeling a tinge of pride to hold it in my hand, all four hundred pages of it, even if it was only the first sixth of the whole magnum opus. Over a couple years, more volumes arrived one at a time. Suddenly I had to allocate half a bookshelf to his work. Unfortunately, I never bothered to read it.

He did have to scamper from one island to another, and bounce from one school to another, a few times. As each college administration grew impatient with his lack of legal paperwork, he would jump ship at the last minute. But he seemed to keep landing on his feet. He started on an island called Saba, then lived briefly on Saint Kitts, then settled on Sint Eustatius and had been there for the past two and a half years. I don't know how long he could have kept the improbable streak going, but it no longer mattered. He'd outrun it long enough.

• • •

Eventually, I detected a white pickup truck on the long road that wound down from the hills. I followed its progress until it finally

pulled into the empty parking lot. A tall man in a painter's cap bounded out and marched toward the building. His pale skin was framed by a thinning mop of white hair and a trim white beard. He stopped and quickly sized me up.

"Look at ya. You look like you got sent to the headmaster's office."

I wasn't sure what he meant and found it a bit unsettling. I tried to smile to project comfort and confidence, but my mouth was cotton-ball dry so my upper lip stuck to my gums and took a moment to release, which must have looked odd. I shook my head and muttered, "I'm fine. Glad to be here."

To which he just offered a pitying smile—presumably less for the loss of my father and more for my awkwardness.

He must have been six-foot-four, at least six inches taller than me. He thrust out his hand, and as we shook, he looked around the airport, then over my shoulder. "Where's your kin?" His Dutch accent sounded oddly formal compared to the patois of the locals.

"There was only one seat on standby," I explained. "They'll hopefully be on the next flight."

"Right. Well," he said, unfazed, as he gestured us toward his pickup, "come along then. There's a lot to tend to."

I threw my bag in the back and climbed into his truck. Duct tape held the handle to the top of the floor-mounted gear-shift, and the dashboard was cracked and faded from the sun. Getting a better look at Luuk's face, I perceived a similar effect on his skin.

He started the engine, and the vehicle lurched into gear. "Where do you want to go first?" he asked then answered his own question. "You should try to speak to Captain Morago at the

police station. He confiscated Joe's computer and mobile." He handed me a thin bifold wallet. "I was able to hide a few things that your dad had in his pockets."

I opened the wallet to reveal Dad's expired New York State driver's license, an ancient social security card, an ATM card, and a piece of paper folded into a tiny square. I stared at the photo on the license, which looked to be from about ten years ago. He looked happy, goofy even, with that big wide grin of his. I was surprised that he even had a driver's license. I hadn't seen him in a car other than a taxi in more than twenty years. I unfolded the little square of paper. It was my father's birth certificate: Herschel Joseph Wohl. Born May 6, 1937. He would have been seventy-one in two weeks.

"Maybe we should go to the funeral home, and at least get that underway, unless you've already spoken to them," I said, shoving the little wallet into my pocket.

He looked at me sideways, and a hint of a smile crept across his face. I stared at him with a mix of confusion and concern.

"You won't find any funeral homes here," he said. "Folks tend to handle those things on their own."

A bead of sweat emerged on my forehead. "Then what, uh, what do we do?"

"Well, to get the body released from the morgue, you're going to need a death certificate, which will need to be filled out by Dr. Merkey and signed by the lieutenant governor."

"Okay," I said. "So, we have to . . ." I trailed off, suddenly feeling confused and overwhelmed. My head began to throb in anticipation of the tasks that lay ahead and the slow, reluctant recognition that I had absolutely no idea of what I was in for. Again, I saw his pitying smile.

"Maybe we just go back to the resort and get you a sandwich. You can put down your bags. And we can figure out a plan." Suddenly he slammed the brakes and honked his horn. A flock of goats had bumbled their way off the steep roadside and onto the pavement. I smiled as they took their time crossing the road, bleating plaintively. One stopped directly in front of the truck and stared at us, cocking his head to the left.

"Welcome to Statia." Luuk smiled sarcastically. He honked the horn repeatedly, and eventually the herd moved on.

A few minutes later we entered what passed for a town. The lush green of the mountain gave way to a surprisingly arid valley. The ground was mostly dirt with small patches of grass, and the few trees were scraggly and parched. The fractured pavement transformed to cobblestone. Small cinder-block buildings with sloped, red clay roofs were haphazardly arranged along the road. A few pedestrians milled here and there; Luuk politely tapped the horn and exchanged a neighborly wave with each. The locals were dark skinned and appeared very poor. I felt conspicuously pale and out of place, especially alongside the tall pale European driving

Luuk pointed to a poorly maintained two-story building with a flag waving in front of it. "That's the police station," he explained. "We'll go back there this afternoon, and you can try to get Joe's stuff out of lockup. And talk to them about permission to dig."

"I don't understand," I said. "Were there suspicious circumstances? Why did they take his stuff?"

Luuk smiled. "Because they can. They probably hope to sell it if no one claims it. You just tell 'em what's what and it'll be fine."

A pair of young women were walking alongside the road, barefoot and dragging a wagon loaded with several five-gallon jugs of water. They waved to us, and Luuk waved back. I tried to join in and gave a pathetic, noncommittal wave.

Luuk's other comment popped back into my mind.

"Permission to dig?" I asked.

"I thought maybe we could bury him at the old Jewish cemetery. But it's been closed."

"There's an old Jewish cemetery here?"

"Ah, Statia's got a rich history, son." He winked but didn't elaborate. "Belinda suggested maybe we could bury him next to Eleanor."

"Who's Eleanor?"

"Belinda's daughter. She died three years ago." He pointed to his midsection. "Cancer."

"Oh, I'm sorry," I said. Then, "Sure, I guess."

That was the first time I'd considered the question of where to bury the body. I wasn't entirely sure if Anais or Toby might want to bring him to Florida where his parents are buried, or to New York, where we would be able visit the grave. I tried to imagine what that would be like; I pictured the rolling hills of Mt. Hebron cemetery in Queens, with its long winding rows of headstones full of familiar Jewish names: Stein, Baum, Katz, Bluestein. I imagined standing at a grave site marked with my father's name, *Herschel Wohl*, on one of those hills crowded with the dead. I felt the cold wind blowing through a gray sky morning. Jetliners low and loud on their way into LaGuardia.

I scanned my body for a trace of feeling. Was there sadness? Loss? Emptiness? But I felt nothing. I could conjure no feeling at all. Just numbness. I pictured myself standing there as the world

went round and the days went on. His absence was meaningless. Insubstantial. Irrelevant.

The road turned back to dirt as the town disappeared behind us, and Luuk outmaneuvered a few more goats by zigzagging onto and off of the bumpy shoulder without even slowing down. The trail curved around and came over a crest, and suddenly the majestic blue of the ocean appeared before us, spreading out in every direction. Luuk made a sharp turn and stopped at a fenced-off driveway. He instructed me to get out and open the gate so he could pull in. I complied in silence. As I opened the door, a breeze hit my skin and I realized there were tears on my cheeks.

CHAPTER 17
THE ALCHEMIST

IN HIGH SCHOOL, I used to bring my friends to visit my dad. We'd be coming to the city for a concert, a party, or to attend the midnight *Rocky Horror Picture Show* at the original 8th Street Playhouse. And we'd stop by his apartment so I could show off my super-cool father who would smoke us out and give us important advice about how to properly inflate a whip-it balloon or which head shop would be best to buy a wooden dugout pipe. And most important: where to score. The popular spot at the time was the sketchy block of 10th street between 1st and A.

"Never, ever buy anything at Washington Square Park," he lectured. "Unless you're looking to buy an expensive bag of oregano."

But it wasn't all about drugs. My father also had a penchant for astrology. I'm not sure when that started, but by the time I was in high school, he was doing "charts" for everyone and anyone. He became semiprofessional, guiding his landlord through a divorce in exchange for a discount on the rent, or giving his pot

dealer celestial parenting advice in exchange for a quarter ounce of Jamaican Green. And naturally, he did Anais's and my charts and monitored them regularly.

It wasn't unusual to receive a phone call from him warning me that "This is not a great week to make important decisions," or "You may be having some extra girlfriend trouble over the next few weeks until Neptune makes its way out of your second house." I never took it very seriously, but whenever I met a girl I liked, I'd always pop the odd questions of what time of day and in what city was she born, so I could report back to him and get his star-guided approval—or warning to stay away.

He explained to me one time how his name had astrological significance. "Herschel was the original name for the planet Uranus, named for the astronomer that discovered it," he quipped professorially. "And as you know, Uranus is the symbol of intuition and change. It's the trickster of the astrological pantheon." Then he'd wink and grin his impish smile.

He had a large brown birthmark that wrapped around the curve of his left wrist. It was hairy and frightened me when I was young. He called it the nebula, explaining that it was actually made up of many little freckles, each a tiny star with its own pull over his life.

Whenever I'd bring a friend by his fifth-floor walk-up to meet him, he'd perform a spontaneous astrology session—inevitably wowing them with inspired and convincing advice and prognostications.

"Do you have a sister?" Dad would inquire of the bassist from my garage band, as he used a well-worn protractor to draw a cryptic arrangement of symbols and figures.

"Yes! How did you know that?"

"It's all written in the stars," he'd say nonchalantly, before taking a deep hit on a joint and passing it to my fifteen-year-old friend. "You used to be close, but you've drifted apart in recent years."

"Yeah. It's true. Wow. This is so trippy!"

Of course it's true! I thought. It's the oldest fortune-telling gimmick in the book: describe the most common, generic situations and relationships, but contextualized to make it seem like you've divined them from some magical source. Still, it never failed to astonish my friends. And I can't deny that I traded on it now and again, bringing people to visit whom I wanted to impress. Not to mention embracing the exotic and sophisticated appearance I earned through my proximity to his charismatic charlatanism.

At the time, I suppose I was as seduced as anyone else, perhaps more so than anyone else. He was, after all, my father. And at that age, I didn't want a disciplinarian or a model for how to succeed in the world. He had already explained, "Authority is just overcompensation for insecurity or spiritual weakness." Instead, I got what seemed like the best of both worlds: a grown-up with access to the things of the adult world, but one who would share those things with me and treat me as a peer, capable of understanding the secrets of the universe that were otherwise beyond the grasp of my teenage life. All I had to do in return was never dare expect actual parental guidance or protection. Also, always keep his secrets.

CHAPTER 18
THE OLD MAN
& THE SEA

A SMALL, FADED SIGN read *Paradise Point Inn*. I felt around the edge of the fence post until I found the lever that released the heavy gate.

"Mind the dogs," Luuk said.

"Dogs?"

I was answered by the deep, hearty bellows of two enormous Great Danes who came bounding toward me as soon as I had the latch lifted and the gate opened a crack. I tried to put my body in the way so they couldn't escape through the opening, but they were nearly as tall as I was and together outweighed me. I braced myself and thrust out my arm to protect my face like I remembered seeing on some TV show—half expecting to sacrifice my forearm to protect my jugular. But they overpowered me easily, and before I could stop them, both of their huge, sloppy tongues were eagerly kissing my face, drooling all over me, and knocking me off balance. Their tails banged percussively on the metal gate.

"LINDA!" Luuk hollered. "Git yer damn dogs!"

A tall fair woman in her sixties with long blond-gray hair half ran to my rescue. "Thumper! Bambi! Don't you dare!" she yelled. The dogs abruptly stopped their love attack and retreated to their master's side. A macaw screeched from nearby, making me jump. Belinda put one hand on each dog's collar and held them still as I approached, though it was clear that if they had wanted to break free they'd have had no problem. Belinda smiled as she regarded me, but then her face went wistful.

"Oh, Joe," she said.

"I know," I smiled, guilty for my familial likeness.

It was strange to hear everyone there refer to him by that name. While I wasn't one of those kids who called his parents by their first names, I still understood his identity as *Herschel*, and that weird disconnect was just one more way the whole experience felt unreal, like I was watching a movie rather than living through it.

The Paradise Point Inn was perched on a dramatic cliff overlooking the windward coast of the island. The parking lot lead to a collection of two large buildings and a handful of smaller bungalows. I had been expecting some sort of boarding house, but I was gathering that this place where he lived was more of a no-frills resort, and he was just one of several long-term residents. One of the large buildings was a two-story ring of single rooms surrounding a small swimming pool, like a roadside motel, and the other was the "main house" where Luuk and Belinda lived. Between the two was an open-air dining patio that overlooked the water. The views were striking. And, being the rainy side of the island, the surrounding landscape was quite lush, rife with giant-leaved jungle plants and a variety of birds.

Dad once wrote me a three-page letter about the many birds endemic to the Caribbean.

Overall, the colors and variety are vastly more impressive than anything on the Eastern Seaboard. Kingbirds and other flycatchers are quite common, and a wide range of warblers and vireos compete with the ubiquitous bananaquits for the insects on the trees around the structures. Shiny cowbirds from South America are increasingly common too. They're brood parasites (like cuckoos), laying their eggs in other birds' nests so the unwitting host mother raises the cowbird chick, even as it outcompetes her own young. The tropicbirds and magnificent frigates are a common sight high in the skies above the harbor. I watch them circle endlessly from the broad patio adjacent to the main house where Luuk and Belinda cook meals for short-term visitors.

There I was, sitting on that same patio, looking out at the water and at the dozens of giant pterodactyl-like birds above the harbor below, just as he had described. What the image brought to my mind though, was vultures circling, waiting to feast on bloody carrion below.

It was hot and I was sweating. I wiped my brow with my sleeve. Luuk stepped over the two giant dogs lying at my feet on the stone patio floor and thrust a beer into my hand, then he sat down across the table from me, put his feet up on another of the chairs, and sighed contentedly.

"That was Joe's favorite spot," Belinda called out. She was preparing me a ham and cheese sandwich in the adjacent open kitchen. I nodded and raised my beer in some kind of invisible salute, though her comment somehow unsettled me. Everything

unsettled me. The place was paradise, and yet I felt like I was in a war zone, jumpy with anticipation of enemy fire.

Looking for a distraction, I took out my flip phone and scanned for a signal. Nothing. I pulled out my laptop. "Is there internet?" I asked.

"Not over the air," Luuk said. "You can use the office computer if you need to, but the connection is pretty sketchy."

I changed the subject, looking to regain some sense of control by focusing on the task at hand. "So, um, I guess we need to buy a casket?" I asked. The word casket suddenly felt bourgeois and pretentious in my mouth. I corrected myself. "A coffin."

"There's no store or anything like that, if that's what you mean. You'd have to go back to Sint Maarten, or maybe down to Saint Kitts. But that'd take a long time." He turned to Belinda. "Maybe Reggie could help. What do you think?"

"I don't understand," I said. "What do people do? How can there be no funeral services anywhere on the island?"

"For what?" Luuk barked.

"I don't know. Whatever it is they charge you ten thousand dollars for."

"You don't want to embalm him, do you?" Belinda raised her eyebrows.

"I don't know. Isn't that more sanitary? Aren't there laws? To like, protect the groundwater or something? How am I supposed to know what to do?"

She brought over my sandwich and sat down beside Luuk, across from me.

"This isn't the States," she said calmly. "You do whatever you believe is right. It's not that complicated."

"Why don't we wait till your brother and sister arrive?" Luuk

offered. "And then you can decide what you want to do. Here," he said, and pulled something out of his pocket. "These were in your dad's nightstand. I took 'em to keep them from being lifted by the cops." He handed me three USB memory sticks, holding my gaze a beat too long as I took them and stuffed them into my pocket.

After I ate, I grabbed my roller bag from the truck, and Belinda led me across the parking lot under the burning sun to one of the bungalows. "This was Joe's," she said, and paused at the door. "You can treat it as your own. Joe was paid through the end of the month, and you can use his food while you're here."

I just stood there. A bead of sweat dripped down from my temple to my cheek. Use his food? How long did she think we were going to be staying?

"Why don't you go in, take a few minutes. I'll leave you alone. When you're ready, just come on back up to the dining area and Luuk will take you back into town."

I nodded and struggled to mutter a thanks, but I found myself just standing there until she again gestured for me to go inside. I walked over and opened the door.

Belinda turned to go, but then added, "Oh, and don't worry, I've cleaned everything up. So just, you know. It's all fine in there."

CHAPTER 19
DESOLATION ANGELS

AFTER MARGO LEFT, Dad's life contracted to what he could afford without her weekly paycheck, which wasn't much. He had to give up the railroad apartment on 6th Street, as the East Village continued its inexorable gentrification. He took up in a hideous dark hole of an efficiency unit on East Houston Street, an area that was still a complete slum. There wasn't room there for me or my sister to stay, and he could hardly afford to even pay for dinner, so I saw him less and less. During my first year in Boston, where I had gone for school, we'd correspond through the mail, and I'd send him my term papers and other writing for his critique and approval, but he never shared very much of what was going on in his life.

One night freshman year I brought home Naomi from Oregon (with whom I shared a rising sign and a short-lived college fling) to visit New York, but instead of meeting with us, Dad lent us his apartment so we wouldn't have to stay with my mom in New Jersey. I appreciated the gesture (and the implicit

encouragement of my getting laid) but was also disappointed that Naomi wouldn't get to meet him and enjoy his clever, eccentric charm. He stayed with a friend or something, and he arranged for the key to be left for us to pick up, so we never even said hello.

Naomi and I arrived at the address on Houston quite late, after a boozy dinner on St. Mark's Place. We followed his instructions to push open the exterior building door where the lock never worked, and we walked through a dark hallway and out through another heavy unlocked door into a poorly lit inner yard. The place was foreboding. We immediately had to step around a splatter of broken glass, and I could see dog shit and smell piss, both too nearby for comfort. I put my arm around Naomi and held her close to me, attempting to exude confidence as I guided her around the knocked-over trash can and its spilled, fetid contents and then back onto the cement path that led down the center of the small yard.

We tried to ignore the handful of people congregated in the darkest corners and nooks of the courtyard. The cherries of their cigarettes provided a rough count of faces: three on the left by a tall metal gate, a couple passing a bottle back and forth in one corner, and one guy standing by himself near a ground floor window that seemed open too wide for such a cold evening. I could feel all their eyes tracking our movements—smelling our apprehension. As we walked, I shivered, belying whatever fearlessness I was trying to fake for Naomi's sake.

We went up to the doorway of the back building as instructed and pressed the button for apartment 2-E. I didn't hear a buzzer, and I wasn't convinced that anything happened. Naomi attempted a shrug, but it came out as a shudder, and I pushed the button again and held it in.

"Shut up already!" came a shout from a window above us and to the right. I released the button and stepped away from the door. A second later we could hear footsteps on a stairway, and a skinny, stubble-faced junkie in a bathrobe pushed open the door.

"You Hershey's kid?" he muttered, though he didn't wait for an answer before handing me a key. "4-C," he said. "Fourth floor, right side."

I took the key, and Naomi and I scurried up four narrow flights of worn-out stairs.

When we entered the apartment, I couldn't believe how small the place was. A twin mattress was pushed up against one corner near a small window, and from the foot of the bed to the other end of the room was only a few feet. The rest of the space was piled floor to ceiling with boxes of books. There was a small bathroom the size of a public toilet stall—and without a door. There was no bathtub nor even a shower.

Naomi remained a good sport, determined not to let our evening be ruined. She immediately unbuttoned her shirt to keep me from spinning off into worrying how my dad could possibly be living in such a place. A moment later, the rest of our clothes were off, and we dove into the tiny bed and held our naked bodies against each other. Our sex was intense, almost feverish—charged by fear and the strangeness of the whole situation.

Afterward, Naomi fell right asleep, but I lay awake a long time and listened to the sirens and barking dogs and the occasional arguments that erupted outside. I wondered if the loud, not-so-distant booms were gunshots. I tensed up with every footstep that passed in the hallway outside the apartment and tried to ignore the unmistakable pitter-patter of rodents scurrying inside the walls.

Later, Dad asked how I had enjoyed the stay. I told him how much fun we had pretending we had our own place in the city. I refrained from asking how he was able to take a shower. I also didn't ask where he had spent the night. I worried that he had been out wandering the streets, or perhaps sleeping at a homeless shelter. If that was his apartment, he certainly couldn't have afforded to spring for a hotel.

He laughed. "Ah, someday you'll be as lucky as me."

CHAPTER 20
THE HOUSE OF THE SPIRITS

WITH BELINDA'S COMMENT about cleaning the place up still ringing in my ears, I pushed through the door and into the bungalow. The curtains were drawn, so it was dark and much cooler than outside. I was immediately struck by the familiar cologne of musty old books mixed with cheap pot and cigarette smoke. It took me right back to East 6th Street and that huge wooden desk of his. I breathed it in deeply.

I looked around at the scant remains of his life. As always, the most prominent things were the books. His cherished collection filled a giant wooden bookcase that covered one wall. A few cardboard boxes remained unpacked: presumably that last shipment from the storage facility in New York.

The place was small—one room with cheap wood paneling on the walls and a cold terracotta-tiled floor. A twin-size bed sat against one wall with a small nightstand beside it. A small writing desk sat across from there, and a skinny sofa sat beside it. A tiny wrought iron mosaic café table with two wire-backed chairs was

tucked between the giant bookcase and a doorway leading to a closet-sized kitchenette.

From the kitchen, a windowed French door lead to a small deck outside. It didn't overlook the ocean but seemed like a pleasant enough place to sit with a cup of coffee. I opened the door, and a pair of tiny yellow bananaquits fluttered away with a bustle of songlike chirps. Feeling the rush of heat flood in, I shut the patio door quickly and located the one other door, which lead to the bathroom—the spot where he died. I paused a moment before I went inside, not sure exactly what I expected to find. I pushed the door open slowly and peered inside. The room was in no worse shape than the rest of the bungalow. A little dank and mildewy, but there was no visible blood or smell or anything to betray what had transpired. Still, the worn toothbrush in a small drinking cup and the capless, near-empty mouthwash bottle told the story of a life interrupted.

The sink counter was messy and disorganized in a way that made me feel like I was invading someone's privacy; the toothpaste was messily overflowing and crusted around the mouth of the tube. The medicine cabinet door was half-open, revealing a mundane assortment of pill bottles, athlete's foot spray, hemorrhoid cream, and a rusty nail clipper.

I went to the toilet and peed. Standing there, I pictured him crawling to the bowl, desperately sick and in excruciating pain, struggling to drag his body to this dirty hole where he could expel the vile bodily fluids that were plaguing him. I tried to push the image out of my head, but it kept swelling back. I imagined his face—yellow, tired, convulsed. I found myself scanning the tiles and the corners of the floor looking for some blood. Some trace. Some proof of this story that I couldn't rend from my mind. My

eyes trained on something—a spot on the wall. But it was just a stain; the toilet brush's rusty wire handle had leaked its dark orange pigment into the worn white bristles, and some of it had smudged onto the wall. I was relieved (and yet strangely disappointed) that it wasn't blood.

Back in the main room, I methodically scanned the desk and bookcase. I didn't really know what I was looking for, but I understood instinctively that I needed to find whatever it was before my siblings arrived. I didn't know what secrets of his I might uncover, but I felt an obligation to locate and expunge them, to protect him from discovery. It was my role, my burden, the price of his love that I somehow agreed to honor in the time before I had continuous memory. I was also looking for a note—a message to us. He clearly knew he was dying, enough to give Belinda instructions. I could only assume he would have left a note for us, to say goodbye. To apologize. To tell us he loved us. To help us understand or make sense of the lives he left us to.

I stared at his desk. There was a tangle of loose cables leading to a big, empty, dust-free rectangle where his computer obviously lived. There were also a few piles of papers: bills and mail, printouts of lectures for his pharmacology class, and pages from a yellow pad with scribbled handwritten notes. I thumbed through it all quickly, pausing at one envelope smeared with a blood-colored fingerprint.

I made a mental note that we would need to go over the bills in more detail later, figure out what debts he owed, and find out what accounts we were going to need to manage and close. I fantasized that he might have been hiding a secret fortune; that some surprising good might come from all of this. Of course, I

knew the more likely reality was that I'd discover some big debt that would now become my problem.

More rummaging finally revealed what looked like a bank statement. It was a few months old, but I was shocked that it looked like he may have had almost twenty thousand dollars saved. It wasn't much in terms of a life savings, but it was almost certainly the most money he'd ever had, at least since he'd dropped out in the early seventies. I was momentarily proud of him until I discerned that the balance was actually listed in Eastern Caribbean dollars, which were about two and a half to one US dollar, making his net worth closer to seventy-five hundred dollars. Barely likely to even cover his funeral expenses.

I went through the desk drawers. In the upper left, where his pot was always kept in the old desk in New York, I found one of those cheap first-generation vaporizers for smoking pot in a healthier way. It was the exact same model I had bought a couple years ago, though I never really used mine. His looked well-worn; the plastic tube that transports the vapor was yellowed and brittle near the connection to the heating unit. I was amused that he would even consider using a tool like that, as he was a consummate joint smoker, proudly unconcerned for the health of his lungs. I felt a flash of pleasure at the thought that he and I had unknowingly chosen the same brand, then immediately shamed myself—for aligning with him, for using drugs, for taking pleasure of any kind, at all, ever. Oy.

There wasn't much more of interest at his desk. Whatever note I was looking for must have been on his computer, which was impounded. We had to get that taken care of as soon as possible. In the meantime, I wanted to see whatever else I could find. I scanned the shelves of the bookcase for papers or anything

that stood out. I scanned through the titles until I was surprised to locate a copy of my own first book, which I had published five years prior. It was a technical how-to about film editing, not something he would have had any interest in reading for its own merits. I guess I must have sent him a copy at some point.

I moved over to the bed. On the nightstand were his reading glasses and a paperback copy of Rudyard Kipling's *Kim*. In those dark final days, he turned to what must have been one of his favorite stories from childhood. To try to find some comfort in Kipling's dulcet mellifluence. I picked up the book. Its spine was deteriorating, and the pages were beginning to fall out. Many of Dad's books were original editions—collected over the course of his life—which made them precious but also often in terrible shape, not least because he had to pack them and unpack them so many times as he relocated again and again.

Beneath the paperback was a small stack of white index cards held together with a rubber band. He had always kept a stash of white index cards and a pen with him wherever he went. That was how he jotted down important notes or story ideas for his novel. I had seen these cards throughout my life: a pile on his desk, a pile next to the toilet, and a pile in the inside pocket of that jean jacket he practically lived in for a decade (until it was so worn and falling apart that Anais made him retire it). I don't think he ever explained, but I understood their importance—inspiration was unpredictable and fleeting, and it needed to be harnessed no matter what the surrounding circumstances. So it wasn't at all surprising to me to find a pile at his bedside there on Statia, but when I picked them up I was stunned by what I saw.

The handwriting was barely legible. I knew my dad's handwriting as well as my own and could identify it better than a

trained police detective. But this wasn't his normal handwriting. It was awkward and messy and drawn diagonally across the card. It read: *Shut down in a cell, alone.* A chill ran up my spine and tingled my scalp. I stared at the card for a moment. Had that been his last thought? Then I flipped the card over. In even more unrecognizable handwriting, what looked like a young child's scrawl, it said: *God. Holy. Good.*

Were these his last fevered words? I sat down on the bed, flummoxed. He was vehemently atheistic and anti-religious his whole life. I was perplexed enough by his request for a Jewish funeral, and now this. Had he found God in the end? What did that even mean?

I stood back up and looked around the bungalow. It suddenly felt unbearably claustrophobic. I stumbled out onto the little patio and raised my hand to block the rays of the midday sun. I put my other hand in my pocket and felt the handful of USB memory sticks that Luuk said he hid from the police.

A moment later I was back inside, sitting at his desk, plugging the first of the drives into my own laptop. This must be where the message I was looking for was hidden. I was sure of it.

CHAPTER 21
INHERENT VICE

THE DRIVE TOOK forever to mount. I clicked impatiently, trying to open it and see its contents before it was fully connected. Probably partitioned in some outdated format, I tsked. Finally it came up, and I scanned the handful of folders listed. The names were cryptic. I suspected it must be some sort of executable—though I couldn't imagine why he'd keep that on a USB stick in his nightstand. Maybe it was a backup start-up disk for some operating system I was unfamiliar with.

I was just about to eject it when I decided to poke a little further. I clicked to open one of the folders. Inside were hundreds of JPEG images. I picked one at random and double-clicked. It was pornography. I was repulsed. That was not what I had expected. The last thing I wanted to discover was my dad's porn. I went back to the root folder. Suddenly the cryptic folder names seemed less obscure: truncated female names with trailing numbers. I opened another folder. It was full of movies. More porn. Why would he have saved this on a memory stick? Why would

anyone back up his pornography collection? What an awkward, unfortunate reality of the digital age.

When I was thirteen, I found a stash of *Hustler* magazines in my dad's bedroom—they weren't exactly hidden—in a basket of magazines next to the magnificent king-size waterbed that he and Margo had somehow installed in their fifth-floor walkup. There might have been a *Rolling Stone* on top of the pile, but otherwise, the smut was right out in the open. I had just recently discovered the delight of masturbation and was ecstatic with the possibilities. I stole one of the magazines, and when I got it home, I found a section where the pages were stuck together. I was revolted at first, but after a while I found myself reluctantly curious about which images my dad must have found so especially compelling.

I wondered if he and Margo looked at the stuff together. They were always very open about sexuality. There was that nudist phase when I was ten or eleven; they encouraged us to join in if we wanted to, but neither of us dared. Still, it was hard to not stare at Margo's breasts or her full bush of red pubic hair as she served me breakfast or sat in the reading chair with the *Times*. She treated my attention as if it was normal and healthy, and I guess in some ways it was, but I will never forget the time she teased me that she knew I would grow to have a really big "cock" because, as she explained with a wink, such things were hereditary.

I clicked open a third folder on the memory stick; this one was labeled "Anai." This folder had text documents in it. I opened one up and began skimming. I was dumbfounded. It was a story about my sister and one of her high school friends hiking to a secret swimming hole. They undress and jump in the water. Then a man appears, and the three of them have sex. It was overly descriptive and erotic. It was terrible, juvenile writing. I scrolled

through the file, growing numb. It was several pages long, with paragraph-long descriptions of the girls' young bodies. Starting on the third page, the text was annotated crudely with photos of young-looking models from clothing ads—not pornographic, but provocative and sexualized by the context.

I slammed my laptop closed. Sitting there, short of breath, I wretched. I gasped. The sweat on my forehead turned cold. I felt like I was looking at the laptop in front of me through a tunnel. I didn't know what to do, what to make of it. I reopened my laptop and looked again at the folder that contained that file. There were dozens more, and I could only assume from the names of the files that they were more of the same. Were these fantasies? Confessions? Was it part of his novel?

Without thinking, I quickly did exactly what I had unknowingly been trained to do. I destroyed the evidence. After deleting all the folders, I reformatted the USB drive just to make sure that the content was fully erased.

With trepidation, I connected the second memory stick. That one contained just a few files: text copies of a few dozen lectures named with the course names and the class number. I put in the third and final stick, and it appeared to be a more miscellaneous backup. I sorted the files by reverse date and found a file saved at 2:33 a.m. on the previous Sunday morning. That would have been mere hours before he died. I opened the file eagerly, still absurdly hoping for a note or some additional clues, but what I found instead was what looked like his manuscript. That was his final act. He was at the gates of death and all he cared about was finishing his stupid book.

I dutifully copied the manuscript and the rest of the drive's contents to my laptop's hard disk. I drafted an email to Marcy and

enclosed the manuscript. I plugged his Ethernet cable into my computer to send the email. It took a while to connect, but after a few tries it seemed to go, and my incoming mailbox filled up with the meaningless junk that was my life back home. I didn't read any of it. Instead, I closed the laptop, and then I closed my eyes. Sitting at that desk, surrounded by his smell, feeling the same confusing mix of duty and disappointment, responsibility, and humiliation that he always evoked in me. How would it be after he was gone? Apparently, it would be exactly like it was when he was alive.

CHAPTER 22
WELCOME TO THE MONKEY HOUSE

AROUND 2:00 P.M., Luuk and I headed back into town on our way to the airport to get Anais and Toby. They had managed to get two seats on the next plane. I thought back to the way Luuk had looked at me when he handed me the thumb drives. Had he looked at them? Did he know? Did he know that I knew? I was still vaguely nauseous but summoned the ability to shove the feelings down into that familiar well.

While the ride from the airport to the resort seemed to take a long time, going the other direction, I realized how small the island really was. We travelled from one side to the other in about ten minutes. At the airport, Anais and Toby made their way through the immigration check, and Luuk and I met them in the parking lot. After a round of greetings and hugs, Anais immediately began thanking Luuk profusely for his help and hospitality.

I explained that there was no funeral home or other services, that the onus was on us to figure out what we want to do and how to do it all ourselves. As I talked, the enormity of the

task ahead became clear to me. I had thought the hard part was going to be the emotional experience, but I was suddenly aware that there was also a real live corpse to tend to, too.

Oddly, annoyingly, predictably, Anais seemed thrilled. "I think it's a glorious opportunity," she beamed. "It's what's been done for thousands of years, before our consumer economy neutered and sterilized every facet of our lives."

There was also going to be the work of tolerating my sister.

Luuk drove us back toward town. There were only two seats in the cabin of the pickup, so Anais sat in the front, and Toby and I climbed into the truck bed with the suitcases. As we drove, we could hear Anais chatting up Luuk.

"Sure talks a lot," Toby said.

"Yeah," I smiled. "You get used to it." He nodded. "I suppose it's worse in a stressful situation like this," I said.

"What stress?" Toby joked. "We're on vacation." He gestured out at the landscape around us, which really was magnificent. Then seeing something moving behind the trees on the side of the road, he blurted, "The hell was that?"

"Goats," I said authoritatively. "Or leopards maybe."

Luuk pulled up in front of the police station and came to a stop in the gravel parking area. There were no police cars, just an old jeep and a few bicycles, plus a couple skinny stray dogs lolling about in a shady spot. The three of us got out, but Luuk stayed in the car.

"Are you coming in?" Anais asked.

"We don't get on," Luuk replied. "Probably better for you this way."

The three of us looked around at each other, a bit hesitant. One of the dogs came over and sniffed around the truck.

Without warning, it was suddenly full-force raining. "Come on. Let's go!" I yelled. And we rushed across the parking lot.

Luuk called after us, "They're probably hoping to sell that laptop, so don't take no for an answer."

Inside there were a few offices and a handful of people milling about, mostly in civilian dress. I leaned into an open room where two young cops were standing over an old metal desk. "Excuse me," I said. "We're looking for . . . Mr. Moranga."

They glowered at me. "Morago. It's Captain Morago," one said curtly.

"Sorry. Where can we find him?"

"Upstairs."

We walked up a dark stairway and heard the unmistakable music of a television soap opera coming from one of the offices. As we reached the top of the stairs, I peered through a partially opened door into a room where a large man was sitting on the corner of a desk facing away from us. He held the receiver of a 1980s-style telephone to his ear, his other hand twisting the thick coiled phone cord around his fingers. A squat tube TV on a flimsy metal stand sat against one wall, its fuzzy signal flickering the telenovela we'd heard from the stairs.

We waited outside the door for a few minutes, but he didn't seem to be talking on the phone he was holding, so finally Toby knocked on the door. "Excuse me," he said.

"Hold it!" the man barked, spinning around to face us. "Stop right there!"

He was towering and muscular, wearing what looked like a military uniform with a row of medals pinned to his chest. Holstered sidearms adorned both hips, and he shook the telephone receiver at us like a weapon.

111

"Who said you could enter?" he growled.

"We, uh, we're . . . nobody said," Toby began.

I took over. "Are you Captain Morago?"

"Yes. I am the captain. State your business."

"I, uh, our father, Herschel Wohl—uh, Joe? Doctor Joe? He passed away, and—"

Morago shushed us with his finger and turned away to speak into the phone. "You must come and speak to the clerk directly. I have no more time for you. Something urgent I must attend to." He slammed the phone into its cradle and turned back to the three of us, suddenly smiling warmly in a disturbing transformation of character. "Please come in," he cooed. He made a show of picking up a remote control and muting the television as if it was some impressive feat of technology.

I continued. "Our father died on Sunday, at the Paradise Point—"

"Yes. I am aware. I am sorry for your loss. Are you visiting the island?"

"Yeah, we came because . . . he died," I explained. "We were wondering—"

"Of course," he interrupted. "You must get the death certificate at the clerk's office on Fort Oranjestraat. Bring it to the hospital and have the attending physician fill it out. Then you must bring it to the census office, where it must be authorized, and then you may bring it to the lieutenant governor's office to have it signed. Then the body will be released."

Anais produced a handful of rubber-banded white index cards and a pen and scribbled down some notes.

"Great. That's . . . thanks," I said. "Also, we were hoping to get his stuff."

Morago's phone rang, and he didn't hesitate to answer. "Captain speaking. Yes." He ignored us. Toby shook his head, frustrated. I tried to keep my cool.

When the captain hung up, I continued. "You confiscated some of his property."

"Yes. Standard procedure," he said. "We must make sure there was no foul play."

Anais interjected. "Oh? Is there suspicion?"

"I cannot discuss that with you at this time," he said, waving his hand. "I'm sure you understand."

We didn't understand, and couldn't take him all that seriously either.

"Do you have any information about the cause of death?" Toby asked.

He threw up his hands dramatically. "These are delicate matters. You must discuss that with the doctor."

We weren't entirely sure what that meant. I continued. "Okay . . . well, we wanted to get his computer and mobile phone. Uh, you did take that stuff?"

"Yes. Everything is safe," he said, crossing his arms.

"It's just that we need to find his contact list." Anais tried to justify the request. "To let them know what happened. It's very important to us. His phone, his laptop."

"You have that stuff?" Toby asked again.

Morago nodded. "I believe there is a password protecting the computer. Do you know the password?"

We looked back and forth to each other and shook our heads. None of us had any idea.

"It is locked up downstairs," he said.

"Great," I said. "That's great. But can we—"

"Come back tomorrow," he interrupted.

"Really? There's no way we can get it now?" I asked.

He shook his head firmly. Then he gestured to his wrist-watch without looking at it. "You must come back tomorrow."

We started to leave, and he called after us. "How long is your stay?"

"Uh, we don't know. We just got here," I said.

"I see. If you need anything, you come right to me. Okay?"

Nodding, we scrambled down the stairs, eager to escape. Outside, the rain had passed, and the sun was quickly drying the ground. The squall quelled the humidity, at least briefly.

Luuk looked at us, incredulous. "Where's the laptop and mobile?"

"Said we have to come back tomorrow," I said.

Luuk shook his head disapprovingly. I felt like we'd some-how failed a test.

"Well, come on then," he said.

CHAPTER 23

ONE FLEW OVER THE CUCKOO'S NEST

LUUK'S TRUCK BOUNCED over the cobblestone streets until he stopped in front of a nondescript office and hopped out. We waited with the sun beating down on us. I wanted to make small talk with Toby but couldn't think of anything to say. I closed my eyes instead. My freaky discovery of a few hours before felt like something I'd imagined. For a moment, I couldn't be certain that it really happened. I hadn't slept, and everything had been so overwhelming. Then the image appeared in my mind of my computer screen showing a photo of a teenage underwear model pasted in the margin alongside a description of my sister's breasts. I opened my eyes and Toby was holding out a bottle of water. I accepted it with a silent nod and took a long swig.

Eventually Luuk exited the building and handed me a crisp, unsealed manila envelope with a single sheet of paper inside. "Death cert," he grunted.

I squeezed the envelope so it bowed open like a fish's mouth and peeked inside. The form was blank. It also appeared to be in

Dutch. Toby looked over, seeing my apparent confusion, but I just shrugged and tucked the folder under my arm.

Luuk got back in the cab and we were off once again, rolling over the bumpy street through the heart of town, dodging a goat here and there, Luuk tapping his horn every time we passed a pedestrian. It was all becoming more familiar. Only a few hours, and already the goats and dogs and waves seemed normal to me.

Toby looked a little green. "You okay?" I asked.

He waved it away. "I'll be alright. My stomach is just . . ." he trailed off.

I cringed. "You want to ride in front?"

He shook his head. "This happens."

After a short drive, we pulled into another gravel parking lot in front of what appeared to be an abandoned hospital. A wide covered courtyard separated two primitive, single-story cement buildings. A faded, hand-painted red cross was visible on the wall facing us. The buildings were old and dilapidated. The concrete ground was cracked and crumbling, with a few rods of naked rebar sticking out wildly like gorgon, rusty snakes. I stared, trying to take it in.

"Well, this place ought to have something for your stomach," I joked.

Luuk led us into the courtyard past a row of concrete benches in what was probably once a nice grassy garden but was now just sunbaked dirt and a bit of trash. He peeked into the window of a locked door. Similar doors were spaced out every ten feet or so, each one leading to a tiny windowless office or examination room. I imagined a charmless Soviet preschool. The lack of humans was disconcerting.

"Hopefully the doctor is around here somewhere," Luuk muttered as he knocked on a few more locked doors.

"This is the hospital?" I finally said aloud. "I thought there was a whole medical school here."

"That's on the other side of the island, but there's no hospital there. It's just classrooms and such," Luuk explained. "Let's just say, when someone gets sick, we take the boat to Saint Kitts."

Anais, Toby, and I stared back at him expectantly.

"Of course, Joe refused," he continued.

What do you mean, of course? I thought, but I kept silent.

Finally, one of the doors opened, revealing a young woman in a nurse's coat. She led us around the corner to another building and into a small exam room. There, she introduced us to Dr. Merkey, a shriveled older man in a threadbare lab coat that looked decades old.

I handed over the folded-up birth certificate and the blank death certificate—a pair of flimsy paper bookends to a life. Luuk stepped outside to smoke his pipe. The three of us crowded over Merkey's shoulder and struggled to follow along as he filled out the certificate of death in Dutch. He wrote excruciatingly slowly, taking a full second or two to form each character. When he got to the section for cause of death, he paused and looked up at us.

"You examined the body?" I asked. He nodded.

"Do you know what killed him?" Toby asked.

"Vell," the doctor began, "dere is so many possibilities." His accent was different than the others we had heard. It was a mix of French and Slovak rounded out with the local island inflection. "Dere is no vay to know for sure." I was reminded of Count Chocula.

"Do you have a hunch?" I asked.

117

"They said he had a stomach infection," Anais added, trying to be helpful.

Toby chimed in, "We heard he was vomiting blood."

The doctor nodded slowly, his pen still hovering above the Cause of Death field.

"Was it diverticulitis?" Anais probed. Merkey shrugged. We were all getting impatient with his vague non-answers.

"To determine ze cause of death vith certainty, ve vould have to do ze autopsy. Zat can be arranged if you like."

We looked around at each other. "How long would that take?" I asked.

"Vell, ve vould have to fly ze body to Curaçao, schedule ze time with ze hospital. It could vell take a few days," he said.

I was still of the mind to get the body into the ground as quickly as possible, and I didn't see the point. But Toby was less sure. "Wouldn't it be good to know what happened?"

"I don't know," I said. "It'll take a lot of time and it's probably expensive. And for what? What difference does it really make?"

But Toby still seemed hesitant. Anais, watching him, softened.

"What do you recommend, Doctor?" Anais asked.

"It is your choice," Merkey answered unhelpfully.

"I don't think we should," I said. "But I want us all to be in agreement. We won't get another chance to revisit this."

Toby nodded, but he seemed unconvinced. "We'll never know what actually killed him."

I flashed to a conversation Dad and I had a few years before. It was around the time he was leaving New York and he was telling me about a skin condition he was suffering from, which had been getting worse. He was lamenting that he'd never be able to afford major end-of-life medical care. He said if he ever got cancer or

something serious like that, he'd take his own life. He bragged that he knew how to do it—the right combination of drugs and so on. I didn't give it all that much thought at the time, but now suddenly I was left to wonder: Was that what happened? Did he kill himself? Was that why he refused to go to the real hospital on Saint Kitts?

I looked to Toby. "You're right," he finally said. "It doesn't matter."

Slowly, one character at a time, Merkey scrawled *onbekend* under cause of death.

"What does that mean?" I asked.

"Cause of ze death is unknown," he explained.

The doctor slowly folded the document into thirds and slipped it into an envelope before handing it back to me. As we got ready to go, he asked us when we planned to return.

"Return for what?" Toby asked.

"To retrieve ze body," he said matter-of-factly.

Toby and Anais both looked to me, but I had no idea. "Well, tomorrow I guess. We're hoping to have the funeral tomorrow afternoon, so . . ."

He nodded.

"Is there someone who . . . prepares it, that we should coordinate with?" I asked, not really sure what preparations were necessary.

"It is ze family's responsibility."

"Right. Of course," I said. "Um, but we've never . . . We don't have any idea—"

"There's a nurse here, Winika. She has ze experience vith zat. She may be able to help you. But you must arrive by two. And have ze paperwork finished, or ze body cannot be released."

I nodded, completely convinced that we were never, ever going to get off of this cursed island.

CHAPTER 24

UNDER THE ROOFS
OF PARIS

WHEN I WAS NINETEEN, Dad invited me to take a three-week trip with him to France. It was the summer of my sophomore year of college, and it would be my first time out of the country. I tried to pretend that it was no big deal when he asked, but inside I was positively giddy. I had friends who had visited Europe for the summer after graduating high school, as was the custom for a certain class of East Coast suburban teenager. I knew one guy who had taken a whole year off to backpack Asia. But my mom didn't have that kind of money, and I didn't have the balls to strike out on my own. I had relegated that fantasy to some eventual future when I was more self-reliant and/or more adventurous.

It would also be the first time in several years that Dad and I would be spending a significant chunk of time together, which I foolishly thought would be great and connective.

When the time came, we boarded a Pakistani Airlines 747 out of JFK on a flight that took off around four in the morning. Paris was just a refueling layover on the way to Karachi, so the

tickets were exceptionally cheap. This was a decade before 9/11, and flying on a foreign carrier meant there were basically no rules. Smoking was allowed, even in the lavatory, and while the frayed seats were equipped with seatbelts, there was no one encouraging us to use them. The plane was quite empty, and we were able to stretch out, each of us taking over a whole five-seat middle row, where we could lay down and try to sleep.

A few hours in, the flight attendants came around in their olive-green and orange uniforms to serve a meal. It was breakfast time, and I was naively confused when we were served lamb curry with jasmine rice instead of eggs or oatmeal. Dad patiently explained that American breakfast traditions were hardly shared around the globe.

When we arrived at Charles de Gaulle, I was loopy with jet lag and getting cranky. Dad showed off his comfort with the foreign city by translating the various signs we passed as we walked through the airport, but when he attempted to address the immigration guard in French, his accent was bad enough that the guy responded in English.

He stopped in front of a tiny vendor's stall in the airport lobby to buy cigarettes. Gitanes Brunes were his favorite, but the Gauloises were cheaper. He asked which I wanted, and I chose the former, so he bought a pack of those for me and a pack of the cheap ones for himself.

When he got the change, he handed me a small wad of fifty or sixty Francs "just in case anything happens." I was impressed by the amount, not yet comprehending the six-to-one exchange rate. I stuffed the cash into my Velcroed fabric travel wallet and took out one of the smokes to give it a try. By the time it was lit, I looked up to see Dad already twenty feet ahead of me, rushing

off, nearly lost in the crowd. I grabbed my giant suitcase and scampered to keep up with him.

I kept my eyes trained on the back of his head and followed him to the entrance of the metro station. He tossed me a token for the turnstile, and as soon as we got to the platform he stepped onto one of the trains without warning just as it started rolling, leaving me little time to hoist my luggage onto the moving car.

He took me straight to the Rive Gauche. As soon as we emerged from the Art Nouveau-styled metro stop, I was blown away by how striking and different it all looked and yet how much it also felt like Greenwich Village. I immediately felt at home. He casually pointed out Notre Dame, the Seine, and a café where Hemingway used to hang out. He sprinted down Boulevard Saint-Michel, and I fought to keep up, though every few feet I wanted to stop and photograph a sculpture, or order a crepe from a street vendor, or gawk at the impossibly glamorous women just going about their banal, quotidian lives. But I knew the drill. Looking like a tourist made you both rude and a potential target—keep your nose to the ground, walk fast, and ignore everyone around you. Still, I couldn't help myself.

He held his nose as we passed Boulevard Saint-Germain, idly complaining about how fashion and commerce was determined to spoil this important historical district. I nodded in emphatic agreement, though it was impossible not to appreciate how picturesque it all looked.

I wanted to stop at a café, but he insisted we first go get a room and put down our stuff. We turned on the Rue Des Ecoles and headed toward the elegant plaza of the Sorbonne, which was swarming with graceful college students, but before we got to

the plaza, we took a quick left down an alley and arrived at a tiny, unmarked guesthouse.

Dad spoke French to the man at the desk and secured us a *chambre pour deux*. Our room was up three flights of stairs so narrow my suitcase wouldn't fit around the corners. We had to hold it sideways and hand it over the banister at each floor level. He ridiculed me for bringing such a big bag while he was making do with a satchel, and half-jokingly threatened to throw it down the stairs behind us.

When we finally got to the room, a vague disquiet crept up my spine. It was tiny—smaller than my college dorm room, and smaller even than that fleapit on East Houston. There were two single cots set a few feet apart from each other, each bare to the stripes of the stained mattress ticking.

"Where's the bathroom?" I asked.

"Down the hall. That's the way they do things in Europe. You share the bathroom with the rest of the guests. It's much more civilized this way. You get to know people, you're not so lazy. Hey, do you know what they call the bathroom?"

I shrugged.

"La doubla-vay-say." He grinned. "The WC, for *water closet*. Isn't that funny?"

"Wouldn't it be the *closet of water*? Don't they put the adjectives second? Say-doubla-vay," I said proudly.

He shook his head dismissively. "No. It's WC."

There was so much I wanted to do and see, but I quickly learned that our entire trip would be regulated by two things: activities that were free, and the irregular geography of tobacco vendors. I had packed a carton of cigarettes in my suitcase and brought them with me from the States. Dad bought his one pack

at a time, which meant that twice a day we had to stop whatever we were doing to go and find a place to buy smokes. On numerous occasions, we missed out on other opportunities to ensure he was *avec le tabac*. For the whole trip, I felt like we were in a sprint, though I wasn't sure why. He seemed skittish, distracted. More than once I caught his face twisted in a dark grimace—though if he saw me looking, he'd quickly wink and switch to his trademark smile.

Of the many museums I wanted to see, I was only able to visit a fraction because the others had expensive entry fees or required a taxi to get to. We went to visit the Eiffel Tower, but Dad insisted that it was much more enjoyable and authentic to appreciate it from the grand lawns at its base rather than from the overly crowded, super-touristy lookout platform at the top. That, and the forty francs per person for the elevator ride up.

He took me to Place Denfert-Rochereau to visit the catacombs. I was enthralled and excited as we descended hundreds of feet to the ancient caverns below the city streets. He explained how, when the cemeteries filled up in the eighteenth century, the city had to disinter thousands of bodies. "But the French being French, they chose to pool all the remains and artfully arrange the skulls and bones into decorative piles and clusters, epitomizing the beautiful but haunting word *macabre*." He rolled the *r* of that last word in an exaggerated way that made me smile.

Despite France's reputation for having the world's finest and most delectable cuisine, he had figured out how to eat on the cheap, and that's what we did. We'd collect a roast chicken from a rotisserie and a fresh baguette from a boulangerie and head out to a nearby park bench. Add a fresh lemon, and you have what he called a *picnic Parisian*.

He'd cut the lemon in half with his pocketknife so we could

squeeze a few drops of lemon juice onto the bread, and then we'd alternate a bite of chicken and a bite of lemony bread. I don't know whether he made up the name, but I confess I felt urbane and cosmopolitan eating like the locals. It was delicious the first time, but that became our evening meal—every night.

And lunch was the same idea, but instead of a *poulet*, we'd get a wedge of brie cheese, and instead of lemon, he'd lift packets of cheap mustard from a street vendor. That was the routine until I just stopped eating. Between that and the endless walking—no one takes the Metro in the Parisian summer heat—I lost ten pounds over the three-week trip.

On our last day before we were to head south, we made our way out to Père Lachaise cemetery to view the famous graves of Balzac, Chopin, Proust, Oscar Wilde, and, most important to me, Jim Morrison. The cemetery was a long train ride from the center of Paris, and we didn't arrive until after 4:00 p.m., leaving us less than an hour until closing. It wasn't much time, as it was a large area and the graves that I wanted to see were spread out.

But before we could go in, Dad insisted on grabbing a pack of Gauloises. The problem was that most of the shops in the area were closed because it was Sunday. So, we wound up walking around the perimeter of the cemetery for more than half an hour looking for an open shop. I grew angrier and angrier until I finally sprinted off away from him, determined to at least get to visit Morrison's grave site before the gates were closed.

We left Paris the next day. At my begging, we splurged and took the TGV to save six hours on our journey to the Cote d'Azur. We rented a room at a cheap seaside motel in Nice. From there we took day trips, including one to Avignon (to traverse the famous *pont*, among other things), and on that particular day we

missed the last train back to Nice because, you guessed it: Dad had to stop and buy more smokes. He was furious that missing the train cost us another night's hotel, but somehow it never occurred to him that it was his own damn fault.

And we fought, constantly, over the opportunities missed because of his poor scheduling, about the repetitive nature of our days, and over many other things. ("Why not, just this one time, buy TWO PACKS AT ONCE?") And he was loathe to indulge in anything that even evoked sightseeing.

"The goal is to feel what it's like to be a local. That's what travel is all about. Doing laundry. Going to a supermarket. Looking beneath the veneer. It's not about getting taken advantage of at tourist traps," he lectured.

"But I want to go to the Louvre! I'm in Paris. How is that too much to ask?"

Three weeks never felt so interminable. I was there for adventure and to explore and to submerge myself in new experiences. He was there to hide out and avoid his debt at home while he figured out what his next move was going to be. I was a thorn in his side—always wanting new activities every day—and he was constantly blunting any thrill or excitement I felt about being abroad.

When I arrived home, I promptly quit smoking. I was so grossed out by the extent and intensity of his addiction that I wanted to distance myself as far as I could from that, and from anything that might resemble aping him or his bullshit values. I set a goal to taper off over a week, and by day three I was done. Forever. I also swore off brie cheese.

And we didn't talk for more than nine months. Just one of many times we took an extended break.

CHAPTER 25
THE SECRET GARDEN

RETURNING FROM THE ISLAND HOSPITAL, we arrived back at the resort, and Belinda and the dogs were at the gate waiting for us. Ignoring my siblings, the dogs again attacked me, covering me with their disgusting mix of slobber and muddy paw prints.

I led Toby and Anais through Dad's door and into the dark living room. I was the expert since I had been there an hour and a half longer than they had. The two of them treaded delicately through the room, taking it all in, examining a detail here or there, just as I had done when I arrived. I became flooded with a reminder of the unpleasant surprise I unearthed and furtively scanned the room to make sure I didn't somehow leave any trace of evidence.

"This is where he was living?" Toby was taken aback by the crowded, dark room.

Anais went straight to the bookcase and ran her hands along the rows of distressed and illegible spines. She began to tear up but smiled. "I always felt like the books were a part of him. You know?"

I nodded. "That smell," I added.

"Yeah," they both agreed in unison. We all shared a smile.

Luuk appeared at the door. "Anais, we've got a second room for you, and we figured the two of you boys can bunk here in Joe's place."

We looked around at each other, and Toby answered first. "Sure. Fine. Cool with me." He looked to me. "Unless you want your own room . . ."

I desperately wished I could have some time and space to be alone, and I wasn't crazy about spending the night in the place where the man died. "No, no. Sure. That's fine," I said.

"That's really generous of you," Anais said to Luuk. "I mean, of course we'll pay for the room . . ." She looked to me for what I guess was permission. I shrugged affirmatively.

"I'll tally everything up and give you all a bill once we're through with everything, if that's okay with you," Luuk explained.

Again, Anais and Toby both darted their eyes to me. How did I get to be the dad? I nodded magnanimously—as if there was any other possible response.

"If it's alright, Linda wants to show you something," Luuk said. "Come on."

We headed back outside, and Belinda led Luuk and the three of us down a path through an overgrown meadow just north of the resort property. The sun had retreated behind some clouds and a light breeze came in off the water, providing a momentary reprieve from the oppressive heat. I closed my eyes and felt the wind cool the back of my neck and my forehead where my skin was wet.

Anais walked beside Belinda a few yards ahead, pontificating about something or another. I closed my eyes, wishing I could

close my ears to my sister's untiring chatter and disappear into silence, even for a few minutes. I slowed my pace to let them get a bit farther ahead, and I trained my ears instead to the crunching of my footsteps on the grass.

On the far side of the meadow we passed through a small patch of trees, where the ground was covered with bramble. My steps grew louder, crushing the sticks and dried leaves beneath me. I plodded through the crumbling remnants of a massive tree that must have fallen many years before. Uninvited, my father's voice suddenly filled my head, explaining the natural processes of how a dead tree feeds the rest of the forest, as if he was narrating his own personal nature documentary. "Termites and rodents and worms all work symbiotically to erode the body of the fallen giant," he lectured in the pedantic but authoritative tone that I both craved and detested, "decomposing it—literally removing its composition—and spreading the bark and the cellulose fibers from the tree's core to create an ideal fertilizer for young saplings. Nature's perfect system to turn death into renewal . . ."

Beyond the small grove of forest, another meadow appeared, and I saw the rest of the group had stopped and gathered at one spot. As I approached, I noticed a modest, flat gravestone embedded in the earth.

"This is my daughter Eleanor," Belinda explained to me as I stepped up.

The date on the stone said 2005.

Anais, the self-trained herbalist, was mid-lecture, picking up where Dad's voice in my head left off, gesturing to the flora around us. "Aboriginals believed agrimony flowers to be a source of protection. And milkweed symbolizes transformation and rebirth—probably because of the association with butterflies and

their metamorphosis—but still, it is a great symbolic endorsement. Oh, Max, I think this is a perfect spot."

Belinda continued. "Joe asked to be buried on the island, and we'd be honored to have him here. He was part of the family as much as anyone."

Yet again, they all looked to me for some kind of final approval. I resented being the de facto authority. Still the man of the house, regardless of my qualifications or lack thereof.

"I don't know. That path is pretty narrow; we're supposed to carry him all the way out here? Wouldn't it be easier to do this in a traditional cemetery? You do have a regular cemetery here on the island, right? Not just that historic Jewish one?" I felt compelled to offer some competing suggestion, though in fact, I really didn't care. "They probably have paved paths and a machine to dig the hole."

"You may be overestimating the level of modern convenience you'll find." Luuk smiled, trying to ascertain the real source of my hesitation. As was I. "Around here," he continued, "no matter where you choose, the family is responsible for everything. Including digging the grave, supplying a marker, pretty much the whole kit and kaboodle. And I think the most sophisticated hole-digging device you're going to find is a shovel."

My body involuntarily began to collapse inward, but Anais lit up.

"I love it. It's like we've gone back in time. Dad would have loved the simple connection with nature, don't you think?"

I looked to Toby for support, but his gaze wisely stayed fixed on the sunlight dazzling the blue sea beyond the cliff's edge. I turned back to Luuk and Belinda, who stood together hand in hand near Eleanor's grave, waiting patiently for me to come to a decision.

Meanwhile, Anais had picked up a fallen milkweed flower's seedpod. Long past its bloom, it was now full of feathery wisps, like a dandelion's. She lifted it to her lips and blew with a calm, blissful kiss, scattering the seeds into the air as if she was making a wish. What could she possibly be wishing for?

I found myself full of rage toward her, which I couldn't explain. Was I blaming the victim? Should I have felt pity? Should the revelation about my dad's sexual fantasies have informed my understanding of who she was? Why she was the way she was? Did it justify the particular, unique way she was broken? Was it supposed to negate how annoying she could be? Did it mean that now I had to be supportive in a way that I never was? I was supposed to carry her even more than I already did?

I was tired of carrying her. I was tired of being the bigger person. Of protecting her. Of protecting him. I was trying to protect everyone except for me. And I was done. I was tired of sacrificing myself for everyone else's needs. I just couldn't do it anymore.

"Fine. Okay. This is our spot," I said.

"Oh, exquisite," Anais cooed.

"Works for me," said Toby.

"Great," Luuk said jovially. "Now let's go build a coffin."

CHAPTER 26
THE INGENIOUS GENTLEMAN, DON QUIXOTE OF LA MANCHA

LUUK DROVE US BACK INTO TOWN, stopping in front of a row of corrugated steel garage doors in what looked like an unmarked storage facility. I had no idea where we were or what we were doing there. Looking around, Anais and Toby seemed equally perplexed. Luuk got out of the truck and banged loudly on one of the large doors. The noise reverberated like thunder. No one responded, so he banged again, and then we heard a muffled voice from behind the corrugated steel. A moment later the door began to roll up, and a slight Rastafarian man slipped out from under the rolling gate. He looked like he had just woken up, even though it was approaching midafternoon.

"For fuck's sake, mon!" the man yelled, but seeing Luuk he calmed down, and he and Luuk exchanged a few words that I couldn't hear. Then Luuk waved us over.

"This is Reggie." Luuk introduced us. "He was a friend of your father."

Reggie shook Toby's hand and gave Anais a polite hug, then he stared at me and a huge smile broke across his face.

"Jah jah, bless!" he exclaimed. "Little Joe!" I smiled and nodded. Then he grabbed me and hugged me fiercely. "Me and Joe was close," he began. "We are all so very sad! We was soul brothers, you know?" He banged his chest.

Luuk translated. "Reggie was Joe's *supplier*."

"Yeah, mon," Reggie continued enthusiastically. "And I build all-a-them bookshelves. He crazy with all-a-them books! But he pay me! He say the books belong here! So I done a good job and build him what he needs."

Luuk jumped in. "Reggie's a woodworker. I thought maybe he could help us out."

I nodded, understanding, but I realized that Luuk expected us to ask him ourselves.

Reggie looked at each of us up and down. "You all his kids." He nodded, and we nodded back. "A terrible, terrible thing has happened, mon. I went to see him on . . . it was Monday. Yah, last Monday. He was no good."

Luuk gave me a look.

"Yes, I know," I said, trying to cut in. "We, uh, we need . . ." I looked to Luuk, who nodded again. "We need a coffin. For his body. Is that something you could help us with?"

Reggie turned deadly serious. "Ah, of course. Of course. It would be my honor."

"Do you know—" I turned to Luuk. "Does he know how to build a coffin? I mean it's got to be—"

Reggie cut me off. "Yah, I build one last year. For my son." He lowered his eyes.

"Oh shit," I said. "I'm sorry."

Anais winced. "Oooh. I'm so sorry!" Toby mumbled an obligatory apology too.

Reggie smiled wistfully. "Yah, it was smaller." He held his arms about four feet apart. "But same, same. I take care of it. It's an honor, for Doctor Joe." His smile widened, proud.

I looked to Luuk, hoping he could help us deal with negotiating a price, but Luuk didn't seem concerned. "Do you want to build it at the resort? We have space there," he offered.

"Yeah, yeah, sure. Good idea, mon," Reggie said.

"We want to have the funeral tomorrow. Is that possible?" Anais asked.

"Oh, I don't know. I can try. Yah?"

We all offered our thanks and each of us hugged him goodbye before retreating to the truck, but then he followed us over and hopped in the back with us. I didn't quite know what was going on, but Luuk seemed to, so I didn't say anything. Reggie, Anais, and I all sat in the back of the pickup, and Toby sat in the front with Luuk.

Luuk yelled out, "One more stop!" before lurching the vehicle into gear.

We wound through several more back alleys and pulled up in front of a small, one-room house with a wooden deck in front and a red clay tile roof with an oversized antenna piercing out of it.

"Radio station," Luuk explained.

I had no idea why we needed to stop at the radio station, but I was grateful Luuk had a plan. Reggie stayed in the truck, and at Luuk's urging, the rest of us headed into the small house.

Inside, a striking young dreadlocked woman with well-worn headphones on sat in a DJ booth. Adjacent to her was a

small recording room with a few mics and musical instruments strewn about.

The DJ waved warmly to all of us and motioned for us to come join her in the booth, but held up her finger for us to wait a moment while she finished reading a weather report from a sheet of paper. "And we can expect a cooling trend by the end of the week as the trade winds make their way to our fair isle. But, in the meantime, we be hot, hot, hot! Enjoy the sunshine and be sure to keep an eye on your livestock."

"What are we doing here?" Toby asked me quietly.

I shrugged.

Anais seemed to know what was going on. "We're gonna broadcast an announcement about the funeral, so people on the island will know when and where it is."

"How did you . . . ?" I asked her, a bit suspicious.

She shrugged, faux-smug, then explained. "Don't be a yutz, Max. Luuk and I discussed it earlier."

"Really?" Toby asked.

"Apparently, people around here listen to the radio."

I wandered into the recording room and picked up a brightly painted maraca. I gave it a little shake, and the DJ brusquely tapped on the glass to silence me. A moment later she finished her report and put on a Jimmy Cliff song.

She invited us all into the booth with her. "Welcome!" she said. "I'm so sorry about Doctor Joe. I'm Chevelle."

We exchanged greetings, and she hugged each of us with sincere tenderness. She explained that we should record an announcement about the funeral, and she would broadcast it a few times that day and the next.

"Is it normal to do this?" I asked.

"Everybody loved Doctor Joe. They'll all want to know about the funeral."

Chevelle set us up in the recording room, and then she retreated back to the booth. The three of us stood there dumbly, and when she cued us, it was Anais who took the lead—and nailed it in a single take:

"Please join us at four p.m. on Thursday, April 24, to celebrate the life and passing of Herschel Wohl, or as most of you know him, 'Doctor Joe.' We'll be gathering at the Paradise Point Inn and walking to the burial site from there. A cold cut buffet will be served afterward." She nodded to Chevelle, who pressed a button and flipped a switch on her soundboard.

"You're a natural!" Chevelle said.

"A cold cut buffet?" I was baffled and suddenly outraged. "Where do you think we are? Scarsdale? There's no fucking buffet. We don't have time. We don't even have a way to . . . Where the hell are we even supposed to get that? Why would we do such a thing? Why do you always have to make things more difficult? We have enough crap to deal with!"

Toby found it hysterically funny. And I could see Chevelle trying to hide her smile too. I was not smiling.

"I don't think providing light refreshments to the guests who are moved to attend our father's funeral is crap, Michael. It's basic human kindness. It's a time-honored tradition that deserves to be upheld. This is what civilization is."

"Well fuck civilization. Fuck cold cuts. Fuck it all."

I stormed out of the radio station, knowing full well everyone was laughing at me, but I couldn't help it. Outside, I tried to take a deep breath, but the humid air and hot sun undercut any relief I might have hoped for. I looked up and fixed my gaze upon

a small power station nearby. Two large windmills were rotating in a loping rhythm, their long blades slicing through the air with surprising force. I watched them go around and around. Imagining their sound, their pulsing, breathing whoosh. A red roof beam behind the propellers was glinting brightly from the sun, flickering on and off with each rotation of the vanes. A puff of steam chugged out of an exhaust valve in the building behind the structures, and for a moment it looked like the windmill was breathing fire. I squinted to blur my eyes and encourage the vision. Here be dragons, I thought. Here be dragons.

As I struggled to regain my cool, I noticed Luuk was by his truck, chatting with a couple of local guys. One was large and muscular, wearing a torn and dirty tank top. The other was very short but also well-built with thick, bumpy hair that radiated out in every direction, making his face look like a bronze caricature of the sun. After a moment, the two guys climbed into the back of the truck and began chatting with Reggie. Luuk saw me and walked over. He was looking at me oddly, and I realized my face was still twisted into a scowl. I switched to a fake smile.

"Who are those guys?" I asked, probably too aggressively.

"Well, in this context, they would be your grave diggers."

"Ah," I nodded, relieved that he was one step ahead of me. "Uh, how much do we need to pay them?"

"Well, kind of a seller's market at the moment, isn't it?" He patted me on the back. "Don't worry. We'll work it out. Everything go okay in there?"

I shrugged, but a moment later Anais and Toby came out and joined us, all smiles. We climbed back into the now crowded truck, shook hands with the new guys, and quickly descended into silence as Luuk jammed the truck into gear. The tires spun

against the gravel for a moment before they gained traction, and we bumped and rattled our way back to Paradise Point.

CHAPTER 27
STILL LIFE WITH WOODPECKER

ANAIS, TOBY, AND I sat on the dining veranda looking out at the sun sinking toward the gorgeous cerulean Caribbean, while Luuk and Belinda cooked. Another couple, guests at the resort, drank wine at one of the other tables. The Great Danes ran back and forth throughout the room. Bambi jumped up to put her forepaws on my lap until Belinda yelled, and then the dog just flopped down at my feet.

Belinda took in the scene. "You must smell like him. They loved Joe."

Next, she fed a bite of carrot to an enormous macaw that perched near the kitchen. The bird was named Maggie, and I asked if she could talk. "She used to speak to Eleanor, but now she just talks in Parrot," Belinda joked. They considered the bird a pet, though she seemed to come and go of her own volition. As if to demonstrate that point, she leapt off her perch with a deafening squawk and lunged into the fan palms nearby.

Meanwhile, Anais lectured about the history of Jews on Statia. As the American revolution was brewing, the British captured the island. They let the French and even the American merchants flee, but they singled out the Jews, imprisoned them, and stole all their possessions. Familiar story, I thought, quietly wishing she would just shut up. But Belinda was deeply engaged, and Toby seemed fascinated too.

After a while, Reggie appeared from the parking area. "Excuse me, Mister Luuk? I be needin' the wood." Luuk and I followed him back down to an area next to the pool that had been cleaned out for him to work. He had a couple sawhorses set up and an old beat-up circular saw was plugged into a wall. A bag of carpentry tools was splayed open on the ground nearby, and there were a few miscellaneous boards of wood, but, as he explained, it was nowhere near enough to make the coffin.

"We need go order from Mr. Frank on Nevis, yah? Take the boat over tomorrow maybe?"

I shook my head. "We really need to get this done and have the funeral tomorrow. Isn't there anywhere on this island to buy lumber?"

The two exchanged looks, but both shook their heads. "No, mon. I's sorry," Reggie said.

I rolled my eyes. This godforsaken island! We couldn't drag this out another day. I just needed to the get the hell out of there before I crawled out of my skin.

I looked around, hoping for inspiration. There was a wooden shed on the edge of the parking area, Could we steal a few boards from there? How much wood do you need for a coffin? I shifted to calculation mode: *Length times width times height cubed.* No, wait, that's volume. My brain churned while another part of me seemed

to float above my body. I realized how ridiculous the whole situation was. How surreal. What was I doing there? It all felt so crazy.

Then, an idea popped into my mind. "What about the bookcases?" I suggested.

"What do you mean?" Luuk asked.

I made a prying gesture. "Use the wood from Dad's bookcases. He won't be needing them, and the next tenant's not likely to have quite so many books, right?"

Reggie smiled and gave a thumbs up. "Yeah, mon!"

Luuk smiled with a shrug and headed back to the dining room to recruit Toby to help. I led Reggie over toward Dad's bungalow. When we arrived, I opened the door, but Reggie hesitated and took a few steps back.

"Come on," I said. "You can come in."

"No, no, I can't be going in there. Outta respect. For the ghosts. You know, mon?"

At first, I thought he was joking, but it quickly became clear that he wasn't. He handed me his cordless drill. "Here. The sideboards are bolted to the studs. I did it that way cuz it was so heavy wit all-a-them books."

I shook my head and almost laughed at his superstition, but I didn't want to appear disrespectful to his belief. Then, just as I reached the threshold of the door, I got an odd chill that made me pause before entering.

"I go git da wagon. You load it up out here, okay, mon?"

Inside, I stood in front of the bookcases, admiring the scale of it all, impressed with Reggie's work. Eight massive shelves covered the width of the wall, stretching from floor to ceiling. Each shelf was made of two hefty, inch-thick, solid wood planks, each about a yard wide and a foot deep. Notched vertical planks

supported the shelves' considerable weight. It was all real hardwood in a range of grain colors and knottiness, giving the whole thing an attractive, rustic quality. I assumed that was more out of necessity than design, but what did I know?

I wasn't sure where to begin disassembling the whole thing, so I started by moving books from the shelves to the floor, taking special care to keep the organization intact, even though there was no plausible reason to do so.

Anais rushed in, with Toby and Luuk a few steps behind. She was distraught. "Are you sure about this?"

"What's the harm?" I asked.

"I like the idea," Toby said. "We were just saying the books are a part of him, what better way to honor that than this?"

Anais eventually came around, and the three of us made quick work of emptying the shelves. I spied that Anais seemed to also attempt to keep the books arranged in Dad's idiosyncratic order. Toby used the drill to remove the vertical boards, which were bolted into the wall, and within an hour we had the whole thing dismantled and moved outside. It was surprisingly heavy and awkward, but Toby, with his bulging arm muscles, easily hoisted three shelves onto his shoulder at once. I was embarrassed that I could only manage one at a time.

The bungalow was a mess. While the books were shelved they seemed orderly and manageable, but now—piled on the floor, on the desk, and all over the rest of the bungalow—the prodigious volume of his collection was apparent. We cleared a path from the sleeping area to the bathroom and agreed to deal with the rest of it later, which reminded me that emptying the bungalow of all his belongings was going to be no small task, physically or emotionally.

CHAPTER 28
THE OUTSIDERS

THE PHYSICAL LABOR made us hungry, so we found our way back up to the dining area, eager but exhausted. When we got there, we were introduced to Dad's best friend on the island, Ralph, and his partner, Robin. Both were expat Americans like Dad was, likely in their late sixties or early seventies. I remember Marcy telling me that Ralph also taught at the medical school.

Belinda served up sautéed whitefish, mashed potatoes, and summer squash, on big plates that we all shared from. It felt more like a home-cooked meal from a friend than something you'd get in a restaurant—not least because Luuk and Belinda sat down and joined us.

I couldn't help wondering how much they were charging us for our meals. Luuk already made it clear that he was charging rent for Anais's room. I much preferred an explicit exchange than some nebulous "favor" they were doing for us, and things like this, sharing a family meal, blurred the lines, which made me uncomfortable.

Anais (blissfully ignorant that there was any money involved)

was overcome with how warm and generous everyone was toward us. "I'm so happy to know he found a place, a home," she began. "He moved around so much, and it really seems like he found a home here. You know? With all of you." She started to cry. "At least for this last part of his life. He had been so lost."

"Thank you, sweetie," Belinda said.

Anais regained her composure. "Sorry." She laughed away her tears. "I just mean to say, this is a beautiful, special place you have here."

I tried to imagine what it would have been like for Dad to live there, the weird mix of a hotel and a boarding house set in the most spectacular of settings but built by hand and with whatever materials they could throw together. It was unique, that's for sure, but I wouldn't have called it beautiful. Everything about the place carried a certain whiff of reclusion, of keeping the rest of the world at bay. It was a place people came to get away from their old lives, their real lives. To hide out, which was exactly what Dad was doing. I looked around at our hosts and the new guests. I wondered what each was escaping.

As the sun's light began to fade, Luuk turned on a string of Italian wedding lights that ran all along the perimeter of the dining area. Everything beyond the deck became inky black in every direction. It felt like we were on a boat in the middle of a vast, vast ocean. We ate our dinner and drank the wine that Ralph and Robin brought. As everyone started in on their second glass, the conversation turned to reminiscing about Dad.

"He would always have one of his adoring students around," Ralph joked.

"I don't know how he got them, but there was Francesca, and Marcy, and Liz . . ." Luuk continued.

Robin jumped in. "There were two Lizzes, remember?" The two older couples laughed. The three of us siblings smiled politely.

"Robin mixed them up once," Ralph explained.

"He'd have these women flying in from the States," Robin started.

"Or Paris!" Luuk interrupted.

"How long was he with Natasha?" Anais asked, referring to the woman who emailed us about his death, but nobody knew. "Hmm," she continued. "He never mentioned her."

"Not to me either," I said, suddenly realizing that we maybe should have invited her for the funeral.

"Oh, he had, to me," Toby interjected. "She was one of his students. She moved to New York, and he wanted me to take her out and show her around, but it fell through."

Sounds familiar, I thought. I darted a look to Anais, but realized she never knew about Dad trying to set me up with Marcy.

"I'll sure miss his cooking," Belinda said. "He was a whiz."

"Oh yeah!" Ralph said. "He was an outstanding chef."

"The two of them would fight over cumin," Robin explained.

"We wouldn't fight," Ralph argued.

Robin contradicted him with a look. Everyone laughed.

"Cumin activates the parasympathetic nervous system, encourages salivation, reduces heart rate, constricts blood vessels—"

"That would take a lot of cumin," Anais said.

"Have you ever tried Joe's chili?" Ralph quipped, getting another laugh out of everyone.

"I never thought he could cook much more than a tuna fish sandwich," I said.

"I remember he made a pretty good omelet," Anais said.

Luuk and Belinda chimed in on cue: "With thyme!" "Yes!" Anais laughed.

"Who puts thyme in an omelet?" Belinda asked.

"And so much of it!" Luuk continued. "He had a—"

"It's still there," Belinda interrupted. "There's a thyme bush right outside his kitchen window. You all should help yourselves!"

"Joe and I used to get into it about conventional medicines too," Ralph continued. "He could go on for hours about the metabolic response to the alkalizing agents in a compound like acetaminophen."

"So could you, darling, and let's not bore them," Robin chided.

"And politics," Luuk added.

"Yes, at least we're all inveterate communists." Ralph smiled and raised his glass.

"Hear, hear!" Everyone toasted to that, though I caught a quiet look of confusion from Toby through the maze of arms and wine glasses. I don't think Toby was all that comfortable calling himself a communist.

"I don't know. Joe had some libertarian tendencies," Belinda chimed in.

"Ah, that's likely just selfishness," I said, trying to maintain the breezy tone.

Toby and Anais smiled, but my joke fell a bit flat among the locals.

"Oh, Joe wasn't selfish," Belinda said earnestly. "He was always so quick to offer his help. And he was so smart about everything. He helped Luuk get rid of the opossums by having us put the coffee grounds over by the window."

CHAPTER 28: THE OUTSIDERS

"He always stayed to help out the students, giving so much of his time," Ralph agreed.

"And with the townspeople too. You saw how Reggie feels about him," Luuk said. "They're all like that." Luuk stared at me with a strange smile. "He may have had some faults, but everyone loved Doctor Joe."

"Oh, Joe, we miss you so," Robin said, tears in his eyes, gently patting Anais's arm.

They all raised their glasses and enjoyed another toast in his honor. I listened to the banter and all I could think was: Who were these people? And who the hell was Joe? They kept saying, *You know Joe!* But I didn't. Had he become a totally different person there, in that last chapter of his life? They certainly didn't sound like they were talking about the Hershel Wohl I knew. I felt like an alien. Like I had shown up to the wrong island. The wrong Earth.

At some point Luuk seemed to notice that the three of us children weren't participating all that much in the love fest. "You all must be bone tired, what with the jet lag and the circumstances and all."

We nodded weakly. That wasn't why we were quiet.

Luuk joined Anais, Toby, and me as we traversed the dark parking area. We were heading to our beds, but we stopped to check on Reggie, who had been hard at work on the coffin. "You wanna maybe give it a rest till the morning?" Luuk asked him.

"Sure, boss," Reggie said.

Anais headed off to her room, and Toby and I headed to Dad's bungalow. When we got inside, I was startled all over again by the piles of books everywhere, forgetting for a moment the bookcase pandemonium of a few hours before. I collapsed onto

the bed. Toby and I hadn't formally talked about who would sleep on the bed or on the sofa, and I didn't want to presume, so I kept all my clothes on. Almost immediately, sleep's ache crept over me. Combined with the wine, I felt like I was wearing one of those lead cloaks doctors drape over you when taking X-rays.

My laptop was connected to the Ethernet cable on Dad's desk, and Toby asked if he could use it to check his email. I had a moment of panic, wondering if there was any possibility I left some trace of my father's turpitude that Toby might discover. Of course there was no way, but I was compelled to make sure. I tried to concoct an excuse for me to get on first. "Let me get on there for a second first to make sure my porn-star friend hasn't sent me any friendly pictures that you're too young to see."

Toby scoffed, but he got his toothbrush and headed into the bathroom. I jumped up, despite my exhaustion, opened the laptop, and tried to log into the internet.

CHAPTER 29
THE MISANTHROPE

I SCANNED THE COMPUTER SCREEN for anything suspicious but found nothing. My email notifications lit up, and despite my exhaustion, I couldn't prevent the Pavlovian response to scan through it. Finally, there was a message from my investor, but it was bad news. He was withdrawing his interest. Something about an impending collapse in the real estate market. I didn't know what the hell he was talking about, but I didn't have the energy to dwell on it. I could add this to my list of false starts and regroup when I got home. If I ever got home. Most of the rest of my inbox was junk, spam, or just meaningless, at least from my current perspective. I had been online dating a lot, and there was a flurry of messages from various prospective dates. I knew better than to scare them off by telling them my father died, so instead I crafted a pithy rejoinder explaining that I was on a fabulous Caribbean vacation, then I copied and pasted that three times.

My romantic life had been a bit of a disaster—mostly a series of too-long monogamous relationships, none of which I really

committed to, save for the first one, which broke my heart. While in college in San Francisco, a flatmate of mine invited her sister from Colorado to visit for a weekend. On her first night there, Kelly and I stayed up the whole night together and bonded in a way vastly more intimate than anything I'd ever known before. She was unbearably cute, with a pixie haircut, a burst of freckles sprinkled across her nose and cheekbones, and a self-conscious smile that invited you in, like she was always sharing a secret. She was Irish (like my childhood crush Mary Ann O'Malley), and being from a big family, her perspective on relationships felt so much healthier and more insightful than my own. I was captivated. And it was mutual. Forty-eight hours later, as she prepared to go back to Boulder, we were already talking about love and our future together.

After she graduated, she moved to San Francisco and we spent seven years together. That was the period of time when I was working the job at the software company that my dad thought was such a betrayal of his values. And also at this time, perhaps coincidentally, his own world had been collapsing in on itself, leaving him financially desperate. He had been evicted (again) and wasn't sure how he was going to survive. A year or so after Kelly and I had moved in together, he called to say he was considering moving to San Francisco. The thought of him coming out to my city, to my safe place, and becoming my burden was more than I could stomach. I didn't know how to tell him, so instead I took it out on Kelly by acting erratically and irresponsibly, and also by growing increasingly depressed.

The software job had grown into a slog; the project that was supposed to take one year had stretched into four, with no end in sight. I became more deeply involved in the intricacies of design-ing software, and I had less and less time to produce my own

films. My job was interesting, but increasingly I began to feel like my dad had been right and that I had indeed given up my artistic dreams for the banal reward of a weekly paycheck.

And all the while, I was worried about Dad. His life was falling apart, and regardless of how much he may have been harming himself, it was dawning on me that, as his son, he might become my responsibility. At one point I tried to explain (in a letter to him) that I feared he was a drug addict, that his relationship to marijuana was, by any objective or rational observation, an addiction. I told him he owed it to himself to at least recognize that fact and see if it might be a cause for some of the problems he was experiencing in his life. He responded with rage.

"You don't know a fucking thing about me!" he wrote. "And clearly you know nothing about the world either. Go ahead and waste your own fucking life kissing corporate ass if you want to, but don't you dare ever tell me how to live mine!"

I was shaken by the wrath I had awoken in him. And not knowing how to respond, I just let it go. When we next talked a few months later, we both ignored the letters, pretending it had never happened, and all seemed to be well.

That would become a pattern. Every time I marshaled the courage to criticize him or express my disappointments, it would follow the same trajectory: I would speak up. He would explode and retaliate with personal attacks. Then, I would withdraw. We'd go a few months (or longer) without talking, and I'd eventually come back to him, pretending nothing had happened. He'd be friendly and eager to share some fascinating observation about art or nature or politics, and we'd be back "on track."

He never moved out to San Francisco, but soon after that exchange was when he asked to borrow five thousand dollars to

help him get back on his feet. I gave him the money, but the whole sequence of events really unnerved me. I didn't care so much about the cash (though it was a significant amount at the time), but I was thrown by his hypocrisy. Taking the money I had earned at the job he claimed was anathema was bad enough, but most disconcerting was the shamelessness with which he asked.

If he really was the selfish asshole that I had begun to suspect him to be, then the entire story of his virtuous role as a divine conduit of truth and art was undermined—he had dispelled the myth I had been relying on to justify and rationalize what other wise looked like pathetic, naked, cowardly selfishness. If that was true, then what else in the world might be true? The entirety of my belief system—my understanding of life and its purpose—was suddenly up for grabs. My depression descended into full-fledged existential crisis. I had lost the ability to trust anyone outside of myself. He was always unreliable, but now he had demonstrated that he was, in fact, destructive and even dangerous.

One day, while driving to a meditation center in Palo Alto, Kelly and I got into an argument. We very rarely fought, but after she let another driver cut us off without reprisal, I became enraged beyond reason.

"You can't just let people treat you like that!" I bellowed.

We parked outside the ivy-covered center of tranquility and calm, and I exploded, screaming at her about things that hardly warranted such vitriol. It wasn't long before she was talking about moving out.

•   •   •

I closed the email program on the laptop. "All yours," I called out

to Toby, and stumbled back over to the bed.

Toby came out of the bathroom and sat down at the computer. I looked over at the light coming from the bathroom and contemplated whether or not I really needed to go in there at all.

"That was a little weird back there, right?" Toby asked, without turning away from the screen.

"Yeah. I know, right?" I said. "Who the hell were they talking about?"

"Was Dad a communist?" he asked.

"I don't think they meant literally, like a follower of Lenin or anything," I tried to explain, realizing that in his youth, Toby might never have been exposed to the Old Left. I knew plenty of proud socialists from living in San Francisco. "He was a hippie. That's for sure. And I think to some people, that's kind of like being a communist."

Toby seemed to accept my explanation, and the conversation ended there. Seconds later, the warm darkness of sleep descended upon me.

CHAPTER 30

NIGHT

I AWOKE WITH A PANIC and grabbed at the ring of icy cold sweat around my neck. My eyes sprung open, and I stared at the ceiling above me. For a moment I couldn't place where I was. The smell of the place, the thickness of the air, and the constant shrill pulse of crickets were all foreign and unexpected to my confounded brain.

After a moment, my eyes came into focus, my ears registered what they were hearing, and my nose recognized that familiar mix of decaying paperbacks and years of pot smoke. It all came back to me: I was on a tiny island in the middle of the Atlantic Ocean, in my dead father's bungalow, while he lay in a morgue somewhere, waiting for me to put him in the ground.

There was no light in the room except for a sliver of moonlight coming in through the window, and so it took my eyes a few more moments before they could transmit any meaningful data to my brain. They fixed on a lightning-bolt-shaped crack that ran across part of the ceiling. I realized that I was looking through

his eyes, seeing exactly what he had seen. I scanned the bungalow: the blue moonlight peeking through the window, flickering
slightly as the window shade wavered in the breeze; the broken
closet door; the way the paint had begun to curl and flake off at
the corner where the wall reached the ceiling . . .

I turned and eyed the nightstand with the copy of *Kim* and
his pile of notecards still right where I had left them. Where he
had left them. I tried to imagine him lying here, just a few days
before. He was here. Right here. Lying here just as I was, in all
his suffering. His gut aching. His brow burning in fever. Vomiting
blood. Choking on his own blood.

I bolted upright. I was lying in his bed. The bed where he lay
dying. The very bed where he was vomiting that blood. My head
on the same pillow where he was sweating and slobbering for
those last few weeks. We didn't even know what it was that killed
him. Probably some tropical micro-bacterial hyper-contagious
and untreatable disease. And I was lying in his bed!

I jumped to my feet and stared down at the mattress, the
impression of my body visible on the blanket. My heart pounded
in my temples. Did they even change the sheets? Why would
someone have even made the bed? And how well could they even
clean around here? I was hyperventilating.

I tried to calm myself down. I needed to go back to sleep. I
took a towel from the closet and placed it over the pillow and put
another one down the length of the bed. I lay back down on top
of the towels and crossed my arms across my chest so none of
my skin was touching the contaminated surface. I tried to breathe
slowly and practice my meditation.

Breathe in. Breathe out. Relax my feet. Relax my ankles.

Why did we decline the autopsy? What was I thinking? Jesus

Christ. I was lying in his bed, and I was going to catch whatever it was that killed him. I was wide awake. There was no way I was going back to sleep. I flipped open my phone to check the time: 2:22 a.m. I could hear Toby breathing restfully across the room. I made my way over to the laptop, carefully tiptoeing around the stupid piles of books that were everywhere. I was still breathing too heavily, but I tried to keep quiet as to not wake Toby. I had to talk to someone. I had to reach out to someone. What if I had contracted a rare, fatal disease? That fucker was trying to take me down with him.

My mind ran in circles. Who could I write to? There was no one in my life that I trusted. I had pushed everyone away. I had learned at a young age that the only way to be safe was to be entirely self-reliant. Dependence on other people was a form of vulnerability, a risk of hurt. Someone to slow you down if you ever had to run. Still, I started writing an email. First to Kelly, though she had married someone else and had two young kids. Then, I changed it and wrote to Debbie, the ex with whom I got the cat. We'd broken up a couple years before, but I could still write to her. I considered writing to Lexi, the porn star, who was the last person I'd been seeing before that trip, but I couldn't confide in her. I thought of addressing it to my mom, but that option was fraught too.

Finally, I skipped over the "To:" field and just started writing. I could decide who to send it to later. I just needed to get my worries out onto the page, so they could escape my head. I wrote about my fear of catching his disease, but realized it would sound crazy. So I tried to give some context to my paranoia: the autopsy we declined and Dr. Merkey's ominous "unknown" declaration; the odd inn/resort/residence/hotel; the coffin made from his

bookcases; Dad's communist friends; and so on. Soon I was writing about my ambivalence about the whole trip. Wondering why we were even there honoring this man with our presence. I wrote about feeling jealous of these people who seemed to know him and love him. People he apparently had treated with decency and respect. I wrote about Toby and how weird it was to have this guy here, my brother. How normal and boring he seemed, and what a relief that was. Maybe he had escaped the crazy, at least a little bit. I hoped for his sake he had.

I started to write about what I found on Dad's computer. But I stopped. No one wanted to hear about that. No one wanted to know that was true. I didn't want to keep the secret, but I couldn't burden anyone else with it. And no matter what, sharing it tainted me. It shouldn't be true, but I knew that it was. He painted me, without me even realizing it. He groomed me to be his fall guy. I stopped and considered writing about the local birds, at which point I recognized that my panic had finally (mostly) subsided to my baseline angst.

When I was ready to pick a recipient and hit Send, I got a network error. The internet was offline. The tether was severed. I was there alone, and there was just no way around it. I was out there in the middle of the ocean with not even the stars to navigate by.

CHAPTER 31
THE METAMORPHOSIS

AFTER KELLY LEFT ME, I finally quit the software job and dedicated my whole being to making an independent feature film. (Interestingly, had I stayed at that job, a decade or so later, my ownership stake would have been worth several million dollars. But forever my father's son, I managed to leave just in time to ensure many subsequent years of financial struggles.) I needed to prove to myself that I could make a piece of art and do something important and worthwhile—something to counter the previous five years when I had traded my soul for someone else's profit. Despite the shattering of my image of my father as such an artist, perhaps I could redeem both him and myself if I could succeed where he had failed.

I had experimented with a number of scripts and finally settled on one that seemed to touch on all my deepest feelings and fears. It was about a software engineer who had a homeless, pot-smoking, astrology-reading father, and how, in his attempt to

save his dad, the engineer let his own life fall apart. Clearly, it was total fiction.

In all honestly, the script was highly fictionalized, but I drew plenty from my real life. One scene, intended to capture the essence of my broken relationship with my father, was based on my trip to New York the year before, to celebrate my birthday with him. It had been a long time since we'd connected, and I felt like it was the mature, adult thing to do to pay him a visit. I was turning thirty, which seemed like an important milestone, and I wanted to spend it with him.

He had been dating Marcy for several years by then, and he insisted on her joining us whenever we got together. I found Marcy's self-pitying, misanthropic energy exhausting, but more importantly I felt that she sapped from him all of his best traits. When she was around, our conversation inevitably became totally focused on her and her woes—injustices for which she miraculously never held any shred of responsibility. When he and I were able to slip into a cerebral debate about big ideas or literature or philosophy (the things I most enjoyed discussing with my father), she would whine impatiently and interject inane or puerile comments intended to derail the conversation.

So this time, on this important birthday, shortly after being dumped by the love of my life, I asked him if he and I could go out together alone, and perhaps Marcy could meet up with us after dinner for a drink or something. That way, he and I could at least have some connective time together. He flatly refused. "If you want to see me, she's going to be there. That's the deal. Take it or leave it."

It was a punch to the gut. I had already booked my flight and wanted to see him, so against my better judgment, I capitulated.

I had requested to go to Elephant & Castle, so I could get their molten chocolate cake for dessert like I remembered so fondly from happier, younger times. But I tried to be the bigger person when the two of them insisted on Shagorika, one of the numberless Indian restaurants on 6th Street between 1st and 2nd Avenues.

Throughout the entire meal the two of them ignored me. They carried on an inane conversation while I sat silently. They laughed at inside jokes without bothering to clue me in. They shared their food without including me or even asking how my meal was. They cooed and snuggled. They performed, perhaps for each other, but also, in some perverse way, for me. I didn't speak a single word the entire meal. I grew angrier and angrier, and then sadder and sadder.

And then, at the end of the meal, they lit up their cigarettes. Dad always insisted on smoking inside restaurants even after the law in New York forbade it. And (at least for the first few years) the proprietors typically acquiesced and brought over an ashtray. I had long since quit smoking and couldn't bear to sit there while they polluted the enclosed space. So, I got up to step outside and escape their fumes.

"Hey, would you mind covering the meal?" he asked. "I'm a little light."

After dinner, I tried to escape into a cab to head back to the bus to New Jersey where I was staying with my mom, but Dad insisted I come back to Marcy's apartment, as she had a surprise for me. Already demoralized and humiliated, I followed along without protest. When we got to her apartment, she revealed the secret: a small, lopsided chocolate cake. No candles or writing, and probably baked out of a box. It had been sitting out since

earlier in the afternoon, and so to add to its troubles, it was visibly dried out. I politely accepted a slice, and then we sat in complete silence for a full five minutes until Dad finally broke in, telling Marcy how delicious and wonderful her cake was.

Then, in the most appalling turn of all, she suggested we put on the TV.

And he concurred.

Part of the Herschel doctrine, repeated endlessly since I was a child, was that television was categorically destructive. Worse than Christ's opiate of the masses, TV was the lobotomizer of civilization, dumbing us all down to be more easily controlled by some unnamed right-wing corporate oligarch. There was nothing more frivolous or crass to him. Televisions, watches, alcohol, owning a car—his list was short but absolute. Or so I thought.

We saw each other once a year at most, and there, on my thirtieth birthday, all I wanted was to spend a little time with my father, and instead I was forced to bear witness to his coddling of this child while she dismantled his very identity. The two of them sat down in front of some sitcom, and I turned and walked out.

It took me a long time to share my screenplay with him. Not only because the character based on him was a homeless, purposeless mess, and that in the story he was dating a miserable younger woman who was an obvious mimic of Marcy, but in the screenplay, I had recreated the whole dinner scene verbatim.

Eventually, I had to send it to him. He had read everything I'd ever written, and I couldn't stop now.

"It's great," he said. "So full of passion!"

CHAPTER 32
BREAKFAST OF CHAMPIONS

WHEN BELINDA ARRIVED, I was sitting in the dining area writing on a notepad. The sun was already hot, though it was probably not even 7:00 a.m.

"Morning, Michael," she said. "Some coffee?" She walked over to the patio's edge and hand-fed Maggie, the macaw, some nuts. The bird purred and clucked loudly as Belinda stroked her feathers.

"Sure. Coffee'd be great," I replied. "Thanks."

I had made a list of all the tasks for the day, and there were a lot of them if we were going to get the whole business done with by four o'clock—which was what Anais had promised in her radio address. I watched Belinda take a large tin of grounds out of the freezer and put a few spoonfuls into the filter box of a tall percolator. She moved with grace and habit, pouring in a pitcher of water and turning the machine on. She filled a dented chrome milk dispenser from a plastic gallon jug and set it on the self-service counter next to a tin of sugar packets. Watching the simple

ritual of it all was somehow calming. She took a half a flat of eggs out of the fridge and set it on the counter next to the griddle and put a bagged loaf of bread beside the toaster. When the coffee was done, she filled a mug for me and placed it near the milk.

"Come for a walk," she said without turning around to face me.

I got up, took my coffee, and followed her. She grabbed a few water bottles and led me down through the parking area and past the buildings toward the field. We reached the grave site in a few minutes, where the two diggers were still hard at work. Were they there all night? I was mortified that I hadn't even thought of them since the day before. They stopped to greet us when we arrived, both covered in soot and sweat. They had made an impressive hole, but it was still only a few feet deep.

Belinda tossed them the water bottles, which they accepted eagerly. "I'll bring out some sandwiches in a little while," she said. They nodded and grunted their appreciation.

I wondered how they knew how big and how deep to dig. Was six feet really necessary? Or was that just a colloquialism? There must be some machine that does this automatically back in the real world, right? Somebody else's problem. One more bit of primeval knowledge we had chosen to forget, to distance ourselves from. Yet, there we were, back in the eighteenth century.

I found myself feeling sorry for these two guys, so desperate for money that they had to work through the night digging a grave. But the truth was they looked neither destitute nor miserable. Maybe they were just regular guys happy to have some honest work. I realized we never agreed to a price and worried for a moment that we were quickly surpassing whatever was left in Dad's bank account. Then I shamed myself for fretting about it.

"Do you think they'll be done by four?" I asked Belinda, immediately feeling stupid for not addressing them directly.

"What do you think, guys?" she asked.

"It's very rocky, so it's slow going. You see?" The short, sunny guy pointed to the pile of excavated dirt. There were some basketball-sized rocks and lots of broken tree roots amidst the soil.

"We'll do our best, Miss Linda," the taller guy said.

When we got back to the dining area, a guest was helping himself to coffee, and Belinda got to work cooking him up some eggs. He and I exchanged pleasantries. He had no idea who I was or why we were there. He probably thought I was a tourist like he was. He didn't know Joe and wasn't going to offer me his condolences or tell me how much I looked like him. Not everyone there knew all of our business. I appreciated the moment of anonymity.

"You're Max?" he asked solemnly. "I heard about your father. So sorry for your loss."

CHAPTER 33
THE GHOST WRITER

I WANDERED BACK to the bungalow to brush my teeth. Anais and Toby were sitting on the floor surrounded by giant piles of books, packing them into shipping boxes they had found in the back of the closet. Anais held one of the volumes of Dad's self-published novel in her hand. "Have either of you read it?" she asked.

Toby shook his head. "He had sent me a copy, but . . ."

"I've brought those books with me on every plane ride I've taken in the last three years, but I don't think I've gotten more than five pages in," I said. "Have you?"

She nodded. "I have." Then she stage whispered, "Honestly, it's not very good."

That revelation upset me, though I wasn't sure exactly why. I suppose I wanted to hold onto the possibility that it could be good. That after everything, perhaps there would someday be a reckoning that redeemed him. And who was she to judge? Could Anais possibly be a fair judge of the book's quality? Though with

her decades of academic study and tens of thousands of read books under her belt, she was far more qualified than I was to assess his work objectively.

On the other hand, I took some comfort in having a confirmation of what I intrinsically believed: there was no "there" there, that all his effort was ultimately in vain. Though that option didn't feel very good either.

"There might be some good stuff in there, at least in a roman à clef sort of way," she continued. "But it's like there's some underlying pain that he suffered that he's just not able to will himself to bring up, and so the whole thing feels like he's beating around some bush. It's kinda sad really."

The hair on my neck bristled.

"Also, he needed an editor. And he was never willing to let anyone have at it."

Toby changed the subject. Catching me up on their earlier discussion, he gestured around to Dad's entire collection. "We thought maybe we could just donate the books to the local library."

"Is there a library on the island?" I asked.

Anais nodded. "I spoke to Luuk about it yesterday. He said we'll probably double the size of their collection."

"Maybe they'll name a wing after him. The Herschel Wohl wing," I joked.

"More like the Doctor Joe wing," Anais corrected.

"That's kinda sad," Toby said. "No one will even know who he was."

"Yeah. Well," she answered, "you get what you give."

I told them that there was breakfast to be had, and the three of us headed back up to the dining area. As we walked through the parking lot, I told them about my mid-night panic, which they

both found hysterical. I laughed too, though I honestly still wasn't sure whether the room was safe. "Why didn't you just wake me up?" Toby asked. "I was right there."

I didn't have an answer. He patted me on the back and laughed again.

"I slept like a baby," he said.

We went through the day's agenda over scrambled eggs made with extra thyme. We needed to go back to the police station to retrieve Dad's computer and mobile phone. There were probably some contacts on the phone that we should reach out to and share the news.

"When was the last time you spoke to Ernie?" Anais asked, referring to Dad's brother.

"*I'm your wicked Uncle Ernie*," I sang. "I don't remember. Maybe twenty years?"

"Me too," she confessed. "He came to my first wedding, but that was in 1988."

"I've never even met him," Toby said, with exaggerated exasperation. "What the hell?"

Maybe my estrangement from Tobias wasn't as odd as I first thought. It was perfectly in line with the rest of the family dynamic. I made a silent vow to try to break that pattern and forge a strong, enduring relationship with this new brother of mine. Then I thought about how infrequently Anais and I talked or saw each other, and I wondered if there was a way it was all already beyond my control, that we were all just living out the stories that were set in motion before we were even born. That was certainly Dad's fatalist view: All of life was presaged in the movement of the stars. His novel was called *The Kind of Life That Was Being Lived*. I was determined to prove him wrong.

I looked over to Toby. I wanted to say something connective and meaningful. I wanted to embrace him and tell him we were in this together—that from now on we would support each other and be there for each other in a way Dad never was. Everything was going to be just a little bit easier, knowing we had each other's backs. That we were a family—for better or worse. But nothing came out. I said nothing at all. I didn't know how to be a big brother. I didn't know how to trust or be trusted. If there was any legacy that this dead man had left, it was one of disconnection. And nowhere was that more manifest than in the non-relation ships I had with my siblings.

The moment passed, and we went back to discussing the logistics of what lay ahead. Anais taught us about the Jewish rituals for preparing a body for burial. It occurred to me, perhaps for the first time in my highly secular life, that religion really may, in fact, have an important practical purpose—it provided guidance for otherwise overwhelming life events like death. And, I supposed, for birth and marriage, and even for the amorphous but critical transition of becoming an adult. When everything feels so unsettled and tenuous, so overwhelming, it can be a relief to have some rules to follow. Maybe those teeming millions were on to something after all.

Back in Dad's room, Anais presented Toby and me with a blue cardboard box that looked like a gift from Bloomingdale's with a dress shirt inside. "This is the *tachrichit*," she said. "The burial garments."

We opened the box to reveal a collection of folded up pieces of loosely woven white muslin. I took one out and held it up. It unfurled and fell all the way to the floor. It was a giant jacket with a deep hood. Definitely one size fits all. Toby took out a pair of "pants." The foot holes were sewn shut.

"There are no pockets," Anais explained. "So there's no way to express wealth or status. Every Jew is buried in this same identical shroud."

"What's this?" Toby asked, holding up a purse-sized bag made of the same material.

"Sometimes the body is in pieces. Or sometimes you only have a little piece to bury."

Toby quickly put it back. I folded up the jacket to put it away. Anais pointed to a satchel of sand in the bottom of the box.

"That's dirt from Israel," Anais said. "To sprinkle in the casket. We don't have to do that, but you can if you want. It symbolizes oneness with Israel . . . or maybe it's about 'from dust to dust' or something. I don't really remember."

We stuffed everything back into the box and put the lid on.

Anais began to tear up. "I've done *taharah* for other families at my synagogue. It's an honor to be able to help with their grief and tend to the people who died. But—" she began to cry fully— "you're not supposed to have to do it for your own family." She talked through her tears. "That's the whole point of having the community around you, so you take care of each other, so you don't have to perform *taharah* on your own family. But we don't have anyone here. And I can't do it. I just can't."

"I know," I said. "You're not going to. Toby and I will do it."

I looked to Toby, who nodded solemnly. Then, as Anais turned away, he flashed me a little grimace, revealing his own hesitation.

"You understand, don't you? I just can't," she sobbed.

I hugged her to me, though it felt more like the appropriate gesture rather than a genuine act of comfort. Like I should have been saying, *there, there*—whatever the hell that meant.

She sobbed into my chest, and I looked over her shoulder at Toby, who stood a comfortable distance away. He and I just looked at each other blankly as Anais sobbed. Both of us projected our feelings onto her. "Do you see how sad *she* is?" We said to each other with our eyes. "I feel so bad for *her.*" Never allowing ourselves to acknowledge the conflicted anguish coursing through our own constricted male veins.

Still, my eyes stung from lack of sleep, my hands and feet tingled from fatigue, and my head throbbed from the heat and the dehydration. I knew what I needed, but I just didn't know how to conjure the tears that might flush me and exhaust me to the point of feeling some relief. So instead, I consoled Anais, patting her head like I would a child. After a moment, she broke away from the hug with a snort.

"You can see why I can't do it!" she said with a pained laugh. "I'd never get through it."

She went on to explain the ritual of washing the body, cleaning it to prepare it for burial, with her characteristic level of detail and thoroughness. For once I was grateful for her compendious knowledge. "You can wipe around the nose and mouth and ears and such, but don't clean inside. You want to try to be as respectful as you can of the body."

Toby and I nodded, listening intently.

"It's part of the practice to gently wash the soles of the feet and the palms of the hands, to remove any perspiration there," she continued. "And then you pour water over the whole body from head to toe, except the face. And then you turn the body over and pour the water over the back too. And be careful because it'll be a lot heavier than you expect. That's where the term 'dead weight' comes from. It'll take both of you to carefully move him."

The whole thing seemed completely normal and ordinary, yet at the same time, I couldn't comprehend that we were talking about manipulating our dead father's corpse.

CHAPTER 34
CAPTAINS COURAGEOUS

WE WENT TO CHECK ON REGGIE. He was finishing up the coffin adjacent to the pool where two young tourist girls frolicked in the water. He had done a surprisingly good job under the circumstances; it looked exactly like a coffin was supposed to—wider at one end for the shoulders, and appropriately deep. As he continued working on assembling the top, he shared his concern that the coffin wasn't long enough to fit Dad. But we assured him it would be okay. Toby tried to keep a straight face as he suggested that I lay down inside to make sure it would fit. I declined, though I was glad to see Toby loosening up a bit. Or maybe, like the rest of us, he was just getting punchy.

Next, we were off to the police station. Our friend the captain was nowhere to be found. First, we were told to wait around for him. We weren't allowed to sit in his office, so we crowded onto the landing at the top of the stairs. After a few minutes, I grew impatient and wandered back downstairs.

"We're here to retrieve my father's belongings," I explained to a cop, who stared at me with a blank look on his face. "Doctor Joe?" I said, gesturing to my face, expecting the same recognition that everyone else on the island seemed to have. Only this time, the guy just stared. "You took his laptop and his mobile and who knows what else," I said. "We need to get that stuff back. Where is it?" I made no attempt to hide my frustration, and that seemed to help me earn some of the guy's deference: He pointed to a room behind me.

Emboldened by that exchange, I barged into that room, where two more cops sat behind a counter. "Captain Morago said we could pick up my father's belongings this morning," I demanded.

"The captain isn't here," the first cop answered.

I called for reinforcements. I stepped outside the room and yelled up the stairs. "Annie, Toby! I think I found it."

They lumbered down the stairs and crowded behind me in the doorway of the room.

"Listen," I said, softening, "Our dad died a few days ago. You guys confiscated his laptop and some other things that belong to us." The cop nodded but didn't make any move to find the stuff. "We need to get our items," I stared at him. "Now."

He looked to the other guy in the room, who shrugged and said something in a thick accent that I couldn't understand at all.

"The captain said it was alright," Toby said gently, playing good cop.

The two cops disappeared into the back of the room for a moment and returned with a huge seventeen-inch Compaq laptop and a cheap little flip phone.

"What is the password?" the cop asked.

"I don't know," I said.

"We have to complete our investigation."

I shook my head. "We don't know. No one knows. But that's our property. Our dad's."

The cop looked to his colleague for support, but that guy just shrugged again. And finally the first cop relented and pushed the equipment toward us. Breaking his stone-face character, he smiled gently. "We're sorry about Doctor Joe."

I nodded, annoyed at their petty power play and how little effort it took to break it. We grabbed the stuff and headed back outside to Luuk's truck. Just as we were exiting the building, Captain Morago appeared and yelled after us. "Excuse me, sir!"

We had gotten what we wanted, and I couldn't see much benefit in having another inane conversation. I thrust the laptop into Toby's hands and hurried Anais and him ahead of me and out of the building. "Just go," I whispered as I stopped to deal with the prickly cop. "We're all set," I said, blocking the doorway with my body.

"Yes. I'm glad we could help," he said, with an unnerving smile. "When is the funeral?"

I was suddenly unsure about whether or not I should tell him the truth. "We're not sure yet," I lied. "Hopefully later today, or maybe tomorrow."

"I heard it on the radio," he said. "Four o'clock. No?"

I smiled, caught in my lie. "Yeah, well, we hope. We don't know if we'll be ready yet. There's still a lot to do."

"I see," he said. Then he just stood there, staring at me.

I pointed over my shoulder. "I've got to . . . go." I bolted out of the building toward the truck. Once again, it was raining heavily without warning. I briefly wondered if it only rained at the police station. I looked up, and the sun was still shining. What an odd little island this was.

I jumped into the truck bed where Toby was holding a plastic poncho over his head. I scooted close to him and he attempted to hold it over both of our heads. Luuk took off. Anais was in the front seat with the computer on her lap, and she was looking at the cell phone. I could feel my cortisol level spike. I needed to get a look at the laptop before Anais or Toby did, to make sure there wasn't anything that they shouldn't see.

Anais's face lit up, and she slid open the tiny window between the cabin and the bed of the truck. "I found Ernie's number," she yelled over the noise of the engine and the tires rolling over the gravel in the rain. "And Dad's phone has service. Should I call him?"

I felt annoyed, but there was no reason to be. Suddenly I was struck by a wave of guilt—not only because it had been several days and we were just now getting in touch with our Uncle Ernie, who had a right to know what happened to his brother, but also because I had left it to Anais to make the call.

I listened to her sobbing as she tried to convey the few facts we had. Toby was lost in his own thoughts, staring off into the bushes along the side of the road as we drove. At least the phone call would keep Anais from opening the laptop, I thought. Then I scolded myself for protecting Dad, even now. Still, I couldn't help myself from scheming about how to make sure I got some time alone with the laptop.

I knocked on the window. Anais opened it. She was still on the phone with Ernie. "Yeah, we're doing it this afternoon. Maybe we can plan a memorial in New York soon." She mouthed to me: *What do you want?*

"Can you give me the laptop?" I asked impatiently. "I want to see if I can figure out the password."

She waved me away and continued her conversation, wiping

some tears from her face. "The island is called Sint Eustatius. Yeah. Statia. Right. Through Sint Maarten." She shut the window and kept talking.

CHAPTER 35
CATCH-22

LUUK PULLED UP in front of a large two-story building with a columned portico and a marble staircase. The rain had stopped, and the heat had resumed. Toby and I jumped out of the back. Anais offered to stay in the truck. "No, come on. You should come with us," I insisted.

She protested but gave in and got out of the car. We made our way into the building, which felt more like a familiar governmental office than anything we'd yet seen there. It was clean, with lots of marble and tall ceilings, though everyone was dressed in T-shirts, jeans, and sandals. And there was no shortage of dreadlocks.

When we arrived at the Lieutenant Governor's office, we were greeted by a secretary sitting at an old-fashioned typewriter outside a closed door. We explained our situation to her and showed her the form, but she shook her head. "He can't sign it until it's been paid," she explained flatly. "You need to pay the fee at the census office on De Ruyterweg," she said, waving her hand vaguely behind her.

"Not in this building?" I asked. She shook her head.

"Can we walk there?" Anais asked.

"Sure," the secretary answered, but then added, "But you need to be back here before we close at noon."

Toby looked at his watch. "That's twenty-five minutes," he said.

All of us jumped at once and ran back toward the staircase, down the marble hallway, and out to the car. Luuk knew where the census office was, but there was no direct route, so we had to go up and around the big hill that I now understood interrupted the otherwise sensible grid of the town.

Toby smiled. "Small town bureaucracy at its finest."

Three goat herds, one pack of feral dogs, and five obligatory neighborly waves later, we arrived at the census office. It only took five or six minutes, but I was already calculating how much time we had to get the signature. I jumped out of the truck and yelled to Luuk to keep the engine running. Toby and Anais stayed in the car.

The census office was a small unmarked storefront nestled among a row of stores on a narrow one way street. I burst through the door and was faced with a row of teller booths behind safety glass like you'd find at a bank. There were no customers, and no one sitting at any of the windows. "Hello?" I called out. "Is anyone here?"

It took a full minute for a fat, wobbly woman with beads strewn through her hair to make her way to one of the windows. She took what felt like another two minutes to get herself situated on the stool behind the window, but my impatience got the best of me, and I began trying to explain our situation before she was ready.

"Hold on!" she scolded. "Gimme a sec."

I waited a few more seconds and began again. "Please!" I said. "I'm in a huge rush. I've got to pay the fee for this form and get it back to the governor by noon."

She took the form through the narrow slot under the safety glass. She studied it carefully. I was sure she was just fucking with me at that point.

"How much is the fee?" I asked. I pulled cash out of my pockets. "Can you accept US dollars?" I had about twenty US dollars' worth of local currency that I got on Sint Maarten, but I didn't know if the fee was going to be more or less than that.

"No US dollars," she said. "It's fourteen guilders and for-ty-five cents."

I was in luck. I picked out two ten-guilder notes, pausing for an instant to appreciate that the bills were decorated with hum-mingbirds rather than dead statesmen. Dad would have approved. I shoved the money through the slot, but she pushed it back at me. "It has to be in stamps."

"What do you mean?"

"You got to buy stamps at the post office and affix them to the document."

I was stupefied. "I don't understand," I said. "I can't just pay you the fee?"

"I'm afraid not," she said with a smile. "You've got to go to the post office. It's just over on Kerkweg. A few blocks away." She waved her hand vaguely behind her, exactly the same way the woman at the lieutenant governor's office had.

I exploded. "Then why did they tell me I had to come here to the census office?"

"You do. I need to stamp the form. But only once you've affixed the fee."

I stormed out of the office and ran back over to the car. Anais had the laptop open. "WHAT ARE YOU DOING?" I screamed.

The three of them turned to me suddenly, shocked and confused by my outburst.

"Did you pay the fee?" Anais asked.

"No. I didn't pay the fucking fee!" I exclaimed, as my exasperation nearly overtook me. I took a deep breath, sighed, and then I explained about the stamps. It all made perfect sense to Luuk, though it hadn't occurred to him before he had brought us to the wrong place.

"Did you get into the laptop?" I asked, afraid to hear the answer.

"No, I can't figure out what his password is. I figured it's probably something astrological. I tried some of the moons of Uranus but—"

Thankfully Toby cut her off. "Let's get to the post office!"

Luuk explained that because of the one-way roads, it would be faster for us to go on foot instead of in the car, and he drew a quick map with a pen on the palm of my hand so we knew where to go. And we were off. We ran around the corner and up the small hill and then turned left onto Rosemary Lane and then left again onto Kerkweg street. Mercifully, the post office was well marked, and when we arrived, huffing and out of breath, we found it was open for business—despite the holiday and the general feeling that God was trying to exhaust our patience. There was, however, a line of locals ahead of us. I looked to Toby who looked to his watch, and then shook his head.

"I don't know. I don't see how we're gonna make it," he said.

Out of time and out of ideas, I started to plead with the other people in line to let us cut. I explained that we were trying to fill out a death certificate so we could have a funeral for our poor father who died and who was supposed to be buried within three days according to Jewish law, but that we're already on day five and—

"Doctor Joe!" the post office clerk belted out with a laugh. "Come here, we take a care of you! You're Doctor Joe's son, yes?"

Finally, my resemblance to the bastard was turning out to be helpful. The clerk sold us the 14.45 guilders worth of stamps, and we rushed out of the post office and back to the census office. But when we got there, impossibly, three locals were now in line. I began to feel woozy and had to sit down. Toby patted me on the back, a little concerned.

Taking my lead from the post office, Toby tried to convince the other customers to let us cut in line, and mercifully they were sympathetic. We gave the fat woman the stamps and the death certificate. She methodically licked each stamp and affixed it directly to the document, taking great care to arrange them neatly. Then she inked up an official seal and marked the certificate, the same way the post office does to show that a letter has been sent. Then, she handed it back to us through the slot in the glass. The fee was now literally glued to the form. The proof of our payment was indisputable. It was a bit convoluted and crazy, but I saw a certain logic to their procedure. In an eighteenth-century kind of way.

We stumbled our way back to Luuk's truck, piled in, and commanded him to race us back to the lieutenant governor's office. It was 11:55 a.m., and I was pretty much convinced that we were screwed, but all we could do was try. Luuk did his best, bouncing over the bumpy road, weaving around the wildlife, all

the while Toby and I held on for dear life in the still-wet truck bed, praying we weren't tossed out and run over.

We arrived at 12:03 according to Toby's watch. I ran as fast as I could toward the governor's office, determined to get the damned paper signed and put this absurd bureaucratic nightmare behind us. I bounded up the stairs two at a time, and for a moment I was back in New York at eight years old, chasing Dad up the stairs at the Astor Place subway station, trying to keep up with him after he sped off the train and onto the platform as soon as the doors opened. I'm trying to keep my eyes on his back, but he begins to get swallowed by the crowd. I fight my way to him, pushing through the people, but once I reach the street at the top of the stairs, he is gone. I look left, I look right, I don't see him anywhere. I'm stuck. Stranded. Alone. What was his fucking hurry? What was he always running from?

I shook off the memory. I saw that the secretary was still there, so I yelled down the hall, asking her to please stay open just a few seconds more. I heard Anais and Toby a few feet behind me trying to keep up, but I didn't look back.

I was struck by the colossal absurdity of the whole business and a wave of levity overtook me. "We have completed the quest, slayed the dragon, and returned with the proof you requested, m'lady!" I said. But neither the secretary nor my siblings seemed to find any humor in my exclamation. She took the form from me, examined it, and nodded.

"This looks fine," she said, "but . . ." She squinched up her face. "I'm so sorry I forgot to tell you that the lieutenant governor was to go to Saint Kitts on official business today. He's just left and won't be returning until Monday next." She winced, anticipating my reply.

My humor drained away along with the color from my face. "Are you kidding me?" I shouted. "Do you know what the hell we just went through? How do you people live on this abominable island?!"

Anais stepped up, pushed me aside, and tried to regain control over the situation. "I'm sorry," she began, "but this is quite urgent. Is there not someone who'd be authorized to sign in the governor's absence? For example, at my work, when my supervisor is away on vacation, or even a mental health day—"

"ANAIS!" I yelled for her to shut up. "Please," I begged the secretary.

"There's a religious imperative," Toby added.

The secretary considered the options and then began apologizing profusely. "I'm so, so very, very sorry." I thought she might cry.

I was beside myself. I remembered that old cliché that people die the same way they live, and this all seemed pretty consistent with that. Dad's death was an enormous hassle and imposition. Not for him, of course, but for anyone who dared to love him.

Just then, Captain Morago came out of the office with another man. He tipped his police cap to us. "I hope you are all enjoying your stay," he smiled. Anais and Toby murmured a polite response, but I just stared in disbelief. Was he somehow behind this? We watched the two of them disappear down the hallway and down the stairs. The secretary again expressed her apologies. Then, I was struck with inspiration.

"Okay. Thank you," I said. I grabbed my siblings' arms. "Come on."

Anais and Toby hesitated, but I implored them with a look, and they let me lead them away from the clerk and back down the stairs.

CHAPTER 36
ILLUSIONS

WHEN WE GOT TO THE LOBBY, I looked around to make sure the coast was clear, then I stopped in front of a large wooden display box at the base of the stairs. Inside there was a framed document. I studied it for a moment. Anais and Toby flanked me.

"What are you doing?" Toby asked.

"You think that's the lieutenant governor's signature?" I asked, pointing to the flowery penmanship at the bottom of the document on exhibition.

"Maybe," Toby said.

"I'm willing to take a gamble," I said.

I took out the death certificate and began examining it, trying to parse the Dutch to figure out where the signature was supposed to go. I found what looked like the right place, and I pulled out my pen. I practiced drawing the signature once or twice on the envelope.

"Max, you shouldn't." Anais tried to stop me.

"If there's one thing I learned from the old man . . ." I began, but didn't really know what I was going to say.

"Laws are just human constructs," Toby finished my thought. "That's what he taught me." He grinned.

"Exactly," I said, tickled by the thread of our connection, even if it was through Dad's felonious philosophy.

• • •

Once, in the eighties, while Dad was working as a document filer at a law firm, he asked me to meet him at the office at the end of his shift. He told me he needed my help with something important. I could tell from the sound of his voice that whatever he had in mind was something fun, and probably illegal. At sixteen years old, nothing could be more exciting.

I took the bus by myself from New Jersey into midtown and then took a cab to the address he gave me. I arrived around six in the evening, but his shift wasn't over until seven so I had to wait around. He stuck me in an unused office and handed me a copy of Samuel Delany's *Dhalgren* to kill the time while he did whatever busywork they were paying him to do.

Once seven o'clock came, pretty much everyone else in the office had gone home, and he came and got me. He asked me if I wanted to smoke out, so we went into a stairwell and shared a joint. Then, talking about the law and the firm whose offices we were desecrating with the skunky scent of Humboldt's finest, he explained, in his earnest way, his perspective on the law.

"You need to make your own rules—your own sense of right and wrong. Where do you think these laws came from? The slave-owning founding fathers? Billionaire landowners leaning on the scales to keep the rest of us down? Following their rules is nothing short of an abdication of your own responsibility."

He put his thumb to his nose and wiggled his fingers. "This is technically illegal in the state of New York."

I laughed, surprised at the absurdity.

"It's also fine for men to walk around without a shirt, but if a woman does it, she'll get a ticket."

"Now that's injustice!" I joked. "Should be the other way around."

He led me down the stairs and to another floor. He stopped at someone's desk, where a few photos of kids and *Ziggy* cartoons were taped to the fabric walls of the cubicle. He casually took a key ring out of the person's desk drawer and led me down another hallway.

"If no one gets hurt, what's the point of a law?"

"Exactly," I said, eager to agree with him. "Like pot smoking."

"Sure. Or prostitution," he said. "That's just a way the Man keeps women from embracing their sexual power."

We turned a corner and he unlocked a door, revealing a large storage closet full of equipment. He scanned through a pile of typewriters and picked out a clean-looking black Selectric III.

"Look at this waste. These are just going to sit here until they're obsolete. Depreciating until they can be thrown away as a loss. Meanwhile, my typewriter at home keeps jamming, and I can't afford to replace it."

He picked up one of the heavy machines and examined the inside to make sure it was functional. "How is that fair? How is that just?" he asked, rhetorically.

We carried the typewriter down the elevator to the lobby, and I hung back with the machine as he invited the security guard outside for a cigarette. They seemed to be friends, so the guard was

easy to distract. I carried the surprisingly weighty device out a side door per my dad's instructions, and a few minutes later he joined me, putting his arm on my shoulder as he whistled to hail a cab.

• • •

I forged the death certificate, capturing the general look and feel of the signature. I was pleased with how well it came out. "What's the worst that can happen?"

I held up the document so they could evaluate my work.

"We all wind up in a Dutch jail cell for the foreseeable future," Anais said mock-cheerfully.

I folded up the form and stuffed it back into my pocket. "Only I'll go to jail. You two know nothing about this," I said. "Come on. Who the fuck is going to know the difference? Or care?" For the first time all day, I felt a sense of power—ill-gotten maybe, but it still made me smile, and Toby and Anais replied in kind. We headed back outside, all grinning in our little familial conspiracy. Luuk was waiting.

"We're all set," I said. Anais and Toby kept their mouths shut.

"You got the signature? Great work," Luuk said. Thankfully, he didn't pry for details.

So back in the car we tumbled, and back across the little island we drove.

CHAPTER 37
THE CALL OF THE WILD

AT SOME POINT, at risk of eviction from yet another apartment, Dad had grown desperate. While his dealer was still willing to trade an eighth of kind bud for a monthly astrological reading, the landlord wasn't so accommodating. Nor was the bodega for food, nor Duane Reade for the expensive medicated ointment he needed for his increasingly chronic psoriasis. He needed cash. And he needed it urgently. He was still counting on his novel to eventually be the windfall that made everything right, but that was still a long way away.

His dealer (who was also one of his only friends) told him that he "knew some people" who could help. After considering his options, Dad reached out. The plan was that he and Marcy would go on a Caribbean cruise, playing the role of happy tourists. When the cruise made its stop at Montego Bay, Jamaica, they would go ashore and someone would meet them and take them for a very special ride.

He didn't tell me about any of this until after they returned from the cruise. And when he relayed it, he made it sound like an exciting, fun, and harmless adventure, though the story still spooked me. Two locals picked them up on the dock and put them in the back of a jeep, and then motored away from the tourists at the pier and drove up the mountain and deep into the jungle.

"Jamaica was Africa," he said. "Once you got out of the resort areas, it was like going back in time. Back to an earlier part of the Earth." He and I were sitting in a café on MacDougal.

He lit a cigarette and continued the story. "This was deep jungle like nothing I'd ever seen before. Houses gave way to huts, and then to the most primitive of structures. The people living there were just animals, surviving in the jungle like the birds and the reptiles and the wild dogs." He exhaled dual dragon plumes of smoke through his nostrils.

There wasn't a lot of time before they had to get back to the cruise ship, and there was a lot to do, so the driver kept the pedal to the floor.

"To call the dirt path we were on a road is generous at best. In some places we were just driving up a steep gully where most of the trees had been washed away. If a thunderstorm came along, which was not unlikely, the path would have turned into a rushing river and washed us all back down to the bay."

Finally, they got to a real structure, a cabin, and as they arrived, a dozen or more men emerged from the surrounding jungle, shirtless but armed with AK-47s. Dad and Marcy were pulled from the jeep and frisked before being led into the cabin and told to strip to their underwear. Marcy was uncomfortable about undressing in front of these armed and dangerous looking men, but she had little choice at that point.

As soon as they were undressed, teams of men descended on them, duct-taping double-bagged kilos of compressed cannabis all over their bodies: a set of bags around their calves, another taped to their inner thighs, a double-thick pack stuffed into the smalls of their backs, and another row around their bellies and chests, and so on. The whole thing took an hour, but these guys were pros and knew exactly how much they could fit in each spot that would remain undetectable once they put their clothes back on.

"It was surprisingly heavy," he said, demonstrating by slouching his body. "I don't know how many kilos they'd loaded us up with, but it took a bit of practice to walk normally once we were fully packed."

They re-dressed and were loaded back into the jeep. Then they raced back down the mountain and were dropped off a block or so from the quay where the cruise ship was moored. At the wharf, bags of souvenirs and trinkets were thrust into their hands, and they merrily reboarded the ship along with the other passengers.

Once they got to their private berth, they unloaded the loot and packed it into their luggage. There was so much pot that they had to throw away much of their clothes and shoes to make room for it. They were concerned that the excess clothing might somehow be conspicuous, so they concocted an elaborate plan to sneak out of their cabin during the night and hurl some of it overboard.

From there, they sipped piña coladas for the remainder of the cruise. There was just one final step to complete. The ship docked in the Port of Miami, and when they disembarked, they had to go through standard US Customs screening. Of course, not every passenger was scrutinized to the same degree. Dad, being a scraggly looking old hippy, might have gotten a bit more attention

than your average passenger, but because he was traveling with Marcy, they were waved through unscathed. I couldn't help but wonder if they assumed she was his daughter instead of his girlfriend, but regardless they passed, and they were home free.

This earned them five grand, not to mention the amazing story, although it was the kind of story you couldn't just tell anyone. And when Dad shared it with me, he made a point of pointing out that he hadn't told Anais or Toby, and that it could just be our little secret. I added it to the collection of secrets he had entrusted me with.

And why not? Sharing secrets with him was at least one way that I could feel like we had a special relationship, and in whatever twisted way, that was appealing. He trusted me, confided in me, and that felt good.

A few months after their exhilarating and profitable mule experience, his coffers began to run low again, and he was invited to make a second trip. The second time around, it was even easier. Now, knowing what to expect, the fear of being caught was reduced, and they breezed through customs again and doubled their ill-gotten gains.

The problem arose when Dad went back for thirds. It was a year later, and this time he didn't have Marcy with him. While everything went smoothly getting in and out of the Jamaican hinterland, when it came time to reenter the United States, he could feel something was different. His pulse raced and he began to sweat. And without the cover of his young sweetheart/daughter, he was apparently much more suspicious looking to the customs agents.

They pulled him out of the line and brought him to a private room for additional screening. Upon opening his suitcase, they found what they'd expected: twenty kilos of highly compressed

reefer. They booked him on felony drug trafficking charges, and he was sent to a federal administrative detention facility in Miami for three days.

This was a little different than the Essex County holding cell where he spent the night so long ago for artful dodgery while I was prancing about as a Dickensian con man in my grade-school class play. In Miami, he was held in a private cell that looked and smelled a lot more like a real prison. He described staring at a set of scratch marks on the cement wall—not hashes counting the days like the movie cliché, but furious, panicked scratches likely made with fingernails. He confided this story with me too, but the tone was more ominous. He was scared in a way I'd never heard before.

I didn't ask for too many details, but I couldn't help but wonder if the cartel he muled for was going to come after him too. After all, he hadn't delivered the drugs as agreed, and these didn't seem like the most understanding or reasonable of business partners. I didn't know if they also were the ones who posted his bail, and perhaps he owed them repayment of that too. Once he was released, he retreated to New York and had little time to figure out how he was going to get out of the country before his hearing, which was scheduled about six weeks later. Unsure of what to do next, he turned to his normal source of guidance: astrology. He did an expansive astrological chart to help him decide where he should live. Scouring the whole globe, he zeroed in on the obscure, tiny islands of the Netherlands Antilles. I don't know if he also consulted the details of their extradition policies.

He boasted about his bold decision to leave as if it was a stroke of inspirational genius, and I suppose it turned out he was right, but at the time, I was worried for him.

"I've received my assignment," he beamed. "Adventure awaits. Something you know nothing about," he teased.

"I'll miss you," I mumbled.

"Ah, you'll be fine." He lit a cigarette, offering me one, though I had quit a decade before. "Just, uh, you know, keep the details from your sister." He winked.

CHAPTER 38
THE IDIOT

ON OUR WAY BACK to the resort from the lieutenant governor's office, Luuk stopped at a small market to mollify Anais's hunger. She and Toby headed into the store, but I stayed behind.

Once they were out of sight, I climbed into the cab of the truck. I finally had a moment alone with the laptop (even if Luuk was sitting there beside me). I opened it up and stared for a moment at a large, bloody palm print smeared beside the track-pad, below the punctuation keys. I tried to wipe it off, but it was quite stubborn. I pressed the space bar to wake the machine up, and I was presented with the password screen. I stared at it for a moment, imagining that maybe the secret code was my birthday, or some combination of the three of ours. I tried a couple of combinations, but all just yielded the error sound. Of course it wasn't one of our birthdays. If anything, it was probably his own. But before I could try that, I accidentally hit the return key while the password field was still empty.

That successfully dismissed the login dialog and the desktop appeared. I laughed, imagining the cops entering all matter of possible passwords and never considering that, in fact, there wasn't any password at all. I was sure there was a metaphor there somewhere, but I didn't have time to ponder it. I scanned the various folders on the desktop, but there was nothing interesting, and there didn't appear to be any pornography, at least not in plain sight. It was mostly work stuff related to his pharmacology lectures, some astrology junk, and some miscellaneous links to web pages and such.

A bit reassured, I performed a search by date to find the last files he touched. Here it would be, I thought. Finally, his last words to us. A goodbye. An explanation, justification, inspiration. Something to help us make sense of the confusion born of his awkward, ill-fitting influence over our lives. Or maybe just an apology for his mistakes and cowardice and poor choices that hurt us so much. Or his appreciation in advance for the nightmare he was putting us through presently. Hell, I'd even have taken a sardonic joke.

But, like Charlie Brown running yet again toward the football held by Lucy, I was the fool. Oh, good grief. The last file modified was the same manuscript document that I had found on the backup disk, and other than that, there were just a few other files in that same folder. None of it personal, none of it addressed to any of us. My stomach sank. This was the last possible place to look. Didn't I know him? Why would he have been any different in his last days than he had been over the seventy years before? Why would he admit failure, or remorse, or weakness?

Luuk had been watching over my shoulder, and I hadn't explained what I was doing, but he was one step ahead of me.

"You know," he began, "your dad was into some stuff. You might want to clear that off before you share it with your sister."

"Yeah. Good idea," I said, unnerved, and unsure what my assent just confirmed or condoned. I shut the laptop. "Later," I said. "You don't have to mention that I figured out the password." I looked at him, feeling that same unsettling conspiratorial weight in my gut. So familiar and so ugly.

"Sure." He nodded. "Here they come."

Luuk took us back to Paradise Point where Belinda had prepared lunch for us. I had no appetite, but when the plate of lasagna landed in front of me I scarfed it down.

I hadn't taken a crap in three days. I began to wonder what goes on inside your guts when it gets all backed up like that. That quickly led to thoughts of intestinal disease and diverticulitis, and I had to stop myself from what I knew would be a dangerous spiral.

We made a plan for Luuk to drop Toby and me off at the hospital while Anais stayed back at the hotel to prepare for the ceremony. But before we headed out, I went back to Dad's room to spend a few more minutes with the laptop, to once and for all locate and eradicate any porn or god knows what else. A few quick searches didn't turn up anything incriminating, and I suspected the best thing was just to wipe the hard drive entirely. Still, I was torn; maybe there was some chance that he had some personal photos or something that should be preserved. But that was just me giving him the benefit of the doubt yet again.

While I was debating, Anais and Toby came in. "Oh, You figured it out!" Anais said, gesturing to the laptop.

"Yeah, it was a combination of all our birthdays," I said, thinking I was making a joke.

But when Toby responded "Really?" a little too excitedly, I realized my joke wasn't funny. For a moment I considered letting it slide, letting Toby hold on to the belief that we were in Dad's thoughts even a little bit. But I was sick of the lying and the deceit. It wasn't my responsibility to protect him, or anyone.

"No," I said. "There wasn't any password at all. I just pressed enter."

Anais picked up an empty yellow legal pad from Dad's desk and set out to make some notes about the ceremony. "My rabbi gave me some suggestions, some passages to recite," she explained. "It's all in the Torah. Does he have a copy of the Torah? He must."

The two of them looked around through the boxes of books that were all over the bungalow. After a moment, Toby found it. "Right here, next to *Bulfinch's Mythology*."

I was still preoccupied with the computer. Before I wiped the drive, I logged onto the internet and reflexively checked my email. There were over a hundred unread messages.

Anais read aloud several Torah passages that she thought might be a good fit for the funeral. By the third one, I'd lost interest. They were all too long, too religious, too cryptic, too something. She kept asking Toby and me to help her decide. For some reason that made me furious. I'd been dealing with all the logistics, holding this whole thing together. The least she could do was figure out which hollow Jewish prayer she wanted to read at the ceremony without requiring my input. I continued to ignore her and cleared the junk out of my inbox.

"What are you doing?" she finally asked, standing over me.

"I'm checking my email," I snapped. "I left a lot of shit in limbo to come down here."

She looked over my shoulder at the screen and saw an

exchange with an OkCupid date. Then she snapped back, "Oh, yeah. That obviously can't wait. While you bury your father. Nice priorities, Max."

"Give me a fucking break!" I yelled, a little louder than I intended. "I'm just checking email and that came up. Most of it was work related." Then, unable to stop myself, I added, "Something you wouldn't know about."

"Fuck you," she said. "Don't you even!"

Toby retreated to the kitchen.

"Jesus fucking Christ, Anais!" I slammed the laptop closed. "You wouldn't even be here if I hadn't laid out the money."

"You offered! Mom was more than happy to lay out—"

"OH PERFECT!" I screamed. "Run to Mom and take her money, right after you go on and on about how much you hate her!"

"Don't even try to pretend you understand," she said, suddenly annoyingly calm. "And what the fuck? What's gotten into you? I'm just trying to plan the ceremony. Is it wrong that I want your input? Do you really not care? Is it more important to make sure you can get laid when you get home? Nice choice of distraction, by the way. Dad would be proud."

I suddenly felt hot. Overwhelmed. Confused. Unsure of what I'd said and how things had suddenly blown up. I wanted to deescalate but I didn't know how. "I'm sorry. You're right," I said, trying to sound conciliatory, but it came out dismissive.

"Whatever," she hissed. And I felt a wrath from her, a vitriol that I didn't know if I'd ever seen before, and it burned. "Get your shit together," she said. "We don't have time for this." She collected her things and headed out the door.

Toby reappeared shyly. "We, uh . . . it's time to go to the morgue."

CHAPTER 39
THE CRUCIBLE

THE HOSPITAL ADMINISTRATOR was a woman in her sixties wearing a Run DMC T-shirt and pink blush that looked comically unnatural on her dark caramel skin. Toby and I sat in front of her desk in a pair of uncomfortable wicker chairs. She asked to inspect the death certificate so that she could authorize the release of the body from the morgue. I rode a little wave of fear, concerned that she would spot the forgery. I avoided looking at Toby as I pulled out the form, careful to hold the envelope upside down to hide the practice signatures on the outside. As she scanned it, I stole a glance at my brother, who was about to burst out laughing. I slowly moved my hand down to the side of my chair, and as surreptitiously as I could, I punched him hard in the thigh.

Luckily, Run DMC didn't seem to notice Toby's grunt. He stifled his smile, and we waited patiently to find out if the counterfeit signature would pass muster. After what felt like forever, she stopped reading and folded her hands over the document.

She looked down at the desk and sighed. Then she stared at us for a long beat. Fuck. She knew. What was I thinking? An island where everyone knew each other? She was used to seeing this guy's signature. I was totally screwed, and I'd involved my innocent brother in the whole thing too. Fuck. I'm such a shit.

"I'm so very sorry for your loss," she said, looking directly into my eyes. "It was a real tragedy. We'll all miss Doctor Joe very much." Then, without missing a beat, she presented us with a three-page handwritten bill that we had to pay before they could release the body.

These people may have been living in the past, but it appeared that they had figured out how to eke a profit by mimicking America's reprobate medical billing system. There was a charge for the ambulance, another for its fuel, and another for Dr. Merkey's time, both when he went out to declare Dad dead at the scene as well as the meeting he had with us the other day. There was a fee for the morgue on a per-hour basis, a cost for the removal and elimination of his clothes (which, she explained, had to be cut off his body and burned to prevent possible contamination or transmission of pathogens), and an endless number of other miscellaneous charges and fees. She walked through the whole thing line by line, justifying and explaining each item, reminding us over and over how they strive to offer the best care possible and how respectful they were of the dead, and so on.

Fortuitously, the prices were at local rates, and the whole thing totaled only 4,456 guilders—just under twenty-five hundred US dollars. I was shocked that the cost was so low. In the States I'm sure the same services would have easily topped ten thousand dollars or more. But there was a hitch: they didn't accept credit cards.

She was willing to accept US dollars in cash, but I only had about three hundred and Toby only had about thirty-five. We also still had to pay Reggie for the casket, and the gravediggers, and who knew what else. This presented us with an impasse. She suggested that we wire money from home, but given the holiday, there was no way that we could get the money quickly. She asked if we could borrow the money from someone locally, but we all agreed it was unlikely anyone would have that much cash on hand, including Luuk and Belinda. She just stared at us, waiting for us to come up with a solution, and seemingly oblivious to the urgency we felt as we got closer and closer to two o'clock, when the nurse who was supposed to help us with the body had to leave. We asked if she could accept partial payment now. She wasn't opposed to that idea, but she was worried that splitting the payment up would lead to confusion later.

"Could we give you an IOU?" Toby offered.

I laughed out loud, thinking he was joking (and maybe he was), but to my surprise, his idea seemed entirely reasonable to her. We were planning to come back to the island in a few weeks to deal with our dad's belongings, and we could bring the cash then. She refused to take the partial payment we offered, insisting that it would be easier if we just paid the full amount all at once when we returned. She didn't even require us to sign the bill or create a formal piece of paper to serve as the IOU. Our word was enough.

When we stepped out of the office, Toby and I look at each other in complete disbelief.

"Did that really just happen?" he asked. We shared a laugh, but it was short lived. There was no longer anything standing between us and the task we were dreading most.

CHAPTER 40
THE UNBEARABLE LIGHTNESS OF BEING

WE WAITED IN A TINY OFFICE for what felt like half an hour, though Toby's watch proved it had only been a few minutes. Finally, a woman came to retrieve us. She was nearly six feet tall with graying hair pulled back tightly into a small bun. She wore a white nurse's coat, but her bare feet were in worn, dirty sandals. "Well, come on, den," she said, and turned to leave.

Toby and I jumped to our feet and followed her, trusting that she was the nurse we were supposed to meet. As we were walking, she introduced herself as Winika. She led us through the courtyard, past the barren garden of dirt and crumbled cinder blocks, and around a corner to the doorway of a small room that looked like all the others, except the door was especially heavy and thick. She unlocked the room and led us inside. It took a minute for my eyes to adjust to the darkness and for my nose to adjust to the peculiar acrid smell. As hot and bright as it was outside, it was strangely cool and dark in there, like the inside of a cave, deep underground.

A large metal table sat squarely in the center of the ten-by-ten room, and an industrial-sized faucet dripped slowly into a shallow pool of dirty liquid standing stagnant in the drain. I was expecting a morgue like I'd seen on television, with a wall full of drawers with cadavers in them. This was a tiny room, and I couldn't imagine where the bodies were stored.

A quiet, shriveled man was suddenly standing among us. He was barely five feet tall and must have been eighty years old. He wore a flannel shirt with the sleeves rolled up and ill-fitting khaki shorts.

"Dis is René. He gone help," Winika explained.

René bowed his head. Toby and I looked to each other, then nodded uncomfortably.

"Go git da box," Winika demanded. "Reggie done brought it. René, show dem."

René led us back into the intense afternoon sun and around a corner, where the casket sat unceremoniously askew on the ground. A handful of young kids were standing around staring at it. René startled me with a loud hissing-whistling sound, successfully scaring the kids away.

The mismatched wooden beams of the coffin resembled a hip modern coffee table. There were rope handles fashioned at all four corners, and a matching lid was resting loosely on top. Two dozen three-inch screws stuck up from the lid's surface. It was nontraditional to be sure, but it had its own eclectic charm.

The three of us lifted it, but it was extraordinarily heavy and René wasn't much help. We struggled to carry it back to the little room. As we entered, Winika pointed to the ground to the left of the metal table. "Right dere." We lowered it to the ground and removed the lid. A white sheet that must have come from the resort was folded up inside.

Winika handed out blue surgical smocks, white paper masks, and purple rubber gloves. We all suited up in silence.

Where's the body?" I asked through my mask.

She pointed to an innocuous stainless steel industrial refrigerator that Toby was leaning against. "He in dere." Toby jumped away from the machine, which elicited a snicker from Winika.

We had left the outside door open after carrying in the coffin, and the group of kids had returned and crowded around the entryway. "What's yer business here, eh?" Winika scolded them. "Doncha have no respeck?" The kids reluctantly skittered off, and Winika slammed the heavy door, again sinking the room into an eerie darkness. She turned back to us. "Well come on."

Toby unlatched the fridge to reveal three shelves loaded with white body bags on metal trays. I then saw that the fridge was six or seven feet deep, extending into an alcove in the room.

"Oooh, dey full," Winika said, more to René than to us. "Is that still Missy Danika? Ain't no one come for her yet?"

I peered into the fridge. "Which one?" I asked.

Winika pulled each tray out a few inches to reach the toe tags on the body bags. "Doctor Joe, yah?" she asked, and we both nodded. She pulled out the middle tray firmly and it teetered almost out of her control. We helped guide it out of the fridge and onto the metal table. The body's shape was visible through the opaque white bag: feet sticking up at one end, belly in the middle.

A cool sweat broke out on my forehead and under my mask. I turned to Toby and asked quietly, "You good?" He nodded.

Winika began to unzip the bag, revealing Dad's face. His hair was matted, and there was dried blood in his beard and on the side of his face. He looked like he was thrown into the morgue fridge with little thought. I recalled the administrator's insistence

that they use "the utmost care and respect for the dead." What a load of crap.

"Ah, they didn't clean 'im up?" Winika tsked and shook her head.

I stared at his face. It had been a number of years since I'd seen him, and he looked older. *Death really ages you*, I thought and smiled to myself beneath my mask. I felt Toby's eyes on me, but I couldn't bring myself to meet his gaze.

Winika continued unzipping, revealing the rest of his body. He was naked except for a white sheet that had been tied around his crotch like a giant diaper. His arms were at his side, and I saw the nebula birthmark on his wrist that was so familiar. If seeing his face wasn't proof enough, the birthmark was the final confirmation that yes, this was indeed my father lying before us, lifeless.

As the zipper extended beyond Winika's reach, Toby took over, revealing Dad's feet, then folding the bag down onto the table. Following his lead, I folded the other side of the bag away so the body was fully exposed. I looked over at Toby, but this time it was he who couldn't raise his eyes.

I looked back down at the body, and timidly I put my gloved hand on Dad's left hand. His hand was curved a little, and my hand slipped perfectly into his. I held it a moment and felt how cold and stiff it was. I reached my other hand over and touched the birthmark, then lifted his arm up and onto his hip. I found some more blood on the palm of his hand, and I was reminded of Anais's instructions. "We uh, we want to clean him," I said, struck with the futility and absurdity of cleaning a corpse, but fortunately, Winika just nodded. "And we have the . . . where is the thing?" I looked to Toby, and he produced the blue box. "We want to put these clothes on him. To wrap him up."

Winika filled a small tub of water and handed us each a washcloth. Then she went to work cleaning the blood from his face. "It's terrible," she muttered, and dabbed forcefully at his face with the cloth.

"Not so rough!" Toby snapped quietly.

She stopped and stared at him incredulously, then she laughed tenderly. "You a good son," she said.

I wiped the inside of his palm to remove the blood there. It took a bit of effort to clean it, and when I dabbed the washcloth into the tub, the ruddy color spread into the water. Toby watched me and then wiped the soles of Dad's feet. I looked over at René, and he was just standing there watching us.

"Did you know him?" I asked.

"Everyone know Doc Joe," Winika answered. "We all gonna miss him so."

Toby helped to lift the other hand, and we wiped that palm together. I looked at Dad's face and I had an urge to touch him there, so I tried to straighten his mustache whiskers, though they resisted my efforts, defiantly sticking askew. I squeezed the washcloth over him, dripping the water across his body, trying to at least symbolically perform the steps that Anais described.

Toby hesitantly reached to untie the diaper, but Winika barked at him. "You crazy?"

He withdrew his hand and looked to me. I shrugged. I was vacillating. I had no interest in seeing or cleaning his genitals. I didn't know if he had shit himself when he died, as I've heard happens to all of us, but if he had, it was clear that no one would have cleaned it up. Still, I thought we should be cleaning his whole body, and I didn't want to be squeamish about it. People shit and people die, and people shit when they die. But ultimately,

what difference did it really make? The cleaning we were doing was symbolic. There wasn't any hygienic reason why we shouldn't bury him with a little extra fertilizer inside the box.

Toby had already moved on and taken out the pants with the feet sewn shut. I lifted Dad's right leg and then his left while Toby struggled to pull the pants up and around his feet. It was a lot harder than I expected. "Can you help?" I asked René, and he jumped in, eager to have something to do. It took all four of us to lift him and scoot the fabric up his legs and over his diapered waist.

"Be careful! Don't wanna spill!" Winika warned.

Next Toby held up the shirt. "How are we gonna do that?" I asked.

"Anais said we're supposed to roll him onto his side." Toby gestured.

Winika objected. "No way. You can't be turning him." She gestured to her midsection. "He done got fluid in dere. We spill it out, gets everywhere. Very bad. Dangerous. We all get sick. Wind up in dere." She pointed to the fridge.

"He's frozen solid," I argued. "What kind of—"

"No way, mon!" She raised her voice. "Don be foolish. He not frozen. That rigor mortis."

René produced a pocketknife. "We can cut?" Winika suggested. "Cut de shirt up de back, then put it over de top an tuck under."

We agreed that seemed like a reasonable compromise, so René and Toby cut the back of the shirt open. We pulled the sleeves over his arms, then rocked the body side to side just enough to tuck the back of the shirt underneath him. It took us a few tries, but eventually we got it on, and I stepped back. I was impressed. He looked like a corpse was supposed to. Mostly.

Then Toby held up the hood.

I voted no on the hood. "Too creepy," I said. He nodded in agreement.

"Okay den," Winika said, wiping her brow. "You boys ready say bye bye?"

I looked at the body once more. *That's my father,* I thought. *For better or worse.* Then I looked at Toby. *That's our father,* I corrected myself. And now we were going to put him into the ground. It was really happening. I took a deep breath in through the mask, waiting to have some kind of revelatory feeling, some emotional epiphany, but nothing came. I conjured the upsetting pornographic discovery. I thought about the secrets he made me keep, the bargain I unwittingly had made. I had a spent a lifetime subverting my own needs for guidance, for boundaries, for a context in which to understand my place in the world. Now, here I was liberated from that unsavory covenant, yet still, again, fatherless.

I'd been terrified of this moment for so long. Not only over the past few days, dreading the actual handling of the body, but for years, waiting for his death. I foreshadowed it in that film I'd made eight years before, including a scene where the protagonist had to identify his father's dead body, and how that had unraveled his entire world, sending him into a tailspin that nearly destroyed his whole life.

But here it was. It had actually come to pass. And there I was, in that dark little room on that dark little island, with Toby and these two strangers—Dad's dead body splayed out before us. I found myself surprisingly glad that we had gotten this intimate time with the body. Flesh and blood and that nebula birthmark, his lips inert, never to form that mischievous smile again. There was no denying it: This was a boundary. This was real.

I looked to Toby and nodded that I was ready to move on. He nodded back.

René had spread out the white sheet to cover the inside of the coffin. The body was very heavy and the position of the table made it difficult, but we awkwardly maneuvered him off the tabletop, gripping the body bag beneath him with all eight of our hands, then slowly lowering him into the box with a minimum of banging around.

I fantasized that we could remove the body bag from beneath him by yanking it quickly, like a tablecloth under a fully set dining table, but of course that only worked in the movies, and when I jerked on the body bag, it barely budged. I accepted that it made more sense to just leave it there. It wasn't like anyone was going to reuse it.

The sheet extended beyond the edges of the casket, and Toby draped the left side over the body, partially covering Dad's face. I picked up the right side and draped it over, fully enclosing him in the white fabric. Toby and I locked eyes.

Toby poured the bag of sand from Israel into the coffin, sprinkling it all the way along the length of Dad's body. Then, we lifted the lid and fit it snugly into place. I had a moment of appreciation for Reggie's design; there was a little lip inside the box that served to both position the lid and to receive the long screws that would secure it.

I was reminded of how Reggie told us he had to make a coffin for his child last year. We didn't even ask what happened.

CHAPTER 41
HARD LAUGHTER

"WELL, THAT HAPPENED," Toby said.

With the box closed, we all pulled off our paper masks. Winika peeled off her rubber gloves and began washing up. I put my gloves in the trash and folded up the blue smock and held it out, unsure what to do with it. Winika bundled them all together and stuffed them into a trash bin.

René offered me a screwdriver. I was exhausted, but I began screwing the lid of the coffin closed. Reggie used long screws, and there were a lot of them. Each one took almost a minute to fully twist in. Toby worked on the other side with René's pocketknife screwdriver. It was ten minutes before the lid was fully sealed. That lid was never coming off. When it was finally done, I sighed and patted the top of the box. "Almost home," I said.

Winika pushed open the heavy door, and once again the hot sunlight poured in. The scattered kids quickly collected at the door, hoping for a glimpse of something morbid, but it was too late. Nothing but a wooden box of remains remained.

The four of us tried to lift the casket, but it was extraordinarily heavy. We raised it a few inches off the ground, but barely. We more or less started dragging it out to the driveway to be transported back to the resort.

"How the hell are we gonna carry it to the grave?" I asked. For some reason that made Toby laugh. I joined in, and then the two of us got the giggles and couldn't seem to stop. Laughing made carrying the heavy box even harder, and we nearly dropped it on my foot, which only made us laugh more. When we finally reached the driveway, Winika, clearly perplexed by our mania, wished us well and got into a car with a man who had come to pick her up. We tried to thank her, but the inappropriateness of our laughing made the whole thing even funnier to me, and I couldn't stop in time to give her a proper thanks. Tears were running down my face, my guffaws utterly silent. I couldn't breathe, which just set Toby off all over again.

Eventually we regained our composure. I thanked René for his help, and he nodded, but then put out his hand. It hadn't occurred to me that that was why he was there in the first place, and that too seemed utterly hilarious. I took out a twenty-dollar bill, which seemed like an absurdly large amount in local terms for how little he had done, but I didn't have any smaller bills. I put it in his hand and he bowed graciously, then spoke for the first time all day. I'd assumed he hadn't been talking because he wasn't comfortable with English, but it turned out he was far more fluent than Winika or most of the other locals we had interacted with.

"So sorry for your loss," he said, with almost no detectable accent. "May he rest in peace." The unexpected clarity of his voice set us both laughing all over again.

• • •

The plan had been for Luuk to arrange for the one hearse on the island to carry the casket back to Paradise Point, but after fifteen minutes of waiting, we began to get worried. Another ten minutes went by, and finally we recognized Luuk's pickup truck heading toward us.

He explained that the hearse had broken down, and we were going to have to transport the coffin in his pickup truck. However, we couldn't lift the thing without more help. We walked out to the road and began waving at passing cars. Of course, the drivers thought we were just saying hi, so we resorted to yelling at them to stop as they passed. It wasn't long before two young men came along, and we were able to enlist their help.

We successfully loaded the coffin, but it was a full foot and a half longer than the truck bed, so we had to leave the gate down and let it hang over the edge while we drove back to the inn. Toby and I sat in the back and gripped the rope handles to keep it from sliding out. Luuk tried to drive carefully, but I became acutely aware of just how bumpy the roads were. One wrong move and the whole thing was going to go careening out of the back of the truck and splatter all over the road.

The hill to Paradise Point was really steep in some places, and at one point I could feel the weight of the box really pulling. I was afraid that it was going to pull my arm out of its socket. Toby and I stared at each other, jaws held tightly shut in our effort. We shared a smile at the absurdity of the situation. And that was right when a stupid goat jumped right in front of the car.

Luuk slammed the brakes, which threw us and the coffin toward the cab—the box banging hard against the fore wall of

the truck bed. Then, just as quickly, he dodged the animal and accelerated, and all three of us hurtled rearward toward the open back. We yelled out in panic; I felt the rope begin to slip through my fingers and I gritted my teeth, sure that I was going to go sailing out of the truck and into the road. I flailed my free arm and barely caught the edge of the spare tire bolted down to the bed. Miraculously, Toby held on. He had one hand on the wall of the truck and one on the rope handle of the coffin, which had slipped nearly halfway out of the back. I saw the muscles in his arms and shoulders straining.

Realizing his miscalculation, Luuk quickly tapped on the brakes again, giving us a gravitational boost and pulling the coffin back in from the precipice. I was able to get a better grip on the rope once again.

"What the hell are you doing?" Toby yelled.

Luuk responded with a cheery "Sorry!" oblivious to the disaster he almost caused.

Somehow, we made it back to the resort without further incident, and Toby and I got a chance to rest our arms.

Anais walked up to greet us. She had changed into a dress, and I was struck with the thought: *Oh shit, we're going to a funeral today.*

CHAPTER 42
THE MISFORTUNES OF VIRTUE

AS WE STOOD THERE in the inn's parking lot, it started to rain again. I was still startled by it, but for once I found it refreshing, even joyous. I looked to the coffin and shrugged. Let the water fall down upon it. Let it fall down on everything. Toby and Anais had already made a run for it, but I slowly, calmly followed them over to Dad's bungalow, letting the rain soak my clothes.

Inside, I toweled my hair and changed into a dry pair of blue jeans and my "nice" shirt, a short-sleeved silk button down in black. I exchanged my sneakers for a pair of black loafers that I'd thrown into my suitcase at the last minute. Even with the rain easing the humidity slightly, a drip of sweat trickled down my side from my armpit to my waist. I rustled through my bag, looking to see if I'd brought any antiperspirant. No such luck.

Toby had changed into a pair of beige khaki pants, a corn-flower-blue dress shirt, and brown dress shoes. It was a clichéd outfit, but he managed to make it look good. He held up a navy tie with yellow polka dots and looked over to me.

I shrugged. "I'm not wearing one," I said.

He held it up to his neck, looking at himself in the mirror inside the room. "I kind of want to wear it just to spite him," he said. I laughed. "What a weird, backward world we live in." He threw the tie back into his suitcase.

Belinda appeared at the doorway holding a length of thick sailing rope. "You all decent?"

I waved for her to come inside. She put the rope down on a pile of books on the desk. "He was such a gentle, beautiful man. You know that?" She shook her head. "You boys are so lucky."

"Thank you," I said.

Toby just grunted.

"I'll see you outside in a few. Don't forget to bring this," she said, patting the rope.

As she left, Anais entered holding some loose papers and a prayer book. Her hair was up, and in her floral printed dress and flat shoes, her whole attire struck me as looking Amish. As if on cue, she dabbed her perspiring forehead with a handkerchief. It was such an antiquated gesture that it made me smile. We actually had been transported back two hundred years in time.

I tried to apologize for the fight earlier. "I get it," she said with a conciliatory smile. "I know it's not about me. Or you. This is hard for all of us." We hugged. She called Toby over, and he joined in. It felt a bit forced, but I appreciated it nonetheless. "We're almost done," she said. "I wish we had some flowers. I just want to do something nice."

Toby stared at her.

"What?" she asked.

Toby shook his head. Then he mustered up his courage and released what must have been pent up since the moment we

arrived. He exploded. "I'm sick of this shit! I can't keep pretend-ing he was some great guy and that we're so 'lucky' and that this day is so sad because he died! It's bullshit! He was an asshole. He totally abandoned me! He abandoned all of us." He swept a tear from his eye before it even reached his cheekbone.

"Oh, well, yeah." Anais smiled. "There's that."

"It's complicated—" I began, but he cut me off.

"No. Whatever. I don't know what went on when you two were kids, but I know about me. He was a fucking jerk. He totally disappeared right when I needed him most. And the fuck if he gave a shit about whether my mom could pay the rent."

"Yeah. Well, that sounds about right," I said.

"You may not be able to count on me for money . . ." Anais quoted.

" . . . but you can count on me for love." Toby and I joined in to finish the refrain. And the fact that we all knew it made us laugh.

"The fuck does that even mean?" Toby roared.

"Well," I said, lowering my voice, "if it's any consolation—"

"What?" Anais asked, a tiny anticipatory smile growing in the corners of her mouth.

"Fucker's dead now," I said.

We all laughed at that. Toby plopped down on the couch, and Anais and I sat down on either side of him, each of us with an arm around him. We sat closer than we had to. Closer than friends would. We sat as family.

"You know, his name, Herschel, was the original name for Uranus," Anais said.

"Astrological demigod of irresponsibility," I interjected. "Fit him pretty well."

"Whenever I hear the word Uranus"—Toby pronounced it *your anus*—"it makes me think of an asshole."

"For good reason," Anais said with a smile.

After a moment, she held out her hand to reveal several scraps of black fabric, each attached to a safety pin.

"I don't know how you'll feel about this," she began, "but one of the rituals at a Jewish funeral is that you tear a piece of your clothing. The idea is to symbolize the way that this change is irreparable. That a death literally tears a hole in the world." She put one of the strips of cloth into each of our hands. "Of course, that was the ancient ritual," she continued. "Now everyone just pins these swatches on and rips them symbolically."

Toby examined the little piece of fabric and began to pin it to his shirt.

"Yeah, okay," I said, annoyed. I took the pin and stuffed it in my pocket. But then, "You know, if you're going to rip your clothes, rip your fucking clothes. It's such bullshit to rip a tiny thing and then throw it away."

"Well not everyone is as macho as you are, Max," she said.

"I'm not being macho. I'm being literal. I don't think his passing makes a permanent hole in my life. More like the opposite; it's a wound that may finally get the chance to heal."

Suddenly, there was a knock at the door. Belinda called from outside. "Uh, guys? We've got a little problem."

CHAPTER 43
A WRINKLE IN TIME

BELINDA WAS STANDING with Captain Morago, in his excessively decorated military-style jacket and crisply pressed pants. "May I again offer my condolences regarding your father, Doctor Joe," the captain began. "But it has come to my attention that you are planning to bury the remains on Salem Hill. Is that correct?"

I looked to Belinda, who nodded and said, "There's more paperwork. You need another authorization form." She crossed her arms.

"We're supposed to begin in just a few minutes," Anais said. "Is that going to be a problem?"

"I'm afraid so," the captain said, and I swore I could see him trying to suppress a smile.

Luuk, standing twenty feet away in the parking lot behind the captain, mimed a strangling gesture, then walked away. Morago took an envelope out of his jacket and handed it to me.

I pulled out a form that was all in Dutch. "We're going to need help filling this out. We don't speak Dutch."

"That's not the thing," Belinda said. "It needs the signature of the lieutenant governor. Like the death certificate."

"No, no, no, no, no," I began to whimper.

Anais threw up her hands. "Seriously?"

"He's not on the island! He's on Saint Kitts! Can't we turn the form in afterward?" Toby asked, trying to remain reasonable.

"It is not possible," the captain said, shaking his head in an exaggerated expression of remorse.

"It's a piece of paper," I said. "Is there any reason that he might not sign it?" I pointed to the bungalow behind us. "You know where to find us. And why didn't you tell us about this yesterday?"

"I'm sorry, but on my island, we must follow the rule of law. And I was unaware that you were planning to bury him in public land."

"Come on," Belinda said. "Let's see what we can do."

Luuk had a six-seat motorboat moored at a small dock down the hill from the resort. "It'll be choppy," he warned, "but we can be back in a couple hours and satisfy that pompous, paper pushing, puss-tard's bullshit."

"What about the body?" I said. We had unloaded the coffin in the shade, but the sun had moved and now shone full force on the wooden box. "We can't leave it out like this." We dragged it into the shade of the building nearby, but I wasn't confident that it was going to last there for two hours without beginning to decompose.

"What difference does it make?" Anais offered. "Rotting is the point. We just want to avoid having to smell the reality of it."

Toby offered a solution. "Let's put him in the bungalow. It's at least a little cooler in there." So, Reggie, Anais, Toby, and I

heaved the box off the ground and scrambled across the parking lot toward Dad's door. When we got close, Reggie reminded us of his religious objection to going inside, so Luuk took his place.

We struggled to squeeze the box through the doorway, rotating the box ninety degrees to fit it plus our bodies through the narrow passage. We could hear the contents shifting inside, which was strangely disturbing. He was in there. We were carrying Dad's body. And the son of a bitch was heavy.

Once we made it through the door, there was simply no place to put it down on the ground, so we maneuvered over to lay the coffin on top of the bed. We got it in place, then stepped away to regard it. A coffin on top of a twin-size bed is oddly symmetrical. Both are specifically designed and built to fit a single human adult, just never at the same time. I thought of vampires.

It was cooler in there than outside, but it was no refrigerator. "Are you sure this isn't going to stink up the whole place?" I asked.

"It's just a couple hours. And the heat of the day has passed. We'll be fine," Luuk said. "But we've got to hurry."

We piled into Luuk's truck. It was a short ride down the hill to the marina. Once there, we jumped out, rushed down the length of the dock. Reggie was waiting there and helped Anais, Toby, and me climb aboard, then jumped on himself. Luuk yanked the starter string to awaken the menacing two-stroke motor. It roared right up, and he wasted no time navigating us away from the pier and into open water.

The engine was so loud that conversation was difficult, so we were forced to relax for a moment and just enjoy the ride. The breeze and the spray of the ocean tempered the hot sun, and I was reminded that we were in a place in the world that people

think of as a vacation spot (at least rich, urban Americans do). I reached my hand over the edge of the boat and dragged my fingers in the perfect turquoise water, making a splash that got Anais wet. She scolded me with her eyes, then turned away annoyed.

A pod of flying fish emerged alongside the boat, riding along with us for several minutes. It was an amazing display that delighted all of us, though Luuk and Reggie had obviously seen it countless times before. Dozens of the six-inch fish launched out of the water and cruised through the air, matching our speed and hovering right at eye-level for five or six seconds before diving back into the water, only to be replaced by another batch. Perfectly aligned to the boat's rate of motion, they appeared to be floating magically in the air just a few inches in front of me. I reached out and tried to touch one, but the fish expertly maneuvered through the air, rolling and twisting to avoid my grasp. It made me laugh out loud. For a moment I was able to be present, to enjoy the sun's warmth and the water's wetness, the fish's crazy behavior and the Earth's magnificence, not to mention the good fortune that we had the wherewithal and flexibility to be there in the first place, despite the circumstances.

I looked over at Toby and Anais, hoping to share my momentary burst of joy, but I was deterred. Toby was looking intently out toward the horizon, his lips pursed together. He looked pained, like he was contemplating death, or more likely that his stomach was turning and he was trying to keep from vomiting. I wished I could offer some sagely salve to unfurrow his brow, but we weren't close enough for that yet. Brothers yes, but still strangers too.

Anais sat with her eyes closed, in a private space that I didn't feel entitled to penetrate. I still felt a morsel of anger toward her,

and then anger at myself for having those feelings. I closed my own eyes and tried to regain the peace I'd felt a moment before. But instead, a pang of terror rose through me like an electric shock under my ribs.

What if the lieutenant governor asked to see the death certificate? He would clearly recognize that I'd forged his signature, not least because he would know that he hadn't signed it. If only I'd realized that before we had left I could have maybe gotten another blank copy of the form, but it was too late for that. Besides—the body was already in our possession. He would know that was impossible without his blessing. Maybe I should have forged the new document too. Or was that just digging an even deeper hole for myself? Had I been operating under such lack of sleep and emotional stress that I'd done something horribly wrong? Was I going to wind up in jail? What the fuck had I let the bastard get me into?

I watched Statia shrink and disappear behind us. We were out in totally open sea. Suddenly I couldn't get enough air into my lungs. I felt dizzy. My hair bristled on my scalp. I rubbed my eyes and grabbed the back of my neck, trying to stave off the ensuing anxiety attack without drawing too much attention. I tried holding my breath to interrupt the panic—like I would to break a bout of hiccups. I closed my eyes and focused on the sound of the motor.

And when I released the air in my lungs and opened my eyes, miraculously, I had survived. Somehow the moment was over. I could just make out the bump of the other island on the horizon, growing rapidly as we approached. Something would work out. I wasn't sure what, but it had to. I was just going to have to have faith.

Soon I could make out cars driving along the coastline road, and then, a few minutes later, I saw people walking along the beach. This island seemed a lot bigger than Statia, and more modern. Before we knew it, we had pulled into a harbor and docked in a sizable marina. As I stepped onto dry land, I felt a moment of wooziness as I adjusted to the lack of movement. But I braced myself and willed my sea legs away. We had too much to do to be off balance. I tried to rush Toby and Anais along, but as usual, my momentum was thwarted.

Because this island was technically a different country, before we could leave the harbor we had to pass through an immigration station, where we waited in a line with tourists and other visitors from surrounding islands. The agents were oblivious to our time constraint, and they seemed to be engaging many of the guests in extended conversations. While we waited, I picked up a tourist map of Basseterre, the capital of Saint Kitts. Luuk explained that the population there was about ten thousand, not including the rest of the island nor the adjoining island, Nevis.

"Compare that to less than three thousand people on all of Statia," he said.

"It almost feels like real life," Toby joked.

Luuk scoffed. "Real life is overrated."

CHAPTER 44

RABBIT, RUN

WE FINALLY GOT our passports stamped, and we were released into the city. Cars, traffic lights, and street vendors livened the road all the way from the marina to the town center. The noise and activity was a bit overwhelming in contrast to where we had been. I could only imagine the reverse culture shock I would feel when I finally saw New York or Los Angeles again.

We agreed to meet Luuk and Reggie back at the boat in forty-five minutes, and we headed off on foot, using a map as a guide. We trekked up the hill toward a park surrounded by a group of government buildings, determined to find our man and get the damned paper signed.

After a minute I noticed that it was just Toby and me, and I looked behind us. Anais had stopped at a sidewalk stall and was chatting up a woman selling dried herbs. I was tempted to leave her and run ahead, but she had the burial document in her purse. "Annie! Come on!" I yelled. But she couldn't hear me. "Damn it," I said to Toby.

"What's she doing?" he asked, appropriately annoyed.

"Sourcing belladonna to poison me with," I muttered and ran back down the hill to grab her, while Toby waited.

When I reached her, I didn't even have to say anything.

"I know, I know," she said, and then thanked the woman as I led her away.

"I know I shouldn't have stopped," she said, "but they've got all these herbs that aren't even legal in the US. Do you remember that witch shop on Avenue A?"

I did. Dad occasionally brought me to this secret herb store near his apartment, a tiny, unmarked, dark room off a basement entrance to someone's flat, where a hippy couple sold Wiccan and occult paraphernalia, as well as a collection of incense and herbs (including some quasi-legal substances like mandrake and acacia leaves). It was the kind of place that could close up and relocate in a hurry if necessary, which I suspect happened with some regularity—though more likely to dodge an intolerant landlord than the vice squad.

Still, it was beguiling. I remember walking through the narrow room, fascinated by the feathers and animal skulls, drinking in the exotic smells and fondling books about the dark arts and Satanism. Dad would chat up the earnest young proprietor woman, using his pharmacological expertise to guide her on the proper temperature to best extract the active alkaloids from a particular herb. And she would listen, fascinated and impressed. I paid attention too, though I may have been more focused on the woman's loose-fitting, braless tank top and the view of her full bush of underarm hair, which I found both repulsive and irresistibly sexy.

"I remember," I said curtly, absurdly jealous that Dad had shared that shop with Anais too. And even more so that she had

later embraced herbalism so fully. The two of them probably were able to bond and connect about it. He and I had nothing. Nothing but secrets. "We just need to get this over with," I said, trying to be patient.

She nodded. "Where's Tobias?"

A rush of people had appeared on the sidewalk ahead of us, and I couldn't see Toby anywhere. "Fuck!" I said. "Are you kidding me?"

I paused to look around. I looked inside the nearby shops, an old-fashioned drugstore and a laundromat. I was about to explode with rage, then Anais spotted Toby on the other side of the street, and he was waving for us to join him. I cut through the moving traffic, not looking back, hoping that Anais was keeping up behind me. When I reached Toby, he was shaking his head.

"You're not going to believe this," he began. "There's some big parade. That's probably why the dude is over here in the first place."

"Carnival," I fumed. Don't these people know we've got actual business to conduct.

"Actually, it's apparently unrelated to Carnival." Toby shook his head then shrugged. I threw my hands in the air.

"Come on. Let's not give up," Anais said. She pointed. "That looks like city hall or something. Let's see what we can figure out."

"What if he asks about the death certificate and who signed it?" I blurted out.

Anais shrugged. "We left it on the other island. We can't worry about that now. Come on." We trudged up the rest of the hill, and as we neared the central square, the crowd thickened. All around us people were congregating for the parade, groups of women in spectacular feathered wings and headdresses, and men

in tribal costumes of orange and red. It was all very impressive, but I didn't have the patience to appreciate it.

Toby had the map and led us through the crowds to the governmental building. We were practically running, and in the heat I was once again sweating through my "nice" clothes. When we reached the building, we climbed the steps and pulled on the large, windowed doors—only to find that they were all locked. "Of course they are," I said. "What the hell were we thinking?"

We collapsed on the steps, accepting our defeat, and watched the people preparing for the parade. A woman came out of the building and Toby jumped to his feet.

"Excuse me!" he said. "I know this is crazy, but we're looking for Lieutenant Governor Berkel from Statia. He's supposed to be here, and we really need to find him."

The woman turned out to be an assistant to the local governor and miraculously knew all about Berkel's visit. "I don't think there's much chance you're going to get to speak to him, though," she cautioned. "He's here as a friend to Commander Thomas. For the festivities." She pointed to a place across the square where a large booth was set up. "He'll likely be in there once the parade starts, but I don't expect you'll be able to see him without an appointment."

"Can't hurt to try," Toby said. And he ran off, instructing us to wait on the steps.

We watched Toby disappear into the crowd. We could hear the marching band practicing their instruments: short bursts of musical phrases, a tuba flourish here, a snare drum rat-a-tat there; three trombones wailed a few notes in near unison before being overtaken by the whistles of cops trying to corral the crowd out of the street.

I looked over at Anais, who seemed quietly content. I realized it was the first time the two of us had been alone together the whole trip. I didn't want to ruin the moment of near peace, but it may have been my only chance to talk to her. Words began to come out of my mouth like bile that I couldn't keep down.

"I, uh, I, um, I found . . ." I stammered. "There was some . . . I need to talk to you about something." She turned and looked at me with a worried look. I mustered my courage. "There was some stuff I found. On Dad's computer. Sort of."

"What?" she asked with great concern.

"It's hard to talk about. There was a lot of pornography."

"Oh, I'm sure," she said with a dismissive smile.

"No, but there was more. There were stories. About you. About you and Lena. You remember Lena?"

Mentioning the name of her high school friend got her attention. "What do you mean?" she asked.

"I don't know how to say it. Erotic stories. Pornographic stories. Detailing things . . . Did he . . . did you . . . ?" I trailed off. My face felt flushed. The heat of the day and the enormity of the secret made blood rush to my head, filling it up like a water balloon stretched to the bursting point. I felt like I was looking at her from farther and farther away through a pinhole, my consciousness shrinking inward, growing smaller and smaller. A familiar cascade of shame rushed through me like I was somehow unwittingly the perpetrator, like I couldn't differentiate myself from him. His panicked lascivious venomous undulating cock-snake helixed around my spine, clinging, constricting, desperately sucking, sacrificing my life force to somehow fortify his own starving soul. My own DNA was half his. Poisoned. Tainted. Despicable. Unlovable.

"Oh, Max," Anais said, smiling gently. I was thrown by her reaction. "How long have you been holding this in?"

I shrugged, gesturing over my shoulder as if to answer her question that way. "Since before. Did he . . . did he molest you?"

"No," she said. "But I'm not surprised." Then, with a twisted smile, "Lena? Really?"

"I don't know, I didn't really read any of it. I just skimmed it to grasp what it was and then I just deleted it all."

She put her arms around me. I was confused as to why she was the one comforting me.

"He was a pervert. You didn't know that?" she said, shaking her head in disgust.

"I don't know. I guess not," I said.

"He never touched me, but there were times, when I was thirteen or fourteen, after this happened"—she grabbed her breasts a bit aggressively—"when I could tell that he was acting weird, or staring."

I could see her remembering. "Jesus, Anais. I'm so sorry," I said.

"I don't know," she said slowly. "I think at some level I appreciated the attention."

"I feel like I was complicit," I admitted. "Or responsible. Like I should have recognized it and intervened," I said. "I'm your brother."

"You were nine years old." She ruffled my hair.

"I guess," I said. "Still . . ." Tears came to my eyes, but I managed to keep most of them from rolling down my cheeks. We sat there side by side, her arm around my shoulder and mine around her back.

"I'm sorry you had to see that," she said. "It's ugly."

"I'm sorry you had to live it."

She nodded, and we fell back into silence, but it was a different silence. Just a tiny bit bigger. "Are you not angry at him?" I finally asked.

She smiled in her odd, conspiratorial way. "I'm furious. Though to be honest, more about the rest of it than his creepy incestuous fantasies." She shuddered. "He was a coward. He didn't take care of us. He never provided. He left us with *Mom*." She shook her head. "I'm furious, but I'm not angry. He doesn't deserve my anger. I'm not going to waste that energy on him. Lord knows I've wasted enough over the years."

I nodded. "But yet, you go through all of this." I gestured around us, indicating the elaborate hassle and unfathomable energy we had spent on this attempt to give him a funeral.

She shrugged. "Yeah. You too. I guess . . . I guess I think it's about responding with love. To his hate or misogyny, to his cowardice, to his inability to love us for real—which of course is just his inability to love himself. I'm going to choose love. To honor him properly in death. Not for him. For me." Then she took my hand and stared at me in *that way*. "I'm doing it for you. For us."

I nodded. But I could feel the queer, conflicting mix of emotions that my relationship with my sister always elicited in me. The intensity of her earnestness left no room for reciprocation, for a dignified reply, for me to have my own feelings. Her magnanimity was somehow voracious, selfish. Like the very affection she was offering intended to envelop me, devour me. To accept it required me to forgo my own feelings, my sense of self.

All at once I was reminded of my relationship with our father. How his love was barbed. To be accepted, to receive his attention, I had to capitulate, genuflect, supplicate. I had to allow

him to feed from me. And while there were times I resisted or stood up to him, he never yielded. And so eventually I'd relent.

I think of the rose, its beauty protected by thorns. Luring in the bees to help it procreate, but anyone else who gets close gets the bloody prickle. Maybe love is just a come-on, a bribe. Maybe Anais came to terms with all this long ago, accepted it and even embraced it herself. Maybe it wasn't even such a tragedy. The killdeer, the cowbird, the creepy firefly—nature is cruel. Brutal. Transactional. Why should I expect human behavior to be any different? No wonder Anais wasn't more upset. For her, his treachery was already baked into the price.

I looked back over at her, but her gaze was now fixed out on the crowd, a half-smile on her lips. I was relieved that I'd relinquished his terrible secret, but alas, I didn't feel much better. It was going to take a lot more than a brief moment of honesty to heal.

Soon, Toby reemerged. From the look of his gait, he hadn't had any luck. The band launched into a fanfare to begin the parade, and the crowd cheered loudly from all directions. I was suddenly concerned that we were going to have trouble getting back to the boat in time, no matter what happened with the governor.

When Toby reached us, he was still holding onto some hope. "He's supposed to be there in that viewing area, but apparently he hasn't arrived yet. Maybe we can just stand there nearby and wait."

"This is crazy," I said. "That's never going to work and we don't have time."

"What else can we do? You want to forge this too?" Anais asked.

"I don't think so. It got by the hospital administrator, but I don't think we should try to pull one over on Idi Amin," I said.

That made them both laugh. "But . . ." I began, an idea forming in my mind. "What if . . . we use *Aikido*?"

"What are you talking about?" Toby asked.

"Use his own weight against him," I said. "A little something the Asshole taught me."

"He taught you Aikido?" Toby asked. "He never taught me shit."

"Nah, he didn't teach me anything practical," I said. "But the concept: It's all about using your opponent's own weight or momentum against them."

Anais and Toby stared at me. They didn't follow.

"What if we convince the captain that he should have the authority to sign the form himself? Isn't he *important* enough? Shouldn't the lieutenant governor trust *him* to make such vital decisions? How could he resist, if we frame it right?"

"Dude, that's a terrible idea," Toby said.

Anais threw up her hands. "Yeah. It's not going to work, but it's better than you falsifying another legal document."

CHAPTER 45
THINGS FALL APART

AS WE APPROACHED THE MARINA, we could see Luuk was pacing back and forth on the dock. Something was wrong. "We're out of petrol," he howled once we were in earshot. The marina gas station was out, so Luuk couldn't refuel the boat; and we didn't have enough fuel to get back to Statia. We had to figure something out quickly, Luuk explained; with the dusk came stormy weather, which would be unsafe to travel through.

And of course, there was also the slowly warming, unembalmed corpse waiting for us back in our bedroom. After a few moments of panic and exasperation, we whipped up a plan for Toby and me to head back into Basseterre, secure a gasoline container, fill it up at a gas station, and carry it back to the boat. We took off. Batman and Robin.

The first gas station didn't have any gas cans. They offered to fill up a few two-liter soda bottles, but we needed at least five gallons. We ran through the streets, asking strangers for help and looking for a store that might sell gas cans. Someone directed

us to a hardware store, but they were out of stock. Desperate and out of ideas, we decided to hire a taxi. A car would be more efficient than running around on foot, and hopefully it would have air-conditioning too. We found a cab pretty quickly, and the driver was happy to help. He drove us to another hardware store, but they were also out of stock. Who would have thought a fuel container was such a hot commodity?

The driver made a couple of phone calls on his mobile. He told us he had a friend with a couple old gas jugs that he could sell us for cheap. We agreed and the driver set off, heading out of the city and up the edge of a mountain. I began to get a creepy vibe. The landscape grew very rural very quickly, and the few residences were made of two-by-fours and rusty corrugated steel. I flashed to my father's story about Jamaica, then I was jolted back to reality as our driver swerved to avoid a mangy dog running through the road. I looked to Toby, and he was similarly unnerved. Still, we had no choice but to trust the guy.

Finally, the cabbie turned down a driveway and headed toward a small house. A short, heavyset guy wearing a yellow baseball cap stood outside, and he had a big friendly smile on his face. Definitely not an axe murderer. He had two old five-gallon metal gas cans, and he sold them to us for five bucks each. I had no idea if that was a lot or a little in local terms, but it hardly mattered. The cans were not in great shape, a bit dented and rusty in places, but they seemed functional enough, so we threw them into the trunk and raced back toward town.

We were unsure whether we needed diesel or gasoline. I tried calling Luuk, but naturally, I couldn't get through. Our cabbie thought diesel was more likely, but I thought I remembered Luuk saying "petrol," which meant regular gas. I went with my

gut, and we filled up the two tanks. "At the very least, gasoline is lighter than diesel," I joked, "so the gas cans will only weigh thirty pounds each instead of thirty-six."

"How the fuck do you know that?" Toby asked.

I shrugged. My brain liked to do math problems when I was under stress. We filled the canisters up, lugged them back into the cab, and drove down to the edge of the marina, as close as the cabbie could get—and I asked him to wait. We waddled as fast as we could with our unwieldy cargo toward the boat, and I yelled ahead to Luuk, "Gas or diesel? Gas or diesel?" He couldn't understand me. "Gas or diesel?" I said again, then clarified, "Petrol or diesel?" Fucking Europeans.

"Petrol," Luuk confirmed. "Didn't I say?"

"Yes. Great. We just weren't positive," I said, and I waved off the cabbie.

Reggie opened one of the gas containers in preparation. "There's no water in the cans, right? They look a bit dodgy," Luuk said.

"I don't think so," I said, though I had no idea. "Is that a problem?"

The answer was yes. But Luuk didn't elaborate. We were already in grave risk of getting back late or worse, getting stuck out in the big swells in the dark. Reggie quickly slashed a plastic water bottle in half to use as a funnel and poured the fuel into the boat's tank. Even before the reservoir was full, Luuk revved the engine and we made our way out of the harbor and into open water.

While we were off pursuing the signature, Luuk and Reggie had loaded the boat full of supplies, so now there was even less room for us to sit amid fifty-pound bags of onions, potatoes,

flour, sugar, and other rudiments. The little engine seemed to strain under all the added weight, but Luuk opened the throttle all the way up and we powered through.

At first, all seemed fine. The seas were rougher than on the way over, especially as we exited the harbor and crossed a few other boats' wakes. Each wave forced the boat to rear up like a wild horse, only to slam back down again as we crossed through the crest. Toby started vomiting over the side. I scurried over to sit next to him and put my hand on his back as he wretched. "It's gonna be okay," I said. But out ahead of us, I spotted some ominous-looking clouds.

It wasn't long before those clouds were overhead. "What's a little rain, when it's so warm out anyway?" I joked, yelling to be heard over the engine. Luuk and Reggie didn't laugh though. Luuk gunned the motor, and Saint Kitts shrunk behind us, enveloped by the vast, magnificent ocean. I remembered the map that I looked at when I was planning my trip. We really were in the middle of the ocean.

I could just perceive a glimpse of the mountain that was Statia sticking out of the ocean when it first happened: The engine hiccupped a little, and I felt a brief lag in our forward momentum. No one said anything, but after another minute it happened again, and then again.

"Ah fuck!" Luuk barked. "That's water in the line."

I looked to my siblings, and we exchange worried glances. The engine continued to gurgle a bit, and our forward progress abated. I looked at the island in the distance and wondered if I could swim for it if I had to. I doubted it. Maybe Toby could have made it, or Reggie, but definitely not Luuk. And Anais and I were far too soft in the middle for that kind of effort. Reggie

clambered over the bags of supplies to get to Luuk, and they conferred.

"What are we gonna do?" Toby asked Anais and me, his voice hoarse from the puking.

"We'll be fine." Anais said, based on nothing at all.

"Maybe we can send out a Mayday signal?" I wondered aloud.

Reggie maneuvered over to the starboard side of the boat and moved a big lever. "I gone swish over to da reserve tank. We see if that one is more better." The engine stalled out, and the quiet came on all at once.

Luuk looked a bit frantic as he scrambled away from the steering wheel and back toward the aft of the boat where the three of us were sitting. "Out of the way!" he barked. We all darted and moved to clear a path. He yanked the starter cord, but it didn't catch. He tried again, and again.

"We're totally fucked," I said quietly to no one at all. "We're never going to get through this. We're going to die out here, for *him*."

Luuk stopped and wiped his brow. Realizing that we were descending into panic, he tried to calm us down. The three of us were huddled near the driver's seat. "We'll be fine. Don't worry," he said, with a big grin that looked entirely for our benefit. "Let's just give it a minute."

"I'm so sorry," I began. "We had no idea, and we were in such a rush."

"It's not your fault. You couldn't have known," he said. "And hey, it's beautiful out here, right? You could go for a swim, eh?"

We laughed. I looked out into the water. It was crystal clear, and only six feet deep. It actually would be a great time to take

a swim. I wondered if Dad ever got to do any snorkeling here before he died.

He had taught me how to snorkel when I was five, on Sanibel Island. I remember being delighted by the unexpectedly rich world of coral and fish living there all the time, just under the surface of what looked so flat and empty. While we were floating together, peering down through our masks into the expansive world below, I saw a seahorse for the first time. It was the funniest-looking and most improbable thing I'd ever beheld. I laughed through my snorkel and grabbed Dad's hand. "Look!" I tried to say through the foot-long tube. He thought I was pointing to a rock and began pontificating about the Mesolithic substrata of the Earth or some shit, but he was talking through the snorkel too, so he was unintelligible. I kept saying, "LOOK!" and pointing at the beautiful creature as it rolled its spiny tail in and out and reared back its stallion-like head with each rocking motion. Finally, I made him join me above the surface and I described the creature in excited, breathless bursts.

"Oh! That's a seahorse, or *hippokampos*, which is from the Greek: *hippo* for horse and *kampos* for sea monster."

The name pleased me, as that's just what it looked like to me: a horse-sea-monster amalgam. I dove back down to see it again, but it was gone.

I glided through the reef, admiring a school of needlefish and a huge, bright, mushroom-like sea anemone. Suddenly a four-foot barracuda appeared and swam directly toward me, one of the few fish I was taught to stay away from—as if its toothy glare wouldn't trigger an instinctive response from my autonomic nervous system. I popped my head out of the water, pumping my feet to keep me afloat. Probably the worst thing I could have done.

"Daddy!" I yelled. "Help!" But I couldn't see him anywhere. "Daddy?" I yelled again, this time a little panicked. I peeked down under the surface but was too scared to go all the way in, so I stayed above, treading. I was terrified that the predator was going to bite me any second, and the fact that I couldn't view his progress made it that much scarier. I waited for the bite. My thigh? My butt? My foot? Would he rip my penis off? I clenched my teeth, but the attack never came. After a minute, I looked back under the surface long enough to verify that the menacing fish was gone.

A few minutes later I finally located Dad, snorkeling on his own, thirty feet away. I swam over to him, buoyant with adrenaline and newfound invincibility, but he was oblivious. Back on the beach, I tried to relay my story, but he was preoccupied, so I stopped.

I remember a look on his face. It was the same look I saw when we were in Paris. It was a look that he wore often when I was young, and I never understood it at the time, but I knew enough that it meant to leave him alone. Now, in my memory, I recognize it. It was terror. As frightened as I may have been of the barracuda, he was enduring something much more existential. I'll never know what, but I'm beginning to understand that he carried it with him always.

• • •

Luuk gave the engine starter another pull, and it revved up. The reserve tank seemed to be clean of water, and we were back underway. Once or twice the engine hiccupped again, and we all tensed up. But it held up. The sky darkened further and the chop

grew stronger as we got closer and closer to our destination. We arrived at the little dock just as the rain began to fall in earnest.

"We caught a break there," Luuk said. "Maybe that was Joe looking down and giving us just a little push, eh?" he joked, and Anais and Toby laughed their agreement.

Not likely, I thought. But I kept my mouth shut.

• • •

We were all exhausted from the tension, but there was still a body to bury. Clearly we were not going to be able to do it that after noon. It was raining and dark, and we still had to convince the crazy cop to let us proceed. But our more immediate problem was that the coffin was still in the bungalow and we had no plan for how to store it.

We sat with several beers in the dining area, trying to come up with a plan. The two dogs ran back and forth around our legs, and the macaw squawked, taking shelter from the rain with us under the roof.

"What about da Piccolo place? I's got a friend who works in the kitchen dere." Reggie asked.

Luuk scoffed. Belinda came over and sat with us. "Those people are ruining the whole damned island," she said.

"Yah, but they got da big walk-in freezer. Maybe they can hold ol' Joe for da night."

"What is it?" Anais asked. "A restaurant?"

"It's another resort. On the leeward side," Luuk explained. "And there's not a soul on the island who doesn't resent their presence."

Reggie tried to call his friend, while Luuk reached out to

Ralph to see if the University had any options that might help. Both of them came up empty.

"We're just gonna have to do it the old-fashioned way," I said.

"Funeral pyre?" Toby joked.

"That would solve all our problems, wouldn't it?" I said. "No, I think Ol' Joe's just gonna have to camp out for the night and we'll see where we are in the morning."

We wrangled the coffin back out of the room and looked for a good spot. Luuk was a little concerned about disturbing the other guests, insistent that it wasn't visible from the pool or the dining area, which turned out to be quite limiting. Finally, we found a spot near the storage shed where it was at least a little bit camouflaged by the grass and the debris and detritus lying around.

It looked rather pathetic, like a forgotten piece of junk that just happened to be a human being inside a box. It was oddly dissonant to remind myself that it was in fact our father's body we were talking about. But then he never did quite fit in anywhere, so I guess it was just par for the course. Luuk pulled out an old tarp, and we managed to rig it into a lean-to style canopy to at least keep the coffin safe from any rain. Somehow that made it look a little more dignified. But not much.

CHAPTER 46
REMEMBRANCE OF THINGS PAST

WHEN WE GOT BACK to the dining area, Belinda had dinner waiting for us: fried chicken and buttermilk biscuits. Despite the exhausting and intense day, dinner provided me with a wave of new energy, and Toby and Anais seemed to rally too. We headed back to Dad's bungalow to figure out what to do with his belongings. I was worried that the room was going to smell or be somehow contaminated, but there didn't appear to be any such problem.

"No whiff of death or anything," I joked.

"Are you sure you want to sleep in here?" Anais asked. "I'm sure they've got another room you can use."

I shook my head. I wouldn't want to seem like I couldn't handle a little death smell; what's a little rotting flesh aroma among family? Also, I didn't want to admit the depth of my freak-out the previous night. I tossed it to Toby, hoping he would insist we move rooms. But he didn't take the bait. "I'm so tired, I'll be asleep as soon as I put my head down."

So, I constructed an elaborate protective barrier over the bed using towels, clean sheets, and the removable lining of my suitcase. I considered covering the bed with a row of Dad's books but figured that would be too uncomfortable. Instead, Toby and I piled the remainder of the books into boxes while Anais went through Dad's closet.

She held up a few shirts and jackets and offered them to Toby and me. Nothing would have fit Toby, who was smaller and in better shape than Dad was, and while I could have probably slipped right into most of it, I had no interest in wearing a dead man's wardrobe.

I did try on his jean jacket. It wasn't the exact one he wore all the time back in the '80s (with the inside pocket that he taught me was for shoplifting), but it was so worn out that it might as well have been. I put it on, along with a pair of his sunglasses, and I mugged for Anais and Toby. "Jah jah, bless!" Toby joked.

In the back of the closet, Anais discovered an old, well-worn suitcase, the heavy hard-sided kind that people used to drag through the airport with a strap before the days of roller bags. She hoisted it onto the bed, popped its metal latches, and opened it—revealing a treasure trove of photos and memorabilia from the span of Dad's life. Toby and I left the books behind, and we all gathered around the suitcase.

Inside was a pile of rejection letters—from Bantam Books; Penguin; Farrar, Straus & Giroux; and others—all neatly bundled together, though the dates stretched over many years. There were ID cards from a variety of jobs, including NYU, MetLife Insurance, Ringling Bros. Circus, and even Schering-Plough, where he had met Margo a million years ago.

Toby read aloud a well-preserved letter from 1971 when

Dad was invited by the World Health Organization to speak in Greece about some drug experiments he was doing. Anais picked up a faded envelope filled with pictures from his wedding with our mom in 1960. There was also an eight-by-ten high school portrait, and lo and behold, it looked exactly like Toby. "Look at that!" Anais called out and held it up beside Toby's face.

It was uncanny. As much as I, at forty, looked like Dad did at seventy, Toby at twenty-five looked exactly like Dad at eighteen. Seeing that brought me a strange kind of relief. I was eager to share the burden of carrying on the man's legacy, and somehow that helped. Toby was amused by it, but he also seemed a bit unsettled by the resemblance. He walked the picture over to a mirror and stared at himself side-by-side with the photo.

"Now you know how I feel walking around this island," I said.

There were lots more pictures. Another envelope contained snapshots of Dad, Margo, and Toby as a baby. Another one had a handful of pictures of Anais and me from across the years: school photos from elementary school, Anais's graduation from college, a few shots from her first wedding, and even some photos of the trip I took with Dad to France. I uncovered a picture of Anais and me as young kids riding an elephant at Jungle Habitat, a short-lived animal safari in Passaic, New Jersey. I was probably four years old, but I still remember that ride: When Dad lifted me up onto the elephant, it snorted a blast of water right in his ear. It made him laugh like I had never seen.

Another folder contained copies of papers and letters written by Anais and me. There were term papers from high school and college. Why would he have kept all that stuff when he was moving around so much? What a hassle to hold onto a bunch of stupid papers from twenty years ago.

Then I found the letters that I wrote to him ten years before. The ones where I called him out on being a shitty father and a drug addict, and about how much it hurt me when he insisted on including Marcy whenever we were together. The letters that aroused such fury and indignation from him and that forged a chasm in our relationship that never completely healed. The melancholy rose in me. It would have been easier if we hadn't had found all of this. If I could have held onto the fiction that he hadn't given a shit about us and had just left us behind when he started his new life as "Doctor Joe." But the truth was less tidy.

Eventually we got the remainder of his books stored in boxes so we could transport them to the island library the following day. Anais lost at Rochambeau and agreed to stay on an extra day or two to clean out the kitchen and to deal with discarding the rest of his belongings. And I agreed to bring the photos home with me and digitize them all. Toby kept Dad's high school portrait.

CHAPTER 47

AS YOU LIKE IT

I WOKE UP THE NEXT MORNING around six forty-five. I was amazed that I'd slept through the night. I walked past Toby, still blissfully unconscious, to the bathroom. I stood at the toilet barefoot, in the exact spot where Dad's body had lay crumpled. The fear and trepidation I'd felt the first time I stood in that spot had been replaced by an odd normalcy. It was just a toilet, and I needed to pee.

I considered waking up Toby, but instead I slipped on my shoes and headed to the dining patio. The early morning light was magnificent, with a blush of pink visible in the east, while in the west, out over the water, the last dredges of the night remained, and I could make out a few stars struggling to be seen despite the dawn. I once joked with Dad that for someone so dedicated to the stars, New York City was a terrible place to live. The light pollution made even Orion a rare sight. He responded that he didn't need to see the stars to feel their pull. He had *faith*. Still, standing there that morning, I hoped he had appreciated

the ample view of the heavens he finally found on this celestially divined island.

Soon I heard a loud, deep bark. One of the Great Danes appeared at the edge of the patio. After eyeing me from a distance, she lumbered over, ready to attack me with her slobber and terrible breath. "Bambi! Sit!" I said, trying to emulate Belinda's confidence. The dog paused obediently and knelt, lowering her giant jaw onto my lap, her chestnut eyes gazing up toward mine. I stroked the top of her head, and she plopped down beside me.

A few minutes later Belinda, Luuk, and the other dog came over. I lamented that we still needed to get Morago to authorize the burial, and that the longer we waited, the more disgusting that coffin was going to smell. With a little prodding, I got Luuk to tell me about his history with Morago. "When we first got here, about nine years ago, we had this idea to open the inn."

"Was that your background?" I asked.

"No, I was in banking. In Amsterdam. And Linda was in corporate HR."

"We had to get out," Belinda added.

"In a bit of a hurry, if you know what I mean." He winked at me.

Belinda brought over coffee and some store-bought muffins that must have been part of the haul we brought back on the boat from Saint Kitts.

Luuk continued, "Morago wasn't the captain then, just a pain in the ass cop with not enough to do. After we opened, a lot of our first guests were friends from back home, and we started the tradition of the Thursday night dinner, where we make a meal for everyone to share. In those early days we used to serve lobster. We had a guy, Suki, who was a diver and a trained chef. Anyway,

Morago decided at one point that the lobsters were off-limits, that we were violating some environmental rule. He came marching over one Thursday while we were enjoying ourselves, and he began—I'm not kidding—he began confiscating the lobsters." Luuk stood up to demonstrate, stealing our muffins. "Right off of people's plates! So I ran over there and started getting into it with him."

"Meanwhile another guy started loading our food into the back of their truck. And not just the lobsters, but everything," Belinda said.

"So I started screaming at Morago, threatening to put a live lobster in his bed at night, and I was getting pretty heated up so his buddy radioed for backup," Luuk said. His face grew beet red just telling the story.

"We were still new here, so no one knew us yet," Belinda chimed in.

"And, I swear, I held myself back. I didn't clock him. But next thing I know they were cuffing me and dragging me off to spend a night in the jail."

"For serving lobster?" I asked.

He nodded, a silly grin on his face. "But that's not the best part. The best part is that the lobsters they confiscated were taken directly to another party for Morago's brother. It was all because he had promised his brother lobsters, but he couldn't find any." He and Belinda laughed at the memory.

"We found that out because Juanita was there and she's friends with Robin, and, anyway," Belinda explained, "Luuk confronted him about it but he never so much as apologized."

"Yet the mysterious lobster ban was rescinded a few weeks later," Luuk shook his head in disgust. "I try to avoid his presence

to keep me from boxing his ears, or worse." Luuk mimed a powerful double-handed blow to an imaginary head in front of him.

"And to keep from spending another night in jail, dear," Belinda teased.

Soon, Toby and Anais joined us in the dining area, and Belinda cooked up some eggs and sausage. There were a lot of other guests around that morning. I forgot that Luuk and Belinda were still running a business, even while they gave us so much attention and helped in preparing for the funeral. I apologized and told them how much we appreciated all that they were doing.

"Joe was our dear friend," Belinda said. "We're not doing you a favor. We're honored to be able to play such a big role."

Once our bellies were full, we headed back down to the police station. By now the route was familiar to me: up and over the hill through the thick part of the forest, then left at the fallen tree. As we entered the town, a sharp right along a small gully. There was a lot of activity at the police station that morning. Cars and several bicycles filled the small parking lot. We had to park on the side of the road, and once again Luuk opted to wait in the car. The three of us marched toward the building.

"What are you going to say?" Toby asked.

"I'm going to tell him the truth and then appeal to his megalomania," I said.

We pushed through the doors and headed directly upstairs. When we got to the top landing, we found Morago's door closed, and the light inside was off.

"Not here yet," Toby observed.

We headed back to the parking lot and waited. Morago finally arrived on a beat-up old bicycle. Eager to get back to the

decaying body, we accosted him as he dismounted. He was wearing street clothes, and without his uniform, he looked like any other local guy on the island.

"Good morning," I said.

"*Goede morgen*, sir," he replied.

"Unfortunately, we were unable to meet with the lieutenant governor," I began. "We rushed over to Saint Kitts yesterday, but to no avail."

"Yes, I am deeply sorry for the inconvenience," he retorted. He tried to head toward the station door, but we positioned ourselves in his way.

"Right. Well," I continued, "we were hoping that, given the circumstances, you might see fit to allow us to go ahead with the funeral and get the form signed later."

"Yes. I see. However, the law states that the form must be signed before you may proceed with the burial." He began walking quickly around us, but we scuttled along with him. "In point of fact, you should not have even begun digging the grave without this form approved and signed."

"There's a religious imperative to get the body buried as soon as possible. He was supposed to be buried within three days. We're already on day six," Anais said. "We're violating the laws of our people!"

The captain nodded. "Yes. But that is not a reason I should allow you to violate the laws of ours. Two wrongs do not make a right. I'm so very, very sorry," he said, and again began walking around us. "I must get to work."

Anais and Toby looked to me. I sprinted ahead a few feet and essentially blocked the door to the building. Anais and Toby came around and flanked me. "Look," I said, "When the

lieutenant governor is gone, who is second in command? Who's the most powerful man on the island? Isn't that you?"

A small smile crept across his face, but he shook his head.

I pressed on, speaking slowly. "Aren't you the *most, powerful, man*? Someone has to have authority when Berkel is away? Couldn't you sign the form in his absence?" I pulled out the form and waved it in front of him, but he refused to take it.

"I have authority over police matters. But I'm afraid this is an administrative matter."

Toby spoke up, going all in with a bribe offer. "Maybe there is a fee we can pay?" That got Morago to pause.

But then: "We both know you can exercise whatever power you want when it suits you, Homero." Luuk's voice boomed from behind us. "Why don't you just step aside and let these kids bury their damned father?"

We all spun around. Luuk swaggered right up to us, grabbed the paper from me and forced it into Morago's hand. He spoke quietly right into Morago's ear. "Sign the form, or so help me . . ."

"I suppose I may grant a temporary permit," Morago said cheerily.

Luuk led us back to the truck. "Son of a bitch," he muttered.

CHAPTER 48
GOODBYE, COLUMBUS

THE ROPE BELINDA HAD BROUGHT over the day before was huge and very heavy. It was braided nylon sailing line, an inch thick, and there must have been twenty or thirty feet of it. I was still unclear on what we needed it for, but I was trusting that one of these eighteenth-century denizens would know what to do. I coiled it around my arm and looped it over my shoulder. I walked out to where the coffin lay. Luuk had removed the tarp, and so the box was just lying there in the sun, looking so odd, and strangely so banal too.

I flashed to what it must be like working in a funeral home in the States. There, coffins and corpses were just the mundane realities of a day's work. But to the rest of us, for the mourners, death has been taken from us, hidden, sanitized, simplified, reduced to a concept that can be easily compartmentalized and forgotten about. Maybe we had it wrong. Getting your hands dirty is important. Seeing actual blood, decay, stillness. It could be

beautiful in its own way. Maybe we were all just avoiding something that would actually set us free.

Then, I got a whiff: rotting human. There was no ambiguity about that smell. I retched and struggled to keep from vomiting. Maybe formaldehyde had its place too.

Ralph and Robin had arrived, and Ralph stood with Luuk and Reggie in front of the truck while Robin joined Anais and Belinda, who took off toward the grave site, leaving five of us to deal with the heavy lifting. There were only four rope handles; Luuk and Ralph jockeyed around a bit deciding who should hold the fourth handle until Ralph stepped up. I handed the pile of loose rope to Luuk to carry, and we arranged ourselves at the corners of the coffin, waiting for some signal to hoist it up. I realized no one else was going to do it, so I took the lead.

"Okay, on three." We all knelt down so we could use our knees to lift. "Ready? One, two, three!" We heaved at the handles, and somehow this time it was lighter than I expected.

We raised it to about waist level and began to walk. Luuk led the way, carrying the rope. It took us a few moments to get our steps in sync. Toby and Reggie were in the front, and at first they went a little too fast, causing Ralph and me to nearly trip trying to keep up. Then they overcompensated and slowed down too much. By the time we reached the edge of the parking lot and started onto the dirt path, we had more or less found a rhythm.

As we walked, I wondered why we hadn't rearranged ourselves to distribute our lifting strength more evenly. I let my mind explore the mathematical possibilities for several moments, knowing that I was just distracting myself from the pain in my shoulder and forearm. I returned to the idea of how the physical act of carrying, and caring for the body, was a way to distract

oneself from feeling the emotions just under the surface. The logistics of arranging the funeral had given me plenty to worry about other than what was going on in my heart. And in just a few more minutes all of that distraction would be behind us, and there would be nothing between me and the cold reality that my father was dead. That he never apologized. That I didn't know if I could ever forgive him. And now any chance of mutual reconciliation was over.

Let alone the disgust and confusion I felt about his incestuous fantasies about Anais, he had failed as a father in every measurable way. And yet I couldn't dismiss him, forget him, ignore his presence in my psyche. He loomed there, that goofy, yellow-toothed smile doggedly assured of his eventual redemption.

• • •

The last time I saw him alive was five years before. I came to visit him when he had first moved to the Dutch Antilles, shortly after the ordeal with US Customs. We spent five days together, but the conversation never got much deeper than the origins of the rare birds on the island. We even spent one evening debating whether the Who or the Rolling Stones were a more influential rock band. He really was still nineteen. Even though I'd matured to thirty-six. Our relationship had grown so shallow and anemic that I didn't know why I'd even bothered to come. But I wanted to at least speak my truth. While I was too weary to dredge up all the deep sadness and hurt feelings, I felt compelled to at least reiterate how disappointed I was. To tell him that even if he couldn't apologize, I had to know that I'd been heard. I'd promised myself that I would say something, that I wouldn't be a coward like him.

That there was nothing I needed from him anymore, and so I had nothing to lose.

I waited until the last day. That night he cooked a steak by consulting his astrological charts, determining that it would be medium rare just as Mercury moved into Sagittarius (or something like that). Finally, I spoke up. "I don't know my third house from my tenth house and I don't know a trine from a retrograde opposition," I said. "You'd think at least some of it would have rubbed off on me, but I have a conspicuous inability to retain even the most basic aspects." I waited for a response but he was silent. "It'd be weird if it wasn't so obvious what that's about." I laughed gently.

He cheerily pointed out in his professorial calm that it was all predetermined. "We're a lineage of father-haters," he offered sagely. "I hated my father and he hated his. It's no surprise that you hate me. It's not your fault really." Then he patted me on the back—not with condescension, but with a strange, unearned comradery. Then he got up and walked back to the kitchen and lit a cigarette. Just like that, he managed to negate the legitimacy of my feelings and avoid any responsibility himself.

In that moment he extinguished whatever energy I had to tell him off. What was the point? I ate my (overcooked) steak in silence and went to bed. Early the next morning, I boarded a plane back to the States.

• • •

"Motherfuck!" Ralph blurted as he stumbled over the limb of a fallen dead tree. He nearly dragged all of us and the coffin down with him as he flailed and fell to his knees. We managed to lay

the box down without dropping it, and all of us took a desperately needed breather. My hand burned from the rope, and the
muscles in my arm and shoulder throbbed. Sweat poured down
my forehead, and the collar of my shirt was soaked through.

Overcompensating for my pathetic, soft American body, I
forced us all to finish the job. "Let's go," I grunted. "Come on.
One, two, three." Everyone obliged, and we again hoisted the coffin up to our waists, though we were all a lot less stable than before.
We struggled through the rest of the wooded area and out to the
field where I saw Luuk had just joined Anais and the others.

We struggled to lower the box next to the hole in the ground
and opposite the prodigious mound of dirt that the diggers had
unearthed. My foot slipped as I stepped too close to the hole and
the edge gave way, sending dirt and rocks into the pit. I looked
down into the void, and I was impressed at just how deep it was.
The gravediggers were sitting nearby resting, and I wondered how
they even got out of the hole when they were done. It looked at
least eight feet deep.

Robin nursed Ralph's twisted ankle as Luuk uncoiled the
rope and measured its length. He and Reggie used a large knife
and cut it into two pieces. One piece went down through the
forward right handle, under the box, and up through the forward
left handle; the other piece went the same way through the back
handles. This was how the four of us could gently lower the coffin into the hole, then pull the rope out and leave the box behind.
Who needs a mechanical lift?

Finally, everything was ready, and there was nobody there
but the ten of us: Luuk and Belinda, Ralph and Robin, Reggie,
the two gravediggers, and us three siblings. I didn't know if it was
even fair to count the gravediggers since we had paid them to be

there. Reggie too, come to think of it. Luuk had called Chevelle at the radio station to update the funeral announcement, but we had no idea how many people would have heard about the change or could attend at short notice. Luuk was confident that word-of-mouth was strong on the island, but I had my doubts.

CHAPTER 49

THEIR EYES WERE WATCHING GOD

TOBY'S WATCH READ 10:48 A.M. Should we just begin? Should we wait for more people to arrive? Anais wanted to give it a few more minutes. Toby wanted to just get it over with. I found myself unable to express an opinion.

"I guess I just hoped there'd be a few more people," Anais said.

"Everyone loved Joe," Belinda cooed. "Don't you worry. Even if they're not here, they're with us in their hearts."

"How do you want to do this?" I asked Anais.

"I'll say a few things, then I'll tell you when it's time," she gestured to the coffin. "And then I've got a closing prayer. I'll keep it brief."

I smiled at the idea of Anais keeping anything brief. But still, a wave of relief washed over me. A light breeze allayed the heat, at least for a moment, and the skin on my neck tingled as the moisture began to evaporate. I could finally hand over the reins.

This was Anais's element. She produced a few sage smudge sticks and hunted around for someone with a lighter.

We heard some voices in the distance, and soon a stream of people appeared on the path heading toward us. Anais looked at me and smiled, though I didn't share her relief. Part of me was disappointed, seeing the lack of attendance as vindication that he got what he deserved. Over the next few minutes, a good twenty or so people appeared. I recognized many of them: the two women from the airport; one of the cops from the police station, though now dressed in street clothes; Chevelle from the radio station with two children in tow; and many others.

People smiled warmly, and some bowed their heads to us as they approached. A few people laid colorful artificial flowers on the coffin. The gesture was kind, but I couldn't help picturing the nonbiodegradable plastic ornaments outliving the corpse itself, whatever that means. I thanked each of the guests quietly as they passed by. The smoke from Anais's smudge sticks smelled nice, and in its own way created a sense of space around us.

The group spontaneously assembled into neat rows in front of the grave, and when the moment seemed right, Anais began the service, thanking the people for coming. She was about to continue, but then another wave of people appeared on the path. We waited as another twenty or thirty people filed in. Nearly everyone we'd met on the island was there, even Captain Morago, who tipped his police hat as he made eye contact and took his place near the back.

Finally, sensing the time was right, Anais held up a triangle chime and struck it firmly, emitting a piercing but placid tone which successfully signaled everyone to quiet down. I realized she must have brought that from home specifically for this occasion.

I was impressed with her forethought. She really did know what she was doing. She really did understand a whole host of things that I didn't. I had a lot to learn from her.

And then she began. "Wow. Thank you. To all of you, for joining us at this service to honor my father. These are my brothers. That's Michael and Tobias, and I'm Anais. And we are all the children of . . . Doctor Joe, whose real name was Herschel Joseph Wohl, and he would have been seventy-one in a few weeks."

I stared at the ground and felt tears begin to stream down my face. I could do nothing to stop it. I was wearing dark sunglasses, and I pretended the shades could hide my grief from all these strangers. I wasn't sobbing; I wasn't making any noise at all, but the tears came heavy and I tasted the salt as they reached my mouth.

Anais went on. "He was a writer, a teacher, a seeker. He was not a traditional father. He didn't give us many of the things each of us wished he had. But he made each of us who we are today, and I wouldn't change that for anything." She paused and turned to face Toby and me. "I wouldn't trade either of you for anything, either."

Now I was sobbing. I couldn't speak. I barely squeaked out the word "Amen."

My sister continued. "One of the Jewish traditions is called *k'ria*. Each family member rends a piece of their clothing to make a permanent tear, just as our dad's parting makes a permanent hole in our lives. In modern times, these little bits of fabric are used to symbolize that."

She paused and tore the little black swatch attached to her dress, then looked to me. I looked down at the bit of fabric safety-pinned to my shirt. But instead of tearing the swatch, I grabbed the whole thing and yanked it, tearing a hole in my shirt. The sound of the fabric coming apart was oddly satisfying. I looked

over to Toby, who followed my lead and tore his shirt as well. We smiled at each other, and then we looked back to Anais.

"Oh, no, no way," she said. "This is my one good dress. Not happening. Sorry, Dad, but this is Laura Ashley."

I laughed through my tears and a few others in the crowd chuckled too. She regained her composure and asked, "Either of you want to say anything?"

I shook my head. "No, you were perfect," I said, and the tears came again full force.

Toby shook his head in agreement.

"Okay. Then let's—" Anais gestured to the coffin. "It's time."

Luuk and I stood to the left of the coffin, and Toby and Reggie stood on the opposite side of the grave. We collected the ropes and took up the slack until all four strands were taut. Then, slowly we inched the casket over the pit, suspended by our ropes. Again, somehow the lead fell to me, and even though I had no idea what we were doing, I tried my best.

"Okay. On three, we let out one arm's length, then pause, then again." The other men nodded. I counted to three, we all let out a bit of rope, and the coffin began to lower. I gave the call and we lowered another foot. It was moving smoothly and slowly, but as it got farther away our leverage decreased, and it was harder to hold it steadily.

"Come on!" Luuk bleated when I didn't give the next instruction quickly enough, and we all began lowering at different rates. It all went wrong very quickly, and I felt the rope slip through my hands, which had become muddy and slick. The coffin lurched to one side.

"Hold it!" Toby barked, but it was too late, and the coffin dropped the last couple feet, landing with a loud crack as it hit

the rocky dirt below. I looked down, afraid that the box had split open, but at least from the top it all looked intact. Of course, it couldn't have mattered less. Dad merrily rejected such affectations of propriety.

I looked out to the crowd, who had been watching our effort, but no one seemed the least bit concerned, so I tried to play it cool. I wiped my hands on my pants and then wiped the sweat from my brow, unknowingly smearing mud across my face. The excess rope was now trapped under the box, and the four of us struggled in a tug of war with the dead man at the bottom of the hole. Eventually we succeeded, though all of us came away covered in a thick muck of dirt and sweat. Toby smiled and gestured to my dirty face, which I tried to wipe with the sleeve of my shirt, making an even bigger mess.

Anais picked up a shovel. She held the tool upside down and scooped a heap of dirt onto the back of the blade. "Another tradition is that all of us participate in filling the grave. All of us. All of you." She gestured to the crowd with the outstretched shovel. "We each shovel a bit of dirt into the pit, as we are all one community, together repairing the hole left in all of our lives," she explained. "We use the back of the shovel to demonstrate our reluctance."

Then she chanted, "*Al mekomo yavo veshalom.*" She shook the soil over the hole, letting it rain down onto the wood below. The sound echoed loudly, and I was struck by how real and final that act was. "I love you, Dad," she said quietly. "Goodbye."

That made me cry all over again.

When she was done, I reached for the shovel, but she stuck it into the pile of dirt instead. Then she explained professorially, Herschel-ly, "And please don't hand the shovel to the next person

in line. No one should be forced to take on the sadness or grief, or be obligated to perform this task. It is strictly voluntary."

I picked up the shovel and scooped a sizable mound onto the back of the blade. I moved it over the hole in the ground, and I let the dirt fall. I thrust the shovel back into the pile and stood beside Anais. She took my hand. I couldn't look at her, but I gripped her hand tightly and squeezed my appreciation. Toby took the shovel next and quickly scooped the dirt from the pile into the hole. Luuk and Belinda each took a turn, then Ralph, and Reggie, and Robin, and some people from the crowd. The sound of dirt falling on wood became softer as more and more of the coffin was covered.

Anais began reciting the Kaddish. I was surprised that I somehow know the Hebrew, and it gave me comfort to hear it spoken. *"Y'it gadal, v'yit kadash, sh'mei raba . . ."* I joined in, and taking Toby's hand in mine, the three of us stood there as the crowd came forward one at a time.

After she finished the prayer, Anais urged the guests to continue taking turns with the shovel. "Go ahead. Everyone who wants to." The custom was new to them and several giggled or resisted a bit. "It's a big hole, and we need your help," she said.

The line of people seemed endless. There were children and many strangers. I was amazed at how many people had made their way here for this. For him. Anais recited another short prayer in Hebrew that I didn't know, then she switched to English and began Psalm 23. *"The lord is my shepherd; I shall not want . . ."*

Immediately, instinctively, the entire crowd joined in. They all knew this one, and their voices swelled into a haunting and powerful chorus. *"He lays me down in green pastures, and leads me beside still waters . . ."* I thought I'd cried all I could, but that wrecked me. Their voices were vast.

"Though I walk through the valley of the shadow of death, I will fear no evil . . ."

I felt something deep and healing emerging, not just for me or my siblings, but for everyone. We were all connected through this. We were all together in this experience: strangers, siblings, the young and the old. We all know death, even if we don't think we do. And this was not just about this one man's death; it was about all of our lives and all of our deaths.

"And I will dwell in the house of the lord forever."

As we finished the prayer, the group broke into song. It was a hymn and it was all about Jesus, but it made no difference. They had taken over, and we were now just visitors there. One by one, people came up and filled the grave and then touched our hands or bowed their heads and said they were sorry and that Jesus loves us. It was sweet, if a little hilarious.

"This is the weirdest Jewish funeral ever," Toby said, and we all laughed.

I lifted my sunglasses from my eyes and hugged Anais and held her as tightly as I could. "I love you. So much."

"I know. Me too," she replied. I cried into her hair, and she sobbed into my chest. Then, we opened the hug and pulled Toby in with us. The three of us held each other for a long time.

"Excuse me, please," a local man interrupted. It was a young guy holding an old film camera with a big flash on top. "I'm so sorry for your loss. May I please take a picture?" We were perplexed at the odd request. "For the newspaper." We stepped apart and wrapped our arms around each other's shoulders. The photographer snapped a few shots of us, then thanked us and stepped back into the crowd.

After all the people had shoveled, there was still a lot of hole to fill, and without being asked, the gravediggers took over.

But the strangest thing was that everyone stayed until they were done. Not just us, not just his close friends, but everyone. The young kids ran around and played, and the women continued to sing hymns, some of which Anais even knew. Everyone just hung out. After nearly an hour, the diggers finally finished, tamping the dirt down into a familiar-looking burial mound and placing the remaining plastic flowers and other offerings neatly on top. The short, sunny digger came over to me.

"You look just like him. You know?"

"I know," I said with a smile. "Thanks."

CHAPTER 50
THE DIVINE COMEDY

LUUK AND BELINDA URGED US to stay through the weekend, but I insisted that I had to get home to deal with a work emergency. Fortunately, no one asked for details, as I'd have had to make something up. Toby had a more legitimate excuse: He had final exams starting on Monday. Anais had work too, but she'd already made arrangements to stay behind to clean out Dad's bungalow.

I scrubbed the bloody palm print off Dad's laptop and installed a fresh system on the hard disk. We agreed that Anais needed a new computer more than Toby or I did. She was also going to bring home the various papers and other personal items we found, and we gave her permission to use her best judgment about what to keep and what to throw away. I hoped there weren't more surprises hidden somewhere, but there was nothing I could do about it at that point. Belinda was going to keep the kitchen items; his clothes were to be donated to a local chapter of the Red Cross; and then there was his book collection.

Luuk drove us over to the library to discuss the donation. It was a tiny two-room house over near the census office, and it was already overflowing with books. While we waited, I noticed a paperback of *Don Quixote* on the reception desk. I stared at the author's name, from whom my own name allegedly derives. The cover depicted the jousting hero comically befuddled, a looming windmill shadow in the background. Had I spent my life fighting an imaginary foe? Was the joke on me after all?

Finally, the librarian arrived; he was a skinny little guy in his mid-twenties in clichéd, oversized eyeglasses. He introduced himself as Dante. I suppressed a giggle. Maybe *Quixote* wasn't the worst literary namesake you could have.

Then it occurred to me: I wasn't named for Quixote at all. I was named for the author who invented him, Miguel De Cervantes, the genius artist who examined the idea of idealism and how, despite its futility, the best of us can't help but pursue it anyway. Idealism—that might be the one trait I was proud to have inherited from my father. The joke *was* on me. I wasn't named for the tragic, flawed hero; I was named for the writer of the first modern novel—still widely read five hundred years after the author's death. Incredible.

When we explained just how many boxes of books we were donating, Dante's eyes widened. We had joked about naming a wing after Dad, but in reality, they were going to need a whole new building.

After the library, we went to the Winair office, and they had two spots on the 4:20 p.m. flight back to Sint Maarten. Toby and I put our names down and headed back to the resort to pack up our things. Just knowing that I had a seat on a plane that would take me away from the place filled me with such joy that I felt

giddy all the way back to the inn. I eagerly smiled and waved at all the people we passed on the side of the road—only now, I really did recognize most of them. We passed two girls who were at the funeral with their father, an administrator at the university; then, I saw one of the guys who we had flagged down at the hospital to help us with the coffin; we passed one of the cops who we had argued with about releasing dad's laptop; I waved to a woman whom I couldn't place at first, but then I remembered she was the clerk at the census office; and so on. All of our mutual, warm greetings felt genuine, familiar.

Back at Paradise Point, I booked a flight back to LA—never mind that it went through Atlanta, then Denver, and then San Francisco. I also found Toby a flight back to New York that left around the same time. Our transfers would be tight, but at least we'd finally be on our way back home.

In the parking lot, I held Anais tightly as I hugged her goodbye.

"I'm so glad you're my sister. I'm really lucky," I said. She sobbed. I told her I loved her, and we promised to stay in better touch. I hoped it was true, but I couldn't help but wonder how quickly we would drift back to the way things were. It takes a long, long time to heal. She and Toby also shared a long, warm hug. I stepped away to give them a moment. I took the time to again thank Belinda for everything and gave the two giant dogs one last belly rub.

I asked Luuk about the money we owed him. There was the cost of the rooms and the meals, and the boat ride to Saint Kitts, as well as the money he laid out to pay Reggie and the gravediggers, and who knows what else I couldn't even remember. He assured me not to worry. "Island rates are pretty low," he said,

promising to send me a bill when he got around to it. "We're gonna miss having Joe around. But it was nice to at least get to know all of you and see that he passed on his best traits."

As I was packing my bag up, a copy of Dad's book poking out of one of the boxes caught my eye. I picked it up and slipped it into my carry-on. Who knows? Maybe this time I would actually read it.

Shortly thereafter, Toby and I sat together on the tiny eleven-seat plane with the broken seat belts. And before we knew it we were back in the air, looking down on the tiny island of Sint Eustatius surrounded by the endless expanse of blue water. I tried to make out the spot where we had held the funeral, and I saw a field that might have been the right one, but quickly it became so small and insignificant that it was hard to know for sure. It was amazing to know that in one tiny corner of one tiny field, on one tiny island surrounded by a world's worth of ocean, my father now lay forevermore.

It all seemed so insignificant. His whole life reduced to a motionless speck on the surface of the Earth. For all the elaborate cosmic celestial clockworks—the intricate movements and perceived interactions of the many planets measured in minutes of degrees over seven decades that guided the hundreds of millions of decisions and actions and choices and thoughts that his life comprised. . . all of it now rendered silent and impotent.

And I had been so scared.

• • •

When we landed in Sint Maarten, Toby and I only had a few minutes before we needed to run off to our respective gates and return to our regularly scheduled lives.

"I'm glad we got to spend this time together," I said.

"Circumstances sucked," he laughed.

"Yeah, well, this is what we call a silver lining." I hugged him. *Holy shit, I have a brother!* "I'm sorry I haven't been in touch," I said.

I wanted to apologize for missing his birthday, twenty times over. For not being there when he turned five, or when he turned ten, or at his own bar mitzvah. For missing his teenage years, when I could have been a voice from the future, assuring him that he'd get through those hard times. For missing his first love, and first heartbreak, his school graduation, and the other accomplishments that would almost certainly have been better when shared with an older brother. And shit, if I'd been around maybe his athleticism might have worn off on me.

"Let's do better going forward. Okay?" I asked. He nodded.

"We're all we got," he said, trying to make it sound like a joke, but it came out as portentous.

"I love you, Toby," I said.

"I love you too, Max."

He walked away with a wave, and I wondered if things would be different now.

• • •

As I settled in on my plane back to the real world, finally in the familiar safe quiet of being alone, I pulled out Dad's book. Opening the cover, I was immediately struck: The dedication was to us—his children. Maybe I misunderstood so much. What if all that hubris, that grandiosity, that reverence for his "life's work" was all in service of us? Perverted? Sure, when he could have just

sat with us and held our hands. But maybe that was just the only way he knew to express his love— *we* were the "two or three people he hoped to inspire or enlighten or entertain." This was the note I'd been looking for. It was there all along.

I turned the page and began to read. Right away I was drawn in. He wasn't Joyce—though you could tell he wished he was—but under the weight of his literary fancy, it was funny and thoughtful, and most of all, there was no doubt he poured everything he had into it. He had gone for it. And that was something to admire.

As the plane ascended through the clouds and we made our way back toward real life, toward the fantasyland of our modern world, I hardly even noticed the turbulence. And finally, I exhaled.

EPILOGUE
BRAVE NEW WORLD

FIVE YEARS LATER, I was parked in the cell-phone lot at LAX. While I waited, I fiddled with the app on my phone that showed the exact location, altitude, and ground speed of the flight I was tracking—the flight that Toby was on and that was scheduled to arrive in nine more minutes. It alerted me that at approximately three hours and ten minutes into the flight, the plane had made an abrupt altitude shift, followed by a moderate change in ground-speed. I remind myself to ask him if they had some turbulence around then.

It was Friday afternoon, and that Sunday I was getting married.

Anais had arrived the day before. Toby and Julie (now his wife) were arriving in a few minutes, and pretty much everything was in place and ready to go. Anais was co-officiating the cere-mony with my sister-in-law to be, and Toby was going to be one of the chuppah-holders. It was not going to be a very Jewish wedding, but Sarah, my fiancé, was also an ambivalent Jew, and

we had picked and chosen the bits that we liked from the Jewish ceremony.

Sarah was a litigator at an international law firm, which Dad would have hated, but she was also a Leo, which he would have thought was a good companion for me. But regardless of labels or astrological synergy, I was crazy about her. I trusted her. And I jumped in with both feet. After Dad's death, the urgent desperation that had been driving my creative efforts dissipated. I gave up the impossible goal of redeeming his mistakes by achieving my own creative success. And with that onus lifted, I felt so much lighter, so much clearer, so much more myself.

Planning the wedding was one of the first times since his death that Dad's absence had become really apparent. I wished he could have been there, but then again, I never would have gotten there while I was expending so much energy battling him.

I drove around to the terminal, and I spotted Toby exiting the door with a small roller bag and a suit bag over his shoulder. In his short sleeves and sunglasses, he looked more Hollywood than most of the actor-types who usually came through this airport. But his wife was nowhere to be seen. I pulled up and popped the trunk, but still got out and went around back to greet him. We shared a long, warm hug.

"Bro!" he said.

"Bro!" I replied. "Where's Julie?"

"I asked her not to come. Let's not talk about it," he grumbled. "Come on. Let's go."

As we drove away from the airport, I treaded lightly. "You okay?"

"It's nothing new," he started. "I just don't know if I can make it work. It's our fucked-up legacy. No one understands

better than you." Then, catching himself, "Or maybe it's just me. I hope you and Sarah are happily ever after."

"Did you move out?" I asked.

"Temporarily. I don't know. I'm at my mom's. How's Anais?"

Anais was doing great. She had ended the dead-end relationship with Stan, moved to a new city, landed a lucrative and satisfying day job, and was pursuing her own entrepreneurial business, something merging herbalism and social media. She was still her father's daughter, but self-sufficient and optimistic about the future.

"How 'bout the job?" I asked. Toby had recently taken a gig with a top-tier engineering firm.

"I'm not sure if I'm in the right career." He shook his head with a dismissive smile.

Five years later, Anais was thriving. Toby was floundering. I was finally allowing myself to move forward and trust someone enough to get married. You can never predict how a parent's death will affect a child.

Toby and Anais had a warm reunion. Later I was comforted to spy the two of them talking privately under the bougainvillea in our backyard.

The next day we held a rehearsal dinner, which was the first time that all of Sarah's family and all of my family were in the same room together. Hers outnumbered mine five to one, though we arranged the seating so the disparity wasn't so obvious. I just had Toby, Anais, my mom, and one cousin who was able to make the trip from New York. On the other side, Sarah had her happily married parents, her sister with her spouse and three-year-old son, and a stream of aunts and uncles, cousins, and nieces and nephews that seemed to go on and on.

I was excited about joining such a big, healthy clan that finds safety in numbers, despite my training in the opposite.

Both Anais and Toby acted a little guarded when Sarah's sister or father or cousin offered a big, inclusive hug, instantly treating them as if they belonged. Belonging was unfamiliar to us, and I recognized their subtle hesitation. But Sarah's family would have none of it, and they forced both of my siblings to join in, plopping our three-year-old nephew into Anais's lap during dinner and dragging Toby into a drinking game where they poured a shot of slivovitz every time someone says *mazel tov*.

The wedding on Sunday went flawlessly. Anais brought to the ceremony all of the thoughtful sentiment and insight that she was so good at. She found a way to make the ancient Jewish rituals, like standing under a chuppah or breaking a glass, feel modern and relevant and beautiful. Toby's symbolic job of holding up the chuppah took on a more literal role when one of Sarah's cousins leaned a little too heavily on his support pole and nearly knocked the whole thing to the ground.

During the reception, Sarah made a toast. "To all the people who couldn't be here to celebrate with Michael and me tonight." We all raised our glasses to her maternal grandparents, both of whom Sarah was very close to.

And then we raised our glasses to Herschel.

If he had been there, he probably would have come stoned, spent most of the time hitting on Sarah's friends and giving me "advice" about how suffocating marriage can be, but nevertheless I do wish he could have shared in my joy on that special day when I was so filled with the promise and possibilities of the future. Maybe he could have done an astrological chart for our union or pontificated on the historical context of the wedding vows

(though Anais covered that pretty well). Maybe he could have just smiled with those yellow smoker's teeth and wished us good luck. I wished he could have met Sarah, and even more so, that she could have met him—that would have helped her understand so much about me.

But alas, my father was dead, and I would live out the rest of my life without him. For the most part, I didn't miss him. I thought of him occasionally, and whenever I spoke to Anais or Toby I felt his presence.

• • •

It was another year and a half before his absence really hit me again—when we learned that Sarah was pregnant, and that I was going to be a father.

A father.

It wasn't like I wanted his advice on parenting, that was for sure. But it would have been nice just to share my good news. To tell him that he was going to be a grandfather. Despite everything, I think that he might have been tickled by that. But he was gone.

Would it have been better to have lost him to slow sickness? To Alzheimer's? Would it have been better to have not even known that he died? We were so out of touch that I had expected I'd find out long after the fact and get a call and hear that he'd died six months prior. "What a shame," I would say, and go on with my day. I had thought it wouldn't hurt. After all, I'd given up on expecting anything from him. Or so I thought.

I suppose I'll always be furious, but I'm done being angry. Anger is a cry expecting a response, and this subject can no longer respond. The next move is mine. And I can only forgive him now.

Or better put, I can only accept him for who he was. But I must accept all of him because he also made me who I am. The deep belief in integrity that I struggle to live up to every day—that was his. And the infinite curiosity and excitement about the natural world that I look forward to passing on to my own child—that's his too.

And I hope that I can also allow room for the parts I don't admire—even those I despise. Because then maybe I can forgive those things in myself. Like it or not, I probably inherited some of those too. He was flawed. He was broken. He made choices that I would never consider. But I have to love him anyway. The alternative is to remain in a crouch. To sacrifice the rest of my own life on his behalf. He certainly didn't earn that. And that's not the kind of life I'm choosing to live.

ABOUT THE AUTHOR

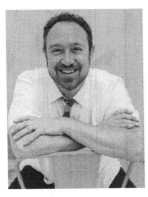 MICHAEL WOHL TELLS STORIES: as an award-winning filmmaker; as an author of more than a dozen non-fiction books about filmmaking; and through curated culinary experiences that reveal the unifying magic of breaking bread. He was one of the original designers of Apple's Emmy award-winning software Final Cut Pro, taught editing at UCLA's Graduate School of Film & TV, and has produced hundreds of hours of online training content. Michael is also the principal baker at Burlesque Buns, a delivery-only bakery focused on traditional Jewish breads and pastries, and he is the founder of Bread Heals, an enigmatic culinary club in Los Angeles.

Made in the USA
Middletown, DE
03 November 2022

13997768R00182

PART IV: THE DRAGON AND THE LOTUS

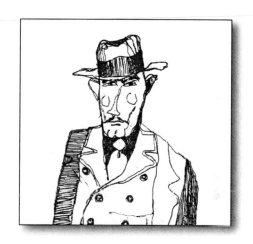

PART ONE
EAST OF WALL STREET

CONTAINING A NEW-YORK MINUTE

New York, New York, October 1929

We're more than happy to move a few sizable stacks of Big Department's rum-running money into penny stocks. He loves the 100%-profit-for-every-penny argument. But this is a colossal miscalculation on the part of my employer. Considering Big Department isn't as toothless as the widows, Aldo actually has to care which stocks he picks. His blue-sky racket's completely cast over.

Poochie makes it clear the Big Department would prefer his shares go up. It only takes a couple days of the market tanking for Aldo Pennebeck's smiling demeanor to disappear. The devil-may-care attitude is gone. Then the market really begins exhaling and it's no accordion making melodies. It's a bellows fanning the flames. Big Department's penny stocks are all losing and Aldo is sweating like one of the damned, as well he should be. To make matters worse, Eva-Maria announces she met some movie producer on the subway who wants to give her a screen test in Los Angeles. I hesitate to object, though I want to. In fact, like some half-wit, I actually *encourage* her, and when she finishes stewing over that fine how-do-you-do, she books a sleeping berth to L.A. without me.

I start thinking about going back to driving full-time but legit, something not too strenuous, like a potato chip route, delivering nice light cartons that no one wants to shoot you for. And I start daydreaming about finding Eva-Maria to convince her she misunderstood me, is all. To kiss and make up. They eat potato chips in L.A., don't they? But before I can pull the trigger, circumstances dance completely out of control.

Wednesday, October 30, 1929, I'm in my redoubt, picking stocks to bet against. I have the *Wall Street Journal* stock page taped to the wall opposite my desk, and I'm flipping darts at it. With my back turned and my eyes closed. Whatever I hit, I'm shorting. What with the market falling through the floor, it's a sure bet. The problem is our floor trader is already drowning in a sea of sell orders and what's the point really in answering the phone? If people want to sell the whole market, they might as well just give it away. People are already calling yesterday Black Tuesday.

That's when Aldo gets a visit from some of our clientele, unannounced and pretty much suddenlike. I hear the outside door close, then heavy footsteps. The floor starts jouncing like it's getting pounded by a ton of falling bricks in shoe leather.

The inner office door closes kind of hard and I hear someone say: "The Department ain't happy, Aldo. The Department ain't happy one bit about them penny-ante stocks you pawned off on us."

"It's a long-term play," Aldo says, fast-talking. "These penny stocks jump around, sure enough, but they're going to make everyone a fortune in the next few months. The market's just going through a little seasonal turbulence ..."

Whatever other malarkey he's about to offer up gets stuffed back down his throat, and the very loud crash that follows has the hair on the back of my neck leaping to attention. I shove my eye up to the pinprick peephole in the door of my well-disguised office. Two gorillas in blue uniforms are storming around Aldo's office as if they're tired of doing time in the Bronx Zoo. A third guy's with them, a giant in a brown suit and Stetson, palming a pistol the size of a cannon. One of the cops makes quick work of Aldo. He blackjacks him and that's that.

The guy in the Stetson throws open a window and the two flatfeet pick Aldo off the floor. He's completely limp, blood's pouring down his face. The poor bastard doesn't know whether he's buying or selling. They rush over to the window and defenestrate him. It's a nightmare— slow, quick, horrible—and Aldo's gone. One of his shoes clips the window frame as he cartwheels out and the window cracks. I've known guys to make stiff demands on the small business owner, but these are extremely tough customers.

When the guy in the Stetson turns around, I get a clear

look. It's Poochie. I try to remember if he ever saw my tiny, back office. I hope I always paid him in the Irish bar.

For Aldo Pennebeck, it's all a dull swirl. He dreams he's playing a game of musical chairs and a polka band is booming and crooning a roomful of oompas. The accordionist rips his accordion in two, the drummer kicks her drums in, and the music stops cold. Like that. He gropes with both hands to claim a chair to settle in, but there is no chair there under him as he sits down on air and there's a whish and a long, long, long, long way…

The next day the papers report he committed suicide. Like three other brokers who couldn't make their margin calls. That's the way they write it up—another broke broker who jumped to his death. When I read the story in the paper, I'm surprised anybody thinks that's what happened. Especially considering his ransacked office. Aldo Pennebeck is the last guy in the world who'd leave a party early. Then again, cops have ways of keeping stuff out of the papers, I'm sure of that.

CHAPTER 2

PICK YOUR POISON

New York, New York, May 1928

But you'll indulge me, I hope, if I throw Aldo's Duesenberg in reverse and back away from his brutal and untimely demise?

A year and a half earlier, I'm at some party, blithely taking it all in. It's a Saturday night. The place is awash in bathtub gin, available *gratis*, and I'm not unhappy to be rubbing elbows with a bunch of swells in Manhattan, not paying too close attention to the troubles I'm already the proud owner of. You know, carefree. I'm riding Poochie's coattails. He's got an in and I'm just kind of crashing along in his wake. Cab Calloway's playing full blast.

Poochie's towering over some sleep-deprived, sharp-cornered guy, who turns and looks in my direction. Then the guy raises his glass and smiles slightly, as if he's grinding his teeth. He looks kind of dazed, like he just walked away from a traffic accident. I push my way through the crowd to join them (and, believe you me, it's some mob).

His smile looks odd, but I think to myself he's making an effort at least, not an unfriendly way to crack the ice. So I grit my teeth back at him and raise the old medicine cabinet. I don't immediately taste my drink, though. I think it wise to give it a sniff. Aldo sees the face I make when I take a whiff and cracks up.

Poochie introduces me as a trusty wheelman, a hundred-percenter, and Aldo begins playing his role as the host of this bedlam.

"What fuel are you drinking, Johnny?"

"I don't know yet. Smells a bit like a gumdrop cocktail. I asked the guy over there to fill it up and he topped it off nicely."

"He wasn't doing you any favors." Aldo holds my glass up to his nose. "I don't want to zing my own liquor cellar, but I wouldn't drink that."

"My car might..."

"Leave Ethel alone. She'll claw your eyes out."

"That's the last thing I need."

"What can I get you? Champagne?"

"Sure."

"Maybe a Scotch?"

"Okay."

"How about a Manhattan?"

"Uh, if you insist."

"Then again, the champagne is ice cold."

The guy won't take "yes" for an answer. "Perfect," I

say, hoping we're going to be done with these preliminaries soon.

He nods to the fellow tending bar and gives a slight shake of his thumb and forefinger. Next thing I know someone's handing me a champagne flute brimming with effervescent gold. Aldo Pennebeck is the outgoing sort, definitely, even in his least exuberant moments. He's a stockjobber who's making money as easily as a bartender draws a pint. A regular knight of the spigot.

"To the pursuit of happiness, Johnny." Aldo likes that idea. That's always his toast, except on rare occasion late at night when he's more likely to mutter: "Let the devil take the hindmost." When it comes to happiness, Aldo's in hot pursuit. "My friends expect me to throw parties now and then, so I throw them. I enjoy it."

"Thanks for not poisoning me."

"Any friend of Poochie's a friend of mine, Johnny." With that, Poochie nods at no one in particular and turns back toward where the hard liquor is to be had.

Have you ever noticed how people like going on about the good old days? When I taste Aldo's champagne, I see their point. I don't know much about them myself. I'm too young for good old days. I wasn't even old enough to drink when Prohibition hit in 1919. I take another sip and Aldo looks at me coolly for a couple seconds, apparently weighing whether to confide in me.

"Poochie tell you about our night on the rainbow?" I give him my professional *je n'en sais rien* look. "Poochie's not much of a talker," I say. In my previous line of work, feigned ignorance was always advisable.

In a low voice, Aldo says: "He and I went to some

three-tap-joint in Chinatown and hitched up some
reindeer. We do a taste and I start getting jittery." Aldo
goes positively vague as he thinks back on that. His
mouth tightens, disgusted. "I try drinking some saké. It
makes me sick to my stomach. Someone passes me some
reefer. I figure it might help, what the hell, and take a
few puffs. Next thing I know I'm feeling dizzy. I'm
reeling. My head feels like it's doing the shim-sham-
shimmy. Next a Chinaman offers me some dream gum. I
wash it down with more saké." He narrows his eyes and
looks like he's still suffering. "The whole room starts
breathing. Some skinny Chinese guys are kicking the
gong around. They pass me the bamboo. It's about a
mile long, and I take a couple drags on that, and
suddenly, I can't believe it. Suddenly I feel fine! It was a
fucking alchemical miracle! The perfect combination!
The capper is some girl in pink silk leans over me and
slips a glass of champagne in my hand. It was the
darnedest thing." He lowers his voice. "Poochie got me
out of there in one piece. He tells me he flashed a police
tin and carried me out slung over his shoulder. If it
weren't for him, I'd probably have woken up without my
top hat, my watch, or my wallet. I might have pried my
eyes open in the morgue. And for that reason, Johnny,"
he says, raising his voice again, "I'm taking it nice and
easy tonight. But don't let my restraint hold you back.
Knock yourself out. Business can wait. Keep track of that
champagne glass and my boys will keep filling it."

"*Merci*, Aldo."

People are funny that way, telling complete strangers
all sorts of stuff they'd carry to the grave before they'd

tell their wife or their best friend. Especially when they're still half-looped from the night before. On the way to the party, Poochie grunted something about a rough night, but he wasn't given to torrential, cokey outpourings the way Aldo was. A few years back, I talked a blue streak to some strangers myself. After I'd spent a stretch in the hospital. Before I made it back to wherever the hell I am. Living the overexposed life.

I don't know Poochie well, but I know he works for some behemoth named Big Department. I used to drive for business partners of theirs. Then they transferred me to New York and the assignment comes with an introduction to Poochie.

I haven't met this Big Department, but they say he stands out, seeing that he's 6 foot 7 and weighs a quarter ton. Word has it he makes Poochie, a hulking lug himself, look like a little fellow. I learn later that the Department got his name as a cop-impersonator, strong arming criminals in the name of the law. His victims never saw anything but a really big blue uniform. They'd rather pay than go to stir. All he had to do was convince one slop-seller to part with an inventory mistake—a gigantic uniform that was never going to move, because no member of the police department would ever need a uniform his size.

Now Big Department is moving into downtown Manhattan and he figures why not get a toehold on Wall Street? He's greasing enough palms to move whiskey by the trainload. Careening over back roads, one load of brown plaid at a time, is *passé*. He's paid his dues. It's time he starts making some easy money.

RICHARD VOORHEES

When he decides to begin dabbling rather seriously in the stock market, Big Department meets Aldo, and next thing you know, Aldo's managing his rum money. Or maybe I should call it what it is—blood money. Aldo isn't particular. He likes clients flush with cash. Money's pouring through the market and scrubbing it clean is pretty simple. That's how Poochie and I get invited to his bash.

Wall Street is on a real tear and he's on a roll, the kind that makes him and his clients a lot of dough. He's a golden boy, in other words, riding the market aloft, like some kind of balmy, hot air balloon. It makes him popular enough. His parties serve a nice business purpose as well. He tells the folks he invites to bring a friend or two and that way he keeps reeling in the suckers.

To his credit, Aldo is the kind of guy who sees the intrinsic value in everyone. He figures out how much they're worth and how much he can divert to his own account. He loves rich people. Also to his credit, he's charming in a superficial sort of way and he serves real champagne at his parties.

Turns out he just jettisoned his assistant, and business being brisk, can use a chauffeur to run his errands. That's why Poochie steers me his way, knowing my abilities behind the wheel. And with the assurance that I'm alert and reticent, he thinks Aldo will take me on.

I've been something of a drifter in my life. Not exactly a man with a plan. I threw the *I Ching* once to divine my fortune and it foretold that for me "success will be like water running downhill." That's been the way of it. I've followed the contours and slid through doors that opened. To call it "success," though, would be over-stating the case.

The following Monday I go up to Aldo's Park Avenue offices for a formal interview. He asks me how I enjoyed the festivities and tells me Poochie is vouching for my *bona fides*. We chat amiably enough. I tell him a little about myself, that I'm from Montreal originally, that I studied chemistry in college, that I can drive at night. He's easy to get along with, it's true. He's satisfied with my answers, ready to hire me to assist him, but first he has one last test for me. He says it's a reading exam. He pulls out his wallet and hands me a one-dollar bill. He asks me what I see. I start reading this short, interesting document and he's nodding.

"What else do you see?"

"George is looking a little green around the gills."

"Anything else?"

"Not off the top of my head."

"What do you notice about this one?" He hands me a five.

"You tell me. It looks like legal tender."

"How about this one? Or this one?" He hands me a ten and a twenty.

"How would you describe the expressions on the portraits?"

"Inscrutable?"

"Exactly. The gents on American folding money are a tight-lipped bunch. Silent types. They never, ever talk about the company they keep or what they've been up to."

"I've worked for guys like that. In fact, I'm like that."

"Good. Remember—do like the gents on the bills, Johnny. Not a word. If I share information with you, which I may, I have to be able to trust you. Loose talk is the one thing I won't tolerate, not a single slip-up."

"I'm not a talker, Aldo. Poochie must have told you that. I'm more of a listener. And a reader."

"Start reading this stack of stock offerings then, and let me know if you find any good investments."

"Sure."

"And give me back those bills."

The next few days, my responsibilities at Aldo's turn out to be pretty straightforward—read the fine print, follow instructions to the letter, be discreet, step lively, drive fast, don't scratch the paint, don't talk to strangers. It's ironic, of course, that Aldo emphasizes the need for secrecy. That first time I met him he talked and talked and talked. I'm pretty sure he knows how to keep his own counsel, though. The rest is just so much bluster—big talk and small talk.

Every week Poochie calls to hit me up. This is his little side business, putting the squeeze on me. He's oblique in his approach, using a surprisingly soft touch. He calls and invariably asks me: "How's you and me?" He wants to know if I'd like to grab a drink after work. He doesn't really sound as if he's asking, and seeing that he's as big as the Woolworth Building, my mouth gets parched as soon as I hear his voice. I meet him at an Irish speakeasy he knows and have a couple of belts, or three or four, and then he asks me what I'm going to pay with. I lay down enough to cover our tab and he crumples it in his fist and stands up nice and slow. After he adjusts his overcoat and puts his hat on real low, he darkens the side door on his way out and leaves me to pay a second time. I think he pulls the same maneuver on Aldo, just at fancier establishments. He lets me off kind of easy. I get a few drinks out of our *rendezvous* but not much conversation. Most of the time he strikes me as someone entertaining murderous thoughts—reminiscing about guys he's murdered or dreaming about guys he's going to murder sometime quite soon. I figure the best thing is to let the man think.

Aldo has a lofty if cramped pair of offices on the 18th floor on Park Avenue, just uptown from Grand Central Station.

I'm holed up in a tiny side office no one knows about, working the phones. He has a bunch of phone lines, so we can talk on umpteen phones at once—buying and selling, bidding and offering. He could have held the phones together and his customers could have carried on without him, but that was his business—to get in the way of all that money.

CHAPTER 3

A LITTLE DEATH

Aldo was no saint, but I've known worse characters. Gangsters and cops. You don't want to cross either of them. They cut a bloodier swath and use blunter instruments. Aldo was more of a gentleman with a shiv. Before Aldo introduces me to the Wall Street bunco, I made decent money driving for a booze ring, smuggling whiskey into the Lower Forty-Eight. I love books and reading and the life of the mind and all that, but smuggling booze pays considerably better. If you can stand the excitement.

How did I find myself behind the wheel? One night I was pretty much pressed into rumrunning, driving a truck home from some party when I was still a young man. A guy standing by a capsized truck with a flat flags me down. I pull over and his colleague comes around the side of the truck and points a gun at me. I saw there was no use arguing.

"Okay, kid, just relax. You help us out, nothing's going to happen to you."

"Okay."

"This is how it's going to be. We borrow your boiler and you drive. My pal's glasses got smashed when we got acquainted with that tree over there. He can't see a thing. And I see terrible at night."

"Well, there we are."

"Once we load our goods in the back of your truck, we'll continue on our merry way. We don't have far to go."

It wasn't far, but the route was plenty dark. And knowing the guy sitting squarely behind you is armed gives you a queasy feeling, *je t'assure.* When they realize how well I can drive at night, and that I get their cargo delivered without mishap, they offer to hire me. How I got such fine night vision myself isn't a terribly long story, but I find it kind of painful to think about; so let's just say, I came by it through little fault of my own.

When I learn how lucrative night driving is, I decide to make the most of it. I begin moonlighting; except, my

Sometimes the tough guys can barely take it. I go ahead and talk a bit, keep up a running patter to reassure them: *"Il n'y a rien a craindre. Je peux voir parfaitement bien. N'ayez pas peur. J'ai pas envie de mourir non plus."* ("Nothing to be afraid of. I can see perfectly. Don't worry. I don't want to die either.") And when I pull up at our destination, with all of us and the load still intact, half the time they start laughing hysterically they're so relieved.

A doctor explained it to me once. He says my pupils

open wider than other people's pupils. (Say that ten times fast.) The dark doesn't scare me. I'm only lost when there really is *no light at all*. I'm afraid of cops, though, and rumrunners who think I'm getting in their way.

After studying a little chemistry in college, I start distilling ersatz Calvados on the side. My family has some land with apple trees in the country and we used to produce gallons of apple cider every year. With the benefit of higher education, I decide to put some cider in a barrel off to the side and let it ferment. It doesn't take long. Then I run it through my homemade still, *et voilà*, I'm bottling apple brandy. As you may notice, I'm lowering my voice. I don't want to go to jail, which is why I'm speaking easy.

I make the mistake of offering my colleagues a taste and they aren't amused. Lucky for me, they decide I have a knack for distillation, and add it to my official duties. They start calling me Johnny Still, and then just Still. The joke is that it's kind of a big surprise that I'm still working for them. That I'm still alive, in fact, horning in on their business like that. Distilling by day and driving by night, I'm making money and losing sleep. Running on adrenalin mostly.

I'm trying to live exclusively in the present anyway. I find it's a fine discipline—to drive too fast over back roads in the dark. Everything else is beside the point except the matter at hand. Not skidding off roads that only I can see.

CHAPTER 4

PLAYING THE ACCORDION

Aldo likes to spend his evenings in the cleaner speak-easies of Manhattan, sipping gin martinis and drawing simple diagrams for his new acquaintances (well-heeled whenever possible), showing them that the path to easy money passes right through his office on 47th and Park. To say the money is easy is overstating difficult. The cream keeps rising to the top and we just keep skimming it off. He's running a classic stiff-joint.

When Pennebeck starts explaining that some investment can't fail to make money, he is of course thinking of it from his own particular vantage point. People have been making and losing fortunes on Wall Street since dice were invented. It's a moody business. The disinterested would say: what falls down might get up. But sales commissions are a dead certainty. Whether the customer buys dogs and ponies or sells them, Aldo makes a dime or two a share. Which explains his sunny disposition. He's a classic huckster—a damn, half-hearted, well wisher.

I realize that if you spend enough time around the stock market, you will perforce become a philosopher of dialectical materialism. A philosopher and pragmatist *à la fois*. The abiding *modus operandi* one observes is people attempting to outguess everyone else in the world *and* eliminate guesswork, to take the long view *and* the short profits. As for risk and reward, the most successful share the former and reap the latter.

Wall Street's attitude, in short, is: "You take the risk, we'll take the reward." And that's the way it is still. (People are always saying that to me.)

One evening after making a barrel of money unloading a couple of our stock positions, we're out celebrating, quaffing steins of beer in a German speakeasy on 86th street. The house polka band is energetically booming some oompas and Aldo leans toward me and casually points at the balding accordionist who's responsible for a lot of what's passing for musical entertainment.

"What you see there before you is the stock market incarnate, Johnny. That guy with the accordion, stretching it out and squeezing it back together, playing all the stops. He's the fucking U.S. stock market."

"In *Lederhosen*."

"He could use a new outfit. I've heard lots of guys describe the market as a rollercoaster. That's way too simplistic. The market is three-dimensional, like an accordion. Or four-dimensional. Who know? Maybe it's ten-dimensional, when you take into account markets all over the world. Look at that accordion. It's got to expand and contract for any music to be made. Same with the market. It has to keep breathing, sucking new money in, blowing money out." Aldo hoists his glass, "Today it was playing the kind of music that makes me want to do a jig."

"With those two gals who just came in the door."

"For instance."

I raise my beer and propose a standard Gallic toast: "*A tes souhaits.*"

"To another day like today."

"Why not tomorrow?"

"And the day after tomorrow."

Aldo snaps his fingers and when the waiter sidles over, he points at the two women we have our eyes on and makes his universal sign for glasses of champagne. He wants them delivered on his tab. After smiling his most ingratiating smile in their direction, he turns back to me, briefly.

"Problem is this—sometimes a few guys decide to see how far the average investor can be stretched and they end up breaking up the whole concert. It's as if they were to give that accordionist the bum's rush right in the middle of Broadway. Cross-town traffic would flatten him. And when it comes to dancing the polka, people don't dance that well to sirens and horns honking, Johnny, trust me on that."

CHAPTER 5

FRONT RUNNING

Aldo has a lucrative racket he teaches me after I'm with Pennebeck & Associates for a while, and it's a sure winner. Front running. And it's not even illegal.

"You know the expression, 'The devil take the hindmost?' On Wall Street, the devil eats the hindmost. The only place to be is out front, Johnny, if only by a fraction of a second." He goes on to explain to me in detail how front running is done and how exactly we're going to do it together.

Front running is an easy way to gain an advantage, based on information served up by the client. It's not infallible, like the dime-a-share commission racket, but it definitely tilts the odds in our favor. When played right, it lets us buy stocks and bonds for ourselves before the price goes up and sell them before the price goes down.

Say a client calls and wants to buy 1,000 shares of Bell Telephone. Aldo has me place an order for ten shares for us first. As he starts expressing interest in acquiring shares for his client, the price tends to rise. The sharks on the other side of the transaction can smell a large trade in the works and they keep asking a little more, a little more, and by the time he's bought 1,000 shares, our ten have gone up in price, too. If we want, we can sell them to the client ourselves at the highest price he pays.

The feds look askance at front running, so we call it proprietary trading. What we say is that we're trading for our own account.

On the other hand, when a client wants to sell a large block of stock, we jump in front and sell ours first, before the sharks start to wonder why someone wants to sell. Before they start wondering if maybe someone else knows something they don't know. Before the price starts its downward drift or begins to tumble in earnest.

After he lays this all out for me, Aldo tells me about his party telephone line. It turns out to be a real party. He sets me up in a tiny office next door to his where I listen in on his conversations on the party line and buy and sell depending. The clients probably appreciate the fact that he's so careful, repeating the order slowly and clearly, making sure to get their orders just right.

CHAPTER 6

FOXY

One evening, Aldo invites me along to some smashing private party with lots of dames, nice looking gals, plenty of real booze, and Cuban cigars. Not to mention a bunch of Wall Street sharps who are normally found armed with pickaxes, hacking away at the lucrative interstices between the law, taxes, and roulette. The place has a view till tomorrow. Out of nowhere, a tall blonde spins into the room, doing several pirouettes. Then laughing and shrugging a little, she looks behind her and another tall woman, a brunette, does two tight pirouettes herself and tiptoes up to her blonde dance partner and takes her by the arm. With everyone's attention, they saunter in unison across the apartment toward where the bar is being tended by a true knight of the spigot. Aldo knows the brunette.

One of the guys at the party murmurs "Foxy,"

pleading with the blonde, but she ignores him. She and the brunette sail across the room toward a knot of revelers at the bar. It turns out the poor beggar is some fast guy out of luck, a Swedish runner named Ulrich. He's in New York to run the Wanamaker Mile at the Millrose Games. They're on the outs for some reason. Another drunk guy calls out "Foxy!" and I think to myself, "At least we all agree on one thing."

I work my way over in due time and make bold to talk to her. She is almost as tall as I am which makes it easier. We exchange some of the basics. Her name: Eva-Maria. Mine: Jean-Yves. Her home: Stockholm. Mine: Montreal. When I tell her I'm from the snowy north, she lights up: "Do you ever go see the isockyteem?" When I figure out what she is getting at, I admit that I used to play ice hockey. Her reason for coming to NY: to study ballet. Modern dance, in fact. Mine: business, pleasure. How long's she been here: six months. Me: a year. Where's she live: Queens. Me: Brooklyn. What is she drinking: Champagne. Me, too. Would she like another *coupe de champagne?* She just blinks her eyes and smacks her lips as if she is a little kid and I think this Eva-Maria is too damn cute. She's wearing black stockings veined with dark green vines. For a moment I know how Jack and the Beanstalk must have felt.

When I return with the champagne, I ask her what she thinks about all these boors yelling foxy this, foxy that. She laughs a little.

"My last name is Fachsi. They know me, sort of. They think they do anyway."

"My family name's LeFouet."

She finds that funny. "Laughaway?"

"If you want," I say, "but it's LeFouet. It means 'whip' in French."

"Oh!"

They clear a space in the apartment for us to dance and I discover something: dancers can dance gracefully with anyone. She follows along with me and makes me feel as if I'm really dancing. Then for fun she throws in a few extra flourishes to keep it interesting. Still, she seems to enjoy my company. The rest of the party recedes into the distance and in spite of all the hurly-burly, all I can see is her shimmying in front of me. She pointedly avoids Ulrich the rest of the evening, and he drinks himself into a blacker and blacker mood, even with his race only a couple of days off. Some guys would have taken a swing at me, but he's a runner not a boxer. He was considered one of the front runners until his foxy girlfriend started giving him the cold shoulder. It appears likely he's going to be one of the also-rans. At some point, he pulls himself to his feet, pretty tottery, throws on his coat and stalks off with a dour look on his face. Eva flashes me a big, relieved smile when she sees him darkening the door.

CHAPTER 7

THE BACK OFFICE

My new office is cozy, a desk wedged in a coat closet. I exaggerate, but you get the idea. Talk about a "back office." But that's the beauty of our racket. My office is set up behind a hidden doorway. Soundproofed with cork paneling. And if a client ever does hear me scuffling around back there, Aldo complains about mice and the exterminator who's late. I even have a view. My little window looks out on a brick wall about six feet away.

We have a young trader at the Exchange—a guy by the name of Kyle Unterfisch—and I buzz him to make our company trades. He tips us off sometimes, too, about any unusually heavy action. He even has some source in Washington, D.C., who tips him off when some bill is likely to move the markets and that we can act on if we're quick. I never learn the guy's name. We kick some of the gains back and we all toast our success in the evenings.

We even have a printer, Otto Trestlemacher, who can forge a stack of stock certificates in short order if he has one original to work with. A real artist. He can even create stock certificates for companies that are still *in utero*. As a joke, he prints up a bunch of shares in the Brooklyn Bridge. And then later on some crazy lark he sells them to some dupes from Shanghai. We have a good laugh over that one. Aldo punches a pinhole in the coat closet door, a tiny peephole, so I don't barge in unannounced on some "private" financial consultation.

Another responsibility Aldo gives me is to read the obituaries every day to keep track of the city's newly minted widows. I'm the official keeper of the potential clients list. My job is to keep adding names and phone numbers to it. A couple of weeks after the terrible news has broken, Aldo gives them a call about protecting their wealth. Widows are a renewable resource and he's able to drum up a fair amount of business helping them invest their inheritance. Penny stocks are a surprisingly appealing investment for people on a budget. (They're so cheap!)

He tries to interest me in making some of these calls, but I tell him frankly I don't have the stomach for it. Driving blind is one thing; stealing old ladies blind is another. He doesn't insist. He seems to like chatting them up and I think he tells himself that he's going to give them better advice than the next bloodthirsty Wall Street type. Some of his stock recommendations do make his clients money. After all, a rising tide floats all boats. If he'd had a line on orphans with money, he'd have been yammering away at them, too.

Aldo likes the way I work and trusts me. He starts calling me his *factotum*, his "do-it-all." Some days, when the phone is lying asleep in its cradle, he sends me out to gather his necessaries—cigars, bootleg liquor, clean clothes—or maybe to drop off items to clients or pick up a check. Touring Manhattan, Brooklyn, Queens, the Bronx, and Staten Island in his Duesenberg is unforgettable.

Late one afternoon, I'm uptown, dropping in on a liquor importer, with express orders to buy real champagne, cost what it costs. A little kid is hanging around out front. Only a youngster, he's one of these ten-year-olds who looks as if he's ten going on thirty. After the man inside obliges me and I step out, the kid looks at me goggle-eyed. "Hey, mister," he says, "a guy's putting gas in your car."

Seeing that's highly unlikely, I tell him thanks for the information and go to see what the hell is up. It's getting dark and sure enough there's a guy alongside the Duesenberg with a hose running from the gas tank into a gas can at his feet. He's siphoning off my livelihood. I walk up to the yahoo, and I'm pretty surprised at his brass, doing what he's doing before the sun's even bothered to go down.

"Hey, fellah, what do I look like, a gas station?" The guy looks up with wide eyes and starts blustering out some story about being out of gas and late for work and sorry this and he'll pay me that. He thrusts a grimy, scraped hand into his pocket and pulls out what I take to be his life savings, a handful of pennies. Not a nickel to his name. His face is all scraped up, as if he fell down dead drunk the night before. He looks like a half-peeled potato.

"Forget it, buddy. Put the gas back in my car and we'll call us square."

I heave the champagne in the back seat and wait. When he's done replenishing my fuel, I dig a quarter out of my pocket, and much to his amazement, give it to him. "Here. If I were you, I'd take the night off." He shambles off with his gas can in hand, a bit sideways, hunched up as if waiting for the cops to come galloping up his back.

I ease the Duesenberg into motion and can't help pitying the poor devil a little and his miserable racket. Trying to make a living one hot gallon at a time. That kind of skimming will barely get you ten miles up the road.

A classy ride, the Duesenberg. The rear seat is about a city block behind the front seat and it has curtains for the rear windows and a little flower vase on each side, in case you happen to have some fresh-cut flowers you need to stash somewhere. It's quite the front room. I'd be glad to motor around in that work of art all day and some days I do.

When Aldo wants me to run an errand for him by car, he only gives me the Duesenberg key. He has another set of keys that he guards as anyone would. The key to the office, the key to his desk, the key to the liquor cabinet, the key to the safe. He doesn't trust me quite that much.

One day I'm taking the garbage out and when I pour the contents in the dumpster outside, I see a little slip of paper still stuck in Aldo's trashcan. It's a tiny little thing caught on some gum clinging to the inside of the can. It has Aldo's handwriting on it and a string of printed numbers. It looks like the combination to a safe. I'm about to brush it out, too, but I hesitate. Then I hesitate some more. I pocket it instead, just in case. I can't help myself.

CHAPTER 8

PENNY STOCKS

Front running penny stocks is especially profitable. These are stocks issued by tiny companies and the shares trade for less than a buck. The humbler variety of investor is attracted to them, because they're affordable, and these days, everyone wants to own stock. Unfortunately, they're a risky proposition. Nine times out of ten the companies are a confection of smoke and hot air, but if you play it right you can still make a killing.

Aldo and I employ a pretty reliable strategy of talking up these stocks to clients and then selling them fast. Ye olde pump-and-dump. Our advice to clients is to buy stocks and hold onto them for the long term. We're out to make actual money ourselves, however, so we buy them *and* we sell them. Guys like him, and there are more than a few, are known as dynamiters.

Aldo teaches me the patter of how to talk up stocks

with clients. ("The beautiful thing is if you buy a share for one cent and it goes up a penny, you double your money. You make 100% profit if it goes up a single, solitary cent!") I manage to move a fair number of penny stocks that we later sell for a hefty profit.

I don't think some are even companies. They're just names. I don't tell clients that if the shares lose a single, solitary cent, go from one cent to zero cents, they will take a 100% loss on their investment. Why dwell on the negative? I'm peddling hopes and dreams here, not hopes and nightmares.

Creating a syndication is another fine way to manipulate the market. Aldo catches wind of it and begins applying it to penny stocks. The way a syndication works is this: a few wealthy investors put together a pile of money—a syndication—and then they target a stock and begin slowly at first to buy, buy, buy and start to drive the price up. The price movement is duly reported in the newspaper. The reading, unsuspecting public takes note that the stock is moving, and they decide to get in on a good thing. They buy and drive the price even higher. Once the stock becomes unmistakably hot, more outsiders buy in and up goes the price even higher. That's when the members of the syndicate sell, sell, sell and pocket the money of the latecomers, who end up owning a stock on the verge of collapse. A prime example of letting the devil take the hindmost.

If you talk to any Wall Street insider who will talk to you honestly, they will tell you that every last one of these guys is working some scheme, some angle, colluding with other guys to cheat their way to a quick fortune. Every one of them, believe you me. They're all taking advantage of being on the inside looking out. They call themselves investment bankers, traders, financial intermediaries, brokers, market makers. Unmakers is more like it.

CHAPTER 9

FRIENDS

The night I met Fachsi, I slipped her my phone number. The next day, she rings me up, wondering if we could get together for coffee "today or later today?" She says she needs to talk to me about something important. Of course we can meet. That afternoon, she shows right on time, looking a little tired but still, when I think back on it, the kind of company that makes you shake your head in disbelief. Once our coffee arrives, we talk a little of this and that, how fine we are, what fun the party was last night, and suddenly she looks at me quite seriously and says, "I need a friend. Will you be my friend? Do you want to be my friend?" I've never had a heartfelt talk with a leggy, melancholy blonde before about being friends. I am more than willing. I think friendship is the best foundation for a torrid and lasting relationship.

She and I are picking at lunch, the best of friends I'm

thinking, and she suddenly begins crying. I try to comfort her. I reassure her that I'll be her friend, we're friends already, that kind of stuff. We're all alone in a big dining room filled with empty tables, and it's sunny, and the waitress, a middle-aged black woman, notices and begins to sing. She sings a whole song for us while taking a graceful dance turn around the restaurant with her broom.

> *Chacun a son goût, mon beau,*
> *chacun a son goût.*
> For me, it's you,
> for me, it's you.
> To each her own, to each his own,
> some like the fat, some like the bone.
> Some admire Coolidge, some Al Capone.
> Some like all night parties,
> some would rather stay at home.
> There's no accounting for taste,
> on what it's based.
> For some it's a certain face,
> for others a turn of phrase.
> Some like their talk sweet,
> others like it new.
> Some like it *doux,*
> others like it blue.
> *Chacun a son goût.*
> Some like their desserts *salés,*
> some like them *sucrés.*
> Some sweet, some salted.
> They can't really be faulted.
> Some like classical music,

some like jazz;
it depends upon the
taste one has.
Chacun a son goût,
even you.

And there sits Fachsi, looking at me with this grateful smile and sleepy eyes, tears rolling down her cheeks yet cheering up immensely and completely. The most therapeutic song I've ever witnessed. One of the top five. And when we get back on the street, she gives me a huge kiss and then we set out together, arm in arm, real friends.

Might this not have been a little too easy? A stop sign is almost invisible when looked at edge-wise. We've just barely met and here she is beseeching me for my *amitié.* But according to her tale, it isn't that outlandish. She's pretty much alone in a strange country, in a huge city, no family, few friends, and a suitor that doesn't suit her. Trying to make it as a dancer but living off her father's dough. Not exactly a sob story but hard enough. Pretty lost.

Her roommate the brunette is another dancer, a tall, skinny, raven-haired gal named Annemie, who seems to spend every waking moment limbering up. Hours on end stretching her long limbs, simply stretching and stretching and stretching. I can't help thinking about the paradox of dancers: otherworldly and so worldly, straining to turn bones and muscles into poetry and spirit. When Annemie introduced herself at the party, it sounded as if she said her name was "Enemy." Aldo

47

called out "Enemy" at her that first evening and I couldn't figure out what he was going on about.

Annemie is the temperamental sort. High-strung. After draining a few drinks, she likes to break things at parties. A glass here, a bottle there. It seems like an accident at first but after awhile you realize she likes the drama, that she thinks every party can use some livening up and that she knows how to get things jumping. As she dashes her glass, she dances a quick, improvised tap dance, as if someone is shooting the place up and she's nimbly sidestepping the bullets.

CHAPTER 10

A SWEDISH MASSAGE

Aldo and I take these two out to a nightclub later that week and they make quite a splash. Tall, graceful, laughing, flirtatious. Pretty much a whole lot of trouble, since it turns out they both have steady boyfriends, one back in Stockholm, the other running the mile with a hangover. But whatever boyfriends they have are nowhere to be seen. And these gals aren't in Sweden at the moment, and they don't seem to be thinking much about Scandinavia. They seem to be cheering up by the minute, and doing what they can not to go back. All day long they stretch and practice their dancing. And when the evening comes, what do they like to do? Go dancing.

That night we go back to Aldo's place for a nightcap after bouncing around some nightclubs. He has a nice apartment in Greenwich Village with a main floor and an upstairs bedroom that you get to by climbing an iron spiral staircase. The windows on one end of the apartment stretch from floor to ceiling. The adjacent wall has a huge oil painting of some creamy pink nude sprawling across three canvases. He assures us it's a priceless example of Modern Art.

Aldo's in a kinetic state and is out to prove himself the host to outdo all hosts. "What can I get you?" he asks, first Fachsi, then Annemie. "Champagne?"

"Yes!"

"Yes!"

"Maybe you'd like some white wine instead?"

"Okay."

"Or rosé?"

"That could be nice."

"Some Grand Marnier might be better?"

"Uhh…" The two girls are getting worn down thinking about all these choices. "Yes" is never good enough for Aldo.

"Are you sure you don't want champagne? It's been chilling all day…?"

"Yes, yes, yes! Champagne!"

"Okay, then, champagne it is!"

He pulls four crystal champagne glasses out of a cabinet and lines them up. Then he plunges into his icebox, pulls out a bottle of champagne and ostentatiously shoots it off, letting the champagne overflow into the glasses and on the table and floor. We're all laughing at this wild performance and then we clink our glasses and take a taste of Aldo's generosity. It is nice to know someone with a line on real French champagne.

All of sudden, the two girls exchange what can only be described as a mischievous look and begin whispering conspiratorially. Then they turn back to us, eyes glistening with excitement.

"Do you want us to give you a Swedish massage?"

"Have you ever had one?"

"No, never."

"And, yes, gladly."

"Aldo, do you want to be first?"

"It would be churlish of me to resist."

"All right, Jean-Yves. You will be the next."

They lead Aldo off to the bedroom and leave me alone. Those two are really something. I sip my drink and gaze out the windows at the city lights uptown. I can see the Empire State Building thirty blocks north.

Fachsi reminds me of Manon, a girl I fell hard for in Montreal. *Eh, oui.* I do my best to forget Manon, to stick to the present. I'm pretty good at it most of the time, but every once in a while the distant past wells up.

CHAPTER 11

MANON

Mais, non. Manon was the grandniece of my Aunt Simone, a dear, elderly neighbor of mine growing up. My favorite job ever was spending two weeks every summer dusting Aunt Simone's books and talking to her about them. She loved reading and literature and I did, too. Still do. Over the course of her 80 years, she acquired a beautiful library. Not only did she have most of what were considered the great works of literature, she'd read them. Some, many times. So she knew their stories and their secrets.

Every book in her library had its own lineage having been purchased at a specific time, in a specific bookstore, under specific circumstances. Often on a particularly memorable voyage with her husband.

Every Christmas, she gave me a book from her library. She would inscribe it with some anecdote about it to let me know that she loved it but was parting with this treasure because she also loved me. For instance, she wrote: "This little book has been in my library for over 50 years..." Or "I found this volume in a quaint, little bookstore in London, England 20 years ago..." Her books all had a distinctive black and gray nameplate that she pasted into the inside front cover. That way, if she did lend them to a friend, there was a good chance they'd find their way back home.

To receive one of her books as a gift was wonderful on so many levels. There was the book itself, chosen because it was a classic that I probably didn't know yet. She usually chose collections—literary essays, poetry, letters—adding another dimension to the famous books themselves. Then there was the particular leather-bound volume and its craftsmanship. There was the story of how this particular edition came into her possession. There was the striking nameplate and what she wrote to me inside. She and her husband didn't have any children. I loved her like a grandmother or a beloved aunt.

Every bedroom in her house had full bookshelves, as did the living room and the study. But where we did most of our work was on a dark, narrow balcony that ran the length of the high-ceilinged living room and which looked down on a piano and a big fireplace. This balcony was barely a corridor with a single, small window on one end and a long Persian rug on the floor.

We would bring our cleaning materials in there and I would use an old stepladder to reach the top shelves. She would perch on a stool and we would begin.

We would take all the books off a shelf, dust the shelf

itself, and then replace the books one at a time, dusting each one separately. She had oil to preserve the leather-bound volumes and a chamois cloth to burnish them. I learned that we had to do double duty on most of these shelves. She had no room for more bookshelves, but she couldn't resist adding a volume here and a volume there. Most of her shelves now had two rows of books, one in front and one behind. And some had a few books squeezed in lying horizontally on top.

The best part, of course, was she would talk to me about her books as we worked. After dusting for a good stretch, we would stop for tea and cookies or a piece of lemon cake, and we would sit at her dining room table and she would tell me stories. This was the enchanting life of a bibliophile, or I should say, two.

One afternoon I had to take a break to go to the bathroom, only to discover too late that it was occupied. I swung open the door and found her grandniece, Manon, awash in the bathtub. I'd never seen a teenage girl bathe. She was a couple of years older than I was, maybe sixteen or seventeen, and in town visiting her great aunt. I'd never seen anything like her. Glistening round floating breasts. Bright red nipples, dark pubic hair. She shrieked and threw a washcloth at me and sloshed a wave over the side of the tub. I swung the door closed on that noisy treasure trove.

Simone's eyes were sparkling with barely suppressed laughter when I returned. I smiled, too, sheepishly, and shrugged. An honest mistake.

"Now, where were we...?" she asked.

"I think we were working on Trollope."

"That's right." She leveled her calm, loving gaze on me. "Shall we continue?"

We shall indeed. The next time I ventured to use the bathroom, I knocked and there was no answer. I opened the door and Manon was standing there in her bathrobe with a finger to her lips and her eyes commanding me not to make a sound. Then gently she took my arm and pulled me inside, pushing the door to. She gave me the kiss of a lifetime, her lips soft and warm. *Bouleversant.*

My neighbor had whole shelves devoted to the collected works of Dickens, Balzac, Zola, Trollope. She told me that Trollope was so prolific that as soon as he finished writing a book, he would get up the next day and begin page one of the next. She loved Joyce, Proust, Matthew Arnold. She once told me that Arnold's poem, "Dover Beach" came close to expressing her perspective on life. The idea, if I may be so unpoetic as to summarize a beautiful poem in half a line, is that the world is ignorant and violent but that we have one salvation before us, which is to hold tight the people we love and to be true to them.

One afternoon, we're dusting the unabridged journals of Samuel Pepys. I glance in one of the dozen volumes and in some sort of pidgin French he describes how he cornered the maid in the stairwell and gave her a kiss. I tell Simone, too approvingly, I guess. All she says is: "Impotent fool." Manon wanders in, looking bored, acting as if she just wants to say hello to her great aunt. She barely looks in my direction. Then she saunters away again. I make an excuse to take a break from dusting and I push through the swinging door to the kitchen and there's Manon and she gives me a kiss, and she lets a trickle of red wine pour into my mouth. She's discovered Simone's liquor cabinet. All that warms me up impossibly.

Then one day, a week after Manon first appeared, Simone informs me that her grandniece is going back to Toronto that very day. When she's all packed up and ready to depart for the train station, she gives me a goodbye kiss. She pretends to kiss me on both cheeks, the way the French do when they say hello and goodbye. But she misses on purpose and gives me a soft half-kiss on each corner of my mouth. I help her granduncle put her suitcases in his automobile and Manon waves as they drive off. Simone puts her arm around my shoulders as we watch them disappear and we take a break from her beloved books and the encroaching enemy, the antipathetical dust. She's holding a plump tomato. "You know, Jean-Yves," she says quietly, "there are two things in life that money can't buy: true love and fresh tomatoes. Let's make a salad with this one. I just picked it. Doesn't it smell heavenly? I believe it has reached perfection."

CHAPTER 12

NOW IT'S MY TURN

Je me reveille de ce rêve, aigre-doux, a sweet and bitter dream, when Fachsi reappears smiling and beckons to me. I trot along after her and we pass Aldo coming out. He looks like they worked him over just about right. These girls are making me nervous, a little. They have me take off my shirt and lie down on the bed in the guest room. Then they kneel one on either side of me and they begin to count out loud, together, "one, two, three," and then simultaneously they put their hands on my back and begin their version of a Swedish massage. With friends like these, who needs lovers? That's how I really get to know Fachsi and Annemie and how they get to know me.

Bottles of champagne later, Aldo suggests we call it a

night, and heads slowly upstairs to his loft. Annemie looks at us, picks up her glass, and follows him up the stairs to the bedroom, leaving Fachsi and me alone. He has a guest bedroom on the ground floor and a couple of big couches in the living room. We look at each other a few moments. Here we are alone. Then we don't hesitate and we give each other a sweet kiss. And another.

"We can both sleep in the guest room," she says, shyly, "if you want. The couches don't look very comfortable." Before we budge, Annemie comes to the edge of the balcony that looks onto Aldo's living room, stark naked, for a second. She lets the crystal champagne glass fall and it shatters on the floor. Now only her laughter still floats above us.

Fachsi and I sleep together half-clad. But when we're under the covers and the lights are out, we give each other one, two, three tentative, friendly kisses. The next morning we're all suffering the effects of too much champagne. Annemie and Aldo go off to the kitchen to make us breakfast. The morning sun is filling those huge windows. Fachsi and I stand still, close together. Then we lean in and kiss as if for the first time. As if it means something this time, in the warm light of morning. And it does. Just like that she trades one front runner for another, and we start meeting every evening after the markets close. I can't wait for her kiss, though she sometimes jokes, blowing into my mouth, making a loud honking sound. She pretends she's going to give me a kiss and instead gives me a Bronx cheer. The raspberry. The snorting sound the horses in Central Park make.

One December afternoon, we go skating at

Rockefeller Center and we skate pretty well together after a few trips across the ice. We pretend we're traversing all the famous streets of New York on the ice. When we make a long slightly bending run, we say we're heading down Broadway. On our return, we glide along Riverside Drive. When we crisscross those long boulevards, we take a trip down Bleecker Street. Then we slide back along St. Marks. When we pause to catch our breath in the middle of the ice, we find ourselves in Times Square. What is time squared? To think about one period in time and multiply it by the events of another? We're both pretty long and lean. She starts calling me her Empire State Building, and when I hold her in my arms, I call her my Chrysler Building. Park Avenue. Fifth Avenue. Houston. We trace them all. Canal Street. Wall Street. Greenwich. 42nd Street. We end the afternoon with a peaceful promenade around the perimeter of the ice, which we pretend is Central Park. That's one of the best afternoons of my whole wide life. A great New York memory. At that moment, I completely forget all the fast ones Aldo and I are pulling. Fachsi and I are together, enjoying a running gag. The ice is smooth and thin.

CHAPTER 13

SAFE

New York, October 30, 1929

But that, dear reader, is a page torn from antiquity. I'm as interested in ancient history as the next fellow, just not so much my own.

After Aldo's legs disappear out the window, it takes about 30 seconds for Poochie and the flatfeet to ransack his office but good. They take a crowbar to Aldo's desk, which is a locked, heavy, oak number. They crack it open and Poochie stuffs stacks of papers into something that looks like a cross between a briefcase and a steamer trunk. Thank God my office is well disguised. After the storm rages and howls, it suddenly goes quiet. I hear the door slam and footsteps dying away.

When I see the outside office is empty, I get quick about it. I assault Aldo's safe, which is tucked away in a corner of my office. Even though I'm shaking like crazy, I start spinning the dial, first to one number then to the next and the next, and by God, the tumblers tumble. It has a heavy door, well oiled, quiet. I tug it open and empty it, then close it back up and spin the dial.

The contents of the safe are now in my briefcase—walking-around money, stock certificates, a little black book, a loaded gun that he bought when he started working for gangsters, ammo, and other papers that look like they might be worth inspecting. I hide my tracks as thoroughly as I can at a dead run. Aldo's office looks as if it's been hit by a hurricane.

I take the back stairs double-time and ease out the back of the building, heading out a service entry to the street. From there I see Aldo isn't going to be coming to work tomorrow. I hear an elderly woman say: "Why would a handsome young man like that kill himself?" Her companion says, "Look at his nice shoes." A crowd has gathered to agree about how little can be done for him now. The cops, the docs, the morbid, the curious. They all want to know why someone with such a fine tailor would kill himself. Why, indeed?

CHAPTER 14

BIG DEPARTMENT

Ten minutes prior, Poochie and the two cops come out of Aldo's building onto the sidewalk, Poochie carrying a bulging suitcase under his arm. They swagger over to where Aldo bottomed out.

Looking at the dead man, one of the cops says: "Better call an ambulance."

"Or the morgue," says the other.

"Call headquarters," says Poochie. "Tell them to send a street sweeper."

People are crowding up to get a look at the suicide. Poochie and the cops peel off and walk over to an unmarked car. Poochie jams it in gear, and they swing around the corner onto 46th Street, heading toward the East River.

By the time they park on East 103rd, the cops have changed. No more police uniforms. They enter a townhouse, lumber up the stairs to an apartment on the second floor, and let themselves in. They dump the suitcase on the floor. Big Department, the gargantuan gangster they work for, is there to greet them.

"We'll have no more problems with the guy in the white shoes, right, Poochie?"

"No, Department. That guy's done making problems."

"We hit him with a lily."

"But he didn't fly like no angel."

"Why would he?"

"We invested real money with that guy and he thought he could get away with giving us butcher paper. Those penny-ante stocks weren't worth a pretzel. And when you lose a penny a share on a penny-ante stock, it adds up to a big fat nothing."

"A total loss."

"A wipe-out."

"A complete bust."

"I won't put up with that. Ever."

Poochie pops the latches on the suitcase and starts unpacking, piling different stacks of papers on the kitchen table in front of Big Department.

The Department whistles. "Well, well. Look here, boys. Bearer bonds. This'll make up for some of Aldo's malfeasance." Big Department holds a sheaf of paper in a mammoth paw and slowly reads the certificates, following the print with a finger the size of a bratwurst.

"Oh, the piker!"

"What's the matter, Department?"

"We just bought the Brooklyn Bridge."

He licks his thumb and runs it across the paper. The ink smears. He flings the forgeries across the room and they practically paper the place.

"Get our friends from Shanghai on the horn, Poochie. They know these scoundrels. They fell for the same bunco. Wait, what's the name of that guy you got a job with this lowlife?"

"Johnny Still?"

"Yeah, Still. What about him? He must know these Street men. He'll help us ferret them out. Aldo ran his mouth plenty when he was in his cups. No secret was safe with that idiot."

CHAPTER 15

BROOKLYN, USA

As Big Department is suffering this little disappointment uptown, I'm ducking into the garage on Park Avenue where Aldo keeps his Duesenberg. I drive it over to Broadway and down to Chinatown, where I turn onto the Brooklyn Bridge and cross over to Brooklyn. I let the air buffet me, which helps keep my head clear. I'm living in a basement apartment in a Brooklyn brownstone, nice enough, but the neighborhood is no laugh after dark.

A few months ago, they cut down all the beautiful elms that lined the streets, because too many stickup artists were hiding behind them and jumping the yokels on their evening strolls. It makes life a little safer and a lot uglier—all those stumps lining the street.

Due to the reach-for-the-sky nature of the neighborhood, people go out of their way to look tough. You see guys 500 yards away coming up the street, swinging their arms, rolling his shoulders, stomping closer, stomping closer, stomping closer. If you wanted to rob someone, they aren't the victims you're looking for. A lot of guys in the neighborhood walk like that.

One of my neighbors and his wife are classical musicians, love to go into Manhattan to concerts or the opera. Over the years, they work out a way to get home safely after dark. They take a hatchet with them in a paper bag and stash it under the seat at the theater. On the return trip, when they get off the subway and are headed the last couple of long, dark blocks to their brownstone, the woman takes the hatchet out of the bag and carries it out in the open. My neighbor explains: "Muggers seem to think twice when the woman's carrying the tomahawk." Still, everyone I know has been robbed. It's the Wild West where I live and there are a lot of cowboys running around.

When I get close to my place, I stash the Duesenberg around the corner, so as not to arouse unnecessary curiosity on the part of my neighbors. I want to be long gone before anyone is the wiser. Just in case. Who knows if Aldo's clients know about me? Poochie does, I'm afraid.

CHAPTER 16

BARRED WINDOWS

As I come around the corner, I look at all the barred windows on the brownstones. That's all you need to know about my neighborhood. People distrust their neighbors so much they feel safer in prison. Come home. Lock yourself in. Heave a sigh of relief, having survived one more day in the glamour and razzmatazz of the big city. I should have lived in a better place, less dangerous, but every night I find myself buying rounds for Aldo's clients (and Poochie). A guy can easily go broke enjoying success like mine.

At my prison cell of a home, something seems odd. The grate at the base of the front stoop has disappeared. It could have been some stupid kid who did it, kicking the jambs out. Still, I don't like the looks of it. It screams: "Here's the way in, boys. Right this way."

I listen outside but just for a moment and then plunge

ahead, unlocking the metal door and stepping inside. The hall light is on. I'm locking the door behind me when someone yells!

Right next to me, fronting the street is a second door, a wooden door I've taken no notice of until now. As I stare, the doorknob begins turning. My skin starts crawling.

I fumble for Aldo's gun and point it at the door. "Who's there?! Quick! Or I start shooting!"

The doorknob rattles back and forth again a couple of times. I back away, keeping my gun trained on the wooden door and try my own apartment door. It's locked. No unannounced visitors. No trick-or-treaters.

From the other side of the wooden door comes a voice: "Johnny, it's me, Fish. Unterfisch!"

"What the hell! Come on, get outta there."

"The door's locked!"

I fool around with the key and unlock the door. The light from the hallway doesn't want anything to do with this moldy crawl space. It barely dares seep inside. It's dark but I can see a grate lying on the ground and I have a nice view out onto the sidewalk, right about ankle level. A couple beer bottles are lying about.

Out of the darkness comes Unterfisch, our floor trader. On his heels comes Fachsi's friend, Annemie. She's ready to jump out of her skin. Her fur coat looks mauled. Her stockings are tattered. Her eyes are wide and she isn't smiling. Somehow in her red silk dress, she still looks pretty good. A bit smudged but pretty slick.

It goes to show you how quick people are on the uptake in New York. Create a niche and right away people start elbowing their way in.

"You scared the crap out of me. What the hell are you doing in there?"

"Oh, nothing. I always jump in the first rat hole I come across."

"What gives?"

"We were followed. Chased."

"To my place? Who by?"

"Those Asian guys. The ones we sold the Brooklyn Bridge. They invited me and Trestlemacher to The Bean and Briar for lunch. Told me they had another wad to invest. But the subway was jam-packed and I had to wait for like four trains before I could shove my way on. When I got there, Trestlemacher was in handcuffs and cops were shoving him through the crowd and out the door."

"C'mon, no point talking out here."

I let us in my apartment and double bolt the door behind us. I feel better locked in.

Unterfisch is dressed like some well-to-do industrialist—tailored suit, flashy tie (wildly askew), silk shirt, Italian shoes. But an afternoon on the run and a flop in my crawl space and he's coming unglued. He looks as if he's been rolled by a Cuban cigar-maker.

Fish came to a party at my place a few months back, that's how he knows where I live. Made a complete ass of himself. He's one of these polite, quiet guys who gets surprisingly loud and belligerent when he drinks too much. We practically had to throw him out. He kept wanting to come back in until we luckily spotted a cab and managed to cram him in. Some guys just can't hold their Mezcal. I hadn't planned on inviting him over

69

again any time soon, but he was back, big as a carbuncle. I guess he liked my place so much he was willing to break in through the front stoop to get another look.

"I could use a drink. How about you?"

"I just want to flex my toes." Annemie is pacing and prowling around, hugging herself to warm up, stretching like a big-game feline.

"You weren't home and it was getting dark, and this suspicious car came crawling down the street and I just figured it's now or never, we better duck out of sight."

"Hm."

"Through the grate I saw a light under some door. Figured that was the way in. The grate was half broken anyway, kinda crumpled, so I gave it a kick and in we dove."

"Sorry you had to go through all the gymnastics."

"You're sorry. Look at my suit. My tie got caught and I almost swung."

"You found the right place, I'll give you that. A stranger would have plugged you without even opening the door. Especially in this neighborhood."

"Every car that drove by made me very scared," Annemie murmured.

"Don't worry, Annemie. You're going to be all right."

I got three glasses and sloshed some whiskey in them.

"How'd those guys from Shanghai find you? Why'd you agree to meet them?"

"They called and said they had another $10,000 they wanted to invest. Said they wanted to buy more infrastructure. Trestlemacher thought they might like some of the shares in the Manhattan Bridge that he's been working on."

"Jesus. Nobody's that dumb." Unterfisch shrugs, as if to say he isn't so sure.

I refill our glasses and then I ask him if he's heard from Aldo.

"No. He's not answering his phone."

"He won't be."

This doesn't seem to register with Unterfisch.

"I'm pretty sure he's dead. What do you say to that?"

"Fuck."

"Of course. Some coppers showed up at our office and threw him out. Literally. They shoved him out the window. Didn't know I was there. They sapped him first. He might not have known what was happening. I hope he didn't."

"Why didn't you help him?"

"I wish I could have, but there was no way. Trust me. Three huge cops. By the time I knew what was happening, Aldo was doing a swan dive."

"The guy owed me money."

"That's too bad."

"Tell me about it."

"He owed me some back wages, too."

"I guess you'd call him a dead beat."

"We're going to be like that, too, someday. Leaving the bills unpaid."

"How can you talk like that about your friend?"

"Sorry."

"It was a shock, that's for sure. Those cops might as well have been an earthquake, the way they shook the place up."

"What's with the cops? They're on a fucking rampage."

"I'm just here to grab my stuff and disappear before more hatchet-faced guys show."

"What train you taking?"

I thought for a second. "I've got Aldo's car. You can join me."

"Can we swing by my apartment?"

"It's not like we're going on vacation."

"Any room for me?" Annemie asks quietly.

"Sure."

"Aldo had that ocean liner, didn't he?"

"Yeah, it's roomy."

"Let's blow then."

"I've always wanted to see the Midwest."

"Ever been to Chicago?"

"No."

"I've been there and back."

"Like it?"

"Not much. But it isn't New York. It's got that going for it."

"Somewhere the hell out of the five boroughs is a start."

My phone rings but I don't want to answer it. It keeps insisting. Finally, I don't know why, I pick it up.

"Uh-huh… Sure, Poochie… No I didn't go in to work today… Yeah, I talked to him, told him I was too hung over from last night, that I'd see him tomorrow… Yeah, I've got it… I can be there in an hour… okay, okay, okay, so long."

Unterfisch and Annemie eye me.

"I really don't want to see that guy. Let's go."

Unterfisch is tolerable company, when he's not three-sheets-to-the-wind. He's a little younger than I am, but he's been working as a Wall Street trader for several years, and that'll age you. He has the black clouds under his eyes common to the type. It's not just the long hours every day that does it. It's dealing with long stretches of inactivity and boredom and then short bouts of frantic, panic-driven mayhem. Economic hyperactivity. And the culture, what there is of it, consists of lots of boozing and carousing after the market closes. Every night. The fear and greed will wear you down. I remember one night around midnight seeing one of these prematurely old, young fire-eaters standing in the rocking, screaming subway, clinging to a beaten-up briefcase. When the driver suddenly hit the brakes, the guy swung halfway around the pole he was clutching and his briefcase flopped around the pole like a rotten fish. He only very slowly regained his balance and hoisted himself upright. The next trading day was only a few short hours away. If I remember correctly, it was a Wednesday.

I'm hoping Vince is home, not out catting around, but I don't see hide nor hair of him. That's bad luck. It takes me about three minutes to grab my suitcase and throw in the necessary. I put some food from the icebox in a bag with a couple bottles of booze. To be nice, I turn off the heat. Why make life hard for my landlord? He's treated me all right. I usher Fish and Annemie out onto the street, but as I lock the outside door, I fight the urge to leave the key. Who knows? Maybe I'll need it. The place is mine till the end of the month.

We scoot down the street to the Duesenberg. I throw my bags and briefcase in the back seat. I open the passenger door for Annemie to slide in front with me. As she slips in, she looks me in the eye with some urgency and whispers, "How about just you and me go..." and she grabs my hand and squeezes. Unterfisch is okay, but she has a point. I hand him the key to the apartment and say as casually as I can: "Drop this in the mail slot, would you? I'll warm up the car and meet you at the door." He takes it and heads back toward the apartment. I turn the key, the car roars, and I start after him but I keep accelerating. When I come up alongside him, I'm going thirty and all he can do is stand clear. I shout after him: "Use my place! Feed Vince!" Then I turn to Annemie and add: "Unless you already dropped the key in the slot..." Annemie laughs and I regret being such a louse, a little. "He was planning to shove you out of the way, anyway. He told me so." I look in the rearview mirror. It's plenty dark, but I can see the white stick figure of Unterfisch holding a gat. We're already out of range. No point in waking up the neighbors just to let us know how pissed he is to see our taillights. Who knows? He might think twice about using the apartment after all. Vince is good company.

As we turn the corner, I hear a scrabbling sound from the back seat and a "meow." He always was a smart cat, Vince. He must have climbed in the open window or hopped in when we were loading the car. Time for the cat to scat, too. Annemie swivels around and reaches for Vince, brings him into the front seat and starts petting him. He looks alarmed, ready to bolt. After a bit, she kind of tosses him back in the back and rummages around some more in back. She finds a bottle of Canadian Club. She shows me the bottle and smiles.

"Want a nip?"

"Not now, thanks."

She shrugs a little. "I do." She uncorks the bottle and takes a sip. Bottle firmly in hand, she leans back in her seat.

It's a little chancy, doubling back on our tracks, but I figure the best way out of town is to cross the Manhattan Bridge, cut west through downtown on Canal, and squeeze through the Holland Tunnel to New Jersey. Under the Hudson River. Then we can head south and pick our way from there. Tomorrow I'll see if I can't ditch this beautiful eyesore. It's too nice a stolen car to be driving. If you're going to drive a stolen car, you want it to be nondescript. This one, I'm afraid, is exceedingly descript. It shouldn't be hard to sell cut-rate. Everybody is taking a bath in the market. People have to raise dough fast, to try to cover their margins. Why should I be any different?

That first night we find a rundown motor court to stay at. I dump the bags and my briefcase in the room and bolt the door. Annemie is giving the place the once over, not paying any attention to me. I approach her, pass my arms around her waist and try to pull her toward me. She just kind of holds herself away and looks at me coolly, questioningly.

I thought, well, she's not exactly struggling, maybe she'll warm up if I give her a kiss. I lean my tired, unshaven face toward her and try. She turns slightly so that all I find is her cheek. Then she turns back and gives me that cool gaze again. I must admit she is doing a very effective job of giving me the brush-off, without even expending much energy. I push the point, give it one more try, and manage to kiss her on the mouth. She doesn't bother to turn away, but there is absolutely nothing there.

"Having fun?"

"Kind of," I say. "How about you?"

She gives an ironic snort and firmly disentangles herself from my grasp.

"You guys are all alike. I'm not especially interested. In general. We're never going to be more than traveling companions."

"That's all right. I was only playing."

"We can share the bed, if you stay on your side."

"If I don't, it won't be intentional. I'm told I wander in my sleep sometimes."

"Try to keep it to a minimum, okay? I'm beat."

"I'm going to stay up a bit, Annemie. I'm going to read by this desk lamp for a bit, if that's okay."

"I don't mind."

She goes into the bathroom and comes back a few minutes later in her underwear. I make a point not to look much. She takes her time, inspects the sheets and blankets for unwanted surprises. Finally, she climbs in, turns her face to the wall, promptly falls asleep and starts snoring. She made a dent in the whiskey and is down for the count.

I mull things over for a bit, my trying to make a move on her, even though I'm smitten with her friend. What the hell was I thinking? She had the idea to hit the road together and leave the third wheel behind. I thought maybe she meant something by it. It was flattering in a way. But honestly I never really noticed her all that much, when she wasn't breaking something. Fachsi had my attention all to herself. But there I was all alone with a pretty girl and only one bed between us. I guess I started thinking Fachsi's God-knows-where in California. Maybe Annemie and I might have a special connection ourselves? She did grab my hand in the car. I saw her naked in Aldo's apartment, going to bed with him. She didn't seem so categorical then. I guess she just wants a ride, a way to get out of town. And we do know each other. We're almost friends. She and Fachsi and I hit some fun parties. But now she says she doesn't like men, "in general." What's the story with her and Fachsi? That's something more to ruminate on. Those nights where they were practically skipping down the street holding hands, wearing those short flouncy skirts, laughing like little kids. Trying to get New York City to halt in its tracks, which they did. I thought they were just trying to get under my skin for some reason, but maybe not.

The clerk at the front desk thinks Annemie and I are married. Telling him that probably got my overheated mind working along these lines. What an embarrassing combination. Middle-of-the-night-romanticism and what-the-hellism. Look how far it got me. Nowheresville, brother, all the way to nowheresville. Now I have to wonder about Fachsi and her.

For an ethereal dancer, she snores like a coal miner. At

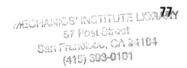

least I can look at this stuff of Aldo's undisturbed. I take out the briefcase with Aldo's papers and start figuring out what my lot in life is exactly. One little detail I take care of right away. I sign the Duesenberg over to yours truly for the tidy sum of $5000. Aldo's scrawl isn't too hard to fake, after I practice it a few times. ("I won the Duesenberg in a crazy poker game one night, straight flush.")

This all sounds pretty *louche*, I know. Fachsi's ditched me and Aldo's dead. He doesn't have any family that I ever heard of. I'm jumping ship and I'm trying not to miss the life raft. Besides, he owes me a couple weeks' pay, plus commissions, plus kickbacks, plus some other considerations that I'm never going to collect.

The first thing I see is a stack of stock certificates. With the market plummeting, they're probably fairly worthless but who knows? I'll try to unload them in Philadelphia, get something for them. I know a broker there by the name of Speckler. I might be able to get in to see him, do some business no questions asked. I'll tell him Wall Street has gone berserk, as if the whole place has closed up shop. That won't be news to him.

Next I find some bearer bonds. These are real beauties. Every six months, you clip a coupon and redeem it for half a year's interest. No one keeps a record of the owner. If you're bearing it, you're the owner. A great way to avoid paying taxes. Seeing that I'm now the lucky man in possession, I'm going to be the one clipping the coupons. Speckler might even buy one or two off of me at the usual discount. I need the cash, trying to start a new life and all.

The next morning, when I locate Speckler's office, he's closed. Annemie trickles off to do a little shopping. I find a pay phone and call him, on the off chance that he simply isn't answering his door. Sure enough. This time when I knock, Speckler lets me in. Speckler is one of these wiry, nervous types. A chain smoker. He used to employ some gorgeous gatekeeper in his office, but she's nowhere to be seen. He's barely survived the initial devastation of the crash. He wants to know where I got all the paper. He lets drop that people are upset with Pennebeck & Associates.

"Aldo didn't print these himself, did he? The ink's not going to run once you leave?"

"Why bring up ancient history? These are commissions I earned when the market was going the right direction."

He takes a pass on the stocks I'm peddling. He can't even get a quote over the phone, orders are so backed up. But he does make me an offer for the bearer bonds. I sell him a half-dozen $500 bonds at a pretty steep discount. He's thinking longer term than I am. I'm thinking coin of the realm.

Speckler says he saw the story about Aldo in the paper. He doesn't understand why he killed himself, either. Aldo sounds like one of the few people who was on the right side of the avalanche. People think he helped start it. One of his sources said that Aldo was shorting National City Bank stock like mad the last few weeks and had guessed right. I tell him I'm heading back to New York and will do my best to oversee the orderly liquidation of Aldo's business. Speckler gives me a half-smile and a little wave of the hand. "Lemme know if I can be of any help, Johnny."

When I get back to the car, there's a note from Annemie saying she's decided to take a boat back to Sweden. She's seen enough of America. Oh, well. I can save some dough roughing it a bit, which I couldn't have done with her along. Aldo's car's as big as a stateroom.

As I'm trying to get to sleep in the back seat of the Duesenberg, I suddenly start thinking about one of my recurring nightmares, a nightmare, unfortunately, that I lived. I'm back at my neighbor's, Aunt Simone's, dusting books, and she tells me her grandniece is back for a visit. I'm standing on the top of that shaky stepladder, reaching down a copy of *Tom Jones*, and I look up and see Manon through the living room window, almost out of sight, getting bent back on her heels, being kissed for all she's worth by some tall, older guy.

I feel lightheaded, the way I felt after drinking the wine from her lips in the kitchen, and instinctively I grope for the wall to steady myself but I don't look at the wall, my eyes are on Manon, and I just thrust my arm deeper into the unresisting air. The ladder tips and I catapult off the balcony. I don't so much fall as spin and the ground swoops up and crack... everything goes white and red and black.

Some dreams are just dumb and some are too real. Here's one that seemed real and really dumb. I'm driving my father's Model T, headed downhill, and the brakes aren't working. I ram my foot down and the brake just collapses all the way to the floorboards and the car is shaking and bumping and then a horse-drawn carriage bolts across my path and I slam into the side of it. I fly through the windshield and land right on my chin in the middle of the road. And I burst out laughing.

That's when I wake up on my back in bed. My mother and father are there. I can't see a thing. There's a heavy bandage over my eyes. But I can hear. I recognize their voices. They tell me how I fell. That I'm going to recover.

Manon actually visits me. When I hear her voice saying hello, I reach up and fumble at the bandage over my eyes. For a second I can see. She's there with her new boyfriend, in uniform, and she smiles at me pretty much as if I'm the little neighbor kid. Her boyfriend must be home from the war. As I stare at them, the room flushes brighter until they dissolve in a cloud of electric dust. I claw the bandage back down over my eyes.

Taking that bandage off too soon screwed up my eyesight but good.

Simone visits me, too. She brings me homemade custard that she took from her oven that morning. And a novel to help me pass the time, one of her favorites, *Barchester Towers*, by good old Anthony Trollope, for when I can read again. She apologizes for bringing me a book when my eyes are bandaged up. But she assures me I'll enjoy it when I can get back to reading. She's such a sweetheart. She stays and reads me the first few chapters.

My cracked skull heals after a few months. I do my share of raving, in and out of the hospital. They tell me I howl in my sleep. Like some ghost! My family tells me the same thing when I'm back home.

Even so, I grow up and go off to the university. I

understand blind rage. Seeing Manon with that soldier, that second time, shocked me as much as landing on my thick head. It practically struck me blind.

My eyesight changes after that. When I finally do get the bandage off, I have to wear sunglasses all the time. I don't care. Otherwise, during the day, everything looks sort of overexposed. When people tell me to look on the bright side, I tell them I always do.

You need someone to lead the way at night? I'm your guy. At night, people look like white line drawings. Like sketches or cartoons. It's almost as if they've been distilled. In fact, I can see when it's pitch dark out. And here's something eerie that I've never told anyone. I think I can even see things in my dreams, things to come. Sometimes I dream images and words that make strange sense later, as if I'm dreaming forward. But maybe that's not so unusual. All the ancients thought their dreams were prophetic.

So much for my career dusting books. Instead, I become a rare commodity, a night driver for people who prefer to move their merchandise after midnight. My job is to make the runs nice and smooth, low profile, so things don't become unnecessarily contentious.

I don't have any moral qualms about helping people quench their thirst during Prohibition. What do they say? A cynic is a disappointed romantic? By the time the machine guns start blaring, I'm in too deep to retire. I know too many of the guys.

I get past my dreams and nightmares about Manon but I never forget her.

In the next few days, I try selling the Duesenberg

twice, thinking maybe I'll travel by train instead, but the used car dealers have too much inventory and too few buyers. All their pitches are in the dirt. I resign myself to holding on to it and getting a better price on the coast. They size me up as a thief anyway, in a rush to dump such a fine automobile. They won't bite unless I really make it worth their guile and while, and I don't. If I can't get a reasonable price for the Duesenberg, I'm going to enjoy driving her a bit longer myself. And I'm not heading back to New York. Or to Chicago. I have another plan in mind. And where I'm going, cars are *de rigueur*. Los Angeles.

CHAPTER 17

MEANDERING WEST

I decide to head west to see if I can't find Eva-Maria. In New York, some guy on the subway (of all places) asks her if she's an actress. Says he knows people. According to her, he's not quite five feet tall. Maybe he is a big shot.

She asks me what I think she should do. Naturally, I want her to tell this new acquaintance of hers to go to hell, but at the same time I don't want to act like some overly jealous ass standing in her way. False pride is what it is. I play it cool, tell her if she wants to go and do it, it could be her big opportunity. I don't lay it on thick. I just leave her dangling with the decision to make on her own. I'm hoping she'll decide not to. She cries a lot and then she goes.

She was exciting and a little overly excitable, in the crazy sense of the word, goofy, inconsolable, at times angry and hysterical. After she leaves, I have two minutes of quiet before I start missing her. Sometimes I think men and women are a kind of mixed metaphor, but I dream of the mixed euphoria.

As I cross the country, I read the papers and track events on Wall Street. I wince at stock quotes that no one can get. The market is stumbling like some drunk falling down the front stoop. A *roué* who's gotten too obnoxious, getting bounced from a party of swells. Head over heels, tumbling all the way to the gutter.

It sounds as if thousands of speculators are sleeping with their heads under the tires of some limo about to be repossessed. And the pagan gods of Wall Street, the gamblers playing craps on the top of the New York Stock Exchange, are still down on their knees, trying to make out the numbers on the pair of dice. I read about other brokers jumping to their deaths and can't help wondering how many were helped the way Aldo was.

Finally, after a couple of months of meandering, I unload the Duesenberg in some God-forsaken town in Arizona. It's a necessary maneuver. Aldo never talked about his family, but somebody might well come forward and claim him. And they might want that car of his, the one that's big as a house. Or a hearse. They might have wanted to use it to trundle him to the cemetery.

The leathery used car salesman makes some deal, dangling a three-year old Hudson limousine in front of me for Aldo's Duesenberg. The Hudson doesn't have any rust, which is one advantage of buying a car that's spent its life in Arizona. It's not such a bad front room, either. And now I have a car title that no one will question. To make my decision to sell the Duesenberg not completely implausible, I insist the guy pay me $75 to go along with the Hudson. That guy will know how to erase all traces of Aldo from his beautiful automobile.

The Hudson limousine is plenty roomy, too, which helps me hold onto much of the money I got from Speckler in Philadelphia. Instead of staying in crummy motor courts, I use my own blankets and pillow and stretch out on the back seat. Vince sleeps in front. Sometimes he curls up next to me. We keep each other warm. With the Hudson, I can moonlight as a limo driver in L.A.

When I start the climb up over the mountains, putting the desert behind me, I begin to enumerate the mishaps the Hudson and I have endured en route from Arizona— a fan belt, an exploding radiator, two blown tires. They are each annoying in their own way, but none is too serious. Really I've been pretty lucky. Not to speak too soon. Quite a swell ride, really. Even with the new radiator, the Hudson tends to overheat. We'll see how it likes Southern California.

As I crest the hills and begin to coast down to the flat, dusty city that spills up and down the Pacific, more and more cars fall in with me, all of us in a big hurry to try our hands at something else. I keep an eye out for a hotel with a vacancy sign and a parking lot.

I find a creaky little hotel to hunker down in, just off Sunset Boulevard, and I begin to think about my future. I figure I should get a "For Hire" sign for the Hudson and see if I can't pick up a few customers. Los Angeles sprawls; you can't really walk from one place to another. You have to drive and I'm betting some people won't feel like it and that's where I'll be able to make a couple bucks.

Once I get my bearings, I start my search for Eva-Maria. I begin with what can only be called trepidation, or you could say a combination of excitement and fear. The kind of hope that makes your breath come short and quick and your heart ache. A diner down the street has a telephone and a telephone directory, and by God, there her name is, listed right there! Look at that! She's come here after all and gotten some sort of toehold, made it into the cast of thousands. I take a deep breath, drop a nickel in the slot, and dial the number. The operator comes on.

"That number has been disconnected."

"Do you have another number for her?"

"No, I'm sorry. There's no other listing for anyone named Fachsi."

I look again at the cover of the phone book. It says 1930. It's the right year. One thing I quickly discover about L.A., though—people move around a lot. In this town, the people come and go, talking of making too much dough.

If you live in a big city like New York or Brooklyn long enough, you feel the tension when day draws to a close and night wraps her arms around things. It gets dark in California, too. Flip off the floodlights and it seems twice as dark at night. And if you're new to the neighborhood, you don't know what you're going to find or what will find you.

A few days of reading the classifieds and I see what I'm looking for: "Driver Wanted. Night shift. Must own car.

Applications accepted after 9 p.m." I'm familiar with
shadowy gigs, these kinds of employers, and I've
punched the clock on the graveyard shift before. At
night the light is soothing and the roads are empty. That
I like. Sometimes you're expected to drive overly fast
given the conditions but that's where you earn your
bread.

The ad gives the name of the company, Granyer
Productions, and an address in Culver City, so I spend
the afternoon washing the meal ticket and throwing out
the newspapers and coffee cups I've been collecting.
This could be my break. Might as well go all out: shave
and plaster down my hair. I consider putting on a tie, but
it doesn't seem like it's going to be that kind of job. I eat
a baloney sandwich for dinner and drive to the address
listed on the want ad.

Modest is the word for the neighborhood. Small
houses, bungalows they call them out here, flat terrain,
no views. I find the building and park right in front. This
might impress them. My limo's as long as a Sunday
afternoon. I like driving and this should be a cinch
compared to tearing back and forth across the U.S.-
Canadian border. Or even navigating lower Manhattan.
Los Angeles is wide open. The streets are long and wide
and straight. Most people don't walk, like I said—either
they drive or take the streetcar.

I find the address and go inside. There's no light in the
lobby but I can make out "Granyer Productions" in the
dark, no problem. What kind of phony name is that,
anyway? Third floor, it says. There are no stairs, just a
little elevator tucked away in the back. I push the button

and wait. It comes soon enough. The doors open so slowly you'd think they'd just woken up. Inside is a kind of accordion door that I slide open. When I hit the button for the third floor, the doors shudder and shut.

There are only three offices on the third floor and I find Granyer's. Could be a costume-jewelry wholesaler. I knock. No answer. I knock again. Still no answer. The office is dark. The whole place seems deserted. I scribble a note on the back of a slip of paper with the hotel's phone number and stick it in the doorjamb. Pretty much a big waste of time. As I'm riding the elevator back down, I'm silently swearing to myself and thinking about what I'm going to do next. It takes too long to get from here to there in L.A. I need to get a job driving for someone soon, to make the running around pay.

When the elevator rattles to a halt back at street level, nothing happens. Swell. The doors don't budge. What the hell, I'm thinking. Here I am in the back of some abandoned building, nobody around, and I'm trapped in the elevator. I hit the Open Door button a couple of times. Nothing happens. Is it time to start yelling? I think to try the L button, which I figure stands for lobby, which is pretty laughable in a dump like this. Like magic the doors suddenly shake back open.

I slip out as fast as I can and run smack into Mr. Granyer Productions himself. He's turned the lobby lights on. He's fairly tall, not old but his hair is completely white. He's got a paunch. He's sweating so much he looks downright sticky. In case he's the guy I'm looking for, I introduce myself. "Charles Granyer," he says and puts out his hand. I give it a quick shake.

89

Clammy, which figures. I tell him I'm here to offer my professional driving around expertise, and that I'm an especially good at night. He lights right up when he hears that.

"Did you bring your car?" He's got some sort of English accent.

"Parked it right in front."

"That's yours?"

"Yes, it is."

He doesn't say anything to that. He just holds his tongue. As his silence keeps on, I feel the need to say something, do some explaining.

"Circumstances change. I sold some stock at the height of the market. Indulged myself. I was lucky. I know guys who lost everything."

"As do I."

He walks over to the curb and hums a little. The Hudson is elegant under the street lamps. After he gives it the walkaround, he turns back and inspects me thoroughly. He seems a little somber as if he remains unconvinced.

"You're from Arizona?"

"That's right.

"What brings you to Los Angeles?"

"I'm looking for my girlfriend. She moved here about a year ago hoping to break into the motion picture business."

"This would be the place. I apologize for not being in my office. I just took a drive with another would-be driver in a Model T. Let's take your motor car for a spin, shall we?"

I later learn that his full name is Charles Blaine Granyer and that his pals at Cambridge used to call him Chilblain.

He stands at the back door of the car and I realize that he's waiting for me to open the door for him, so after a little unprofessional hesitation on my part, I whip the door open, wait for him to settle himself inside, and then firmly shut the door behind him. I'm happy to demonstrate my *savoir-faire*, as it seems to be taking us in the direction I want, which is me landing a paycheck and a way to pay for getting around town while looking for Fachsi.

I observe Charles Granyer in the rear-view mirror. He looks not unpleased. He's enjoying the Hudson, feeling expansive. I'm cautiously optimistic. My competition is rattling around town in a car that rolled out of Detroit in 1915.

"How's she do in traffic on a hot day?"

"Fine." I flick on the electric fan mounted on the side of the dashboard and it sends a thin breeze toward the back seat.

"I need someone I can rely on when I'm entertaining clients. I must be able to concentrate on relaxation. I've never gotten used to driving on the right side of the road. I would be something of a menace if I tried."

"I'm plenty used to it."

"I had to fire my last chauffeur. He took a couple of us down Mulholland Drive and missed a bend. We ended up down an embankment. Blasted car was standing on end. Absolutely vertical."

"Hm."

"We're hanging upside down and he turns to me and you know what he says...? 'Cheers!'"

"Hm."

"We were standing on our heads, like knickers on a clothesline, until some Good Samaritan hauled us out. I was sore for days."

"Nothing like that'll ever happen with me."

"I should hope not. How soon can you start?"

"Soon. When do you need me?"

"Evenings. I'm in the motion picture business myself. I have lots of people I need to entertain after dark. Actors. Actresses. Investors. My previous chauffeur was a *bon vivant*. After they rescued us, the cops booked him for driving with one hand on the steering wheel and one on a martini."

"Ah."

"We tried to tell them we were the ones drinking the martinis. That they'd simply spilled into the front seat when we went down that unfortunate embankment."

"Did they believe you?"

"When they checked his registration, it turned out the limousine wasn't exactly his. He can't do me any good now. I don't need a rickshaw driver."

"What kind of car did he have?"

"He'd borrowed a Lincoln Continental from someone in Kansas City."

"Well, that's a pity."

"This is an exceedingly comfortable car. It is yours, isn't it?"

"Like I said. I was lucky. I rode some stocks to the top and hopped off into this baby."

"Okay, then. If you want the job, you're hired."

"I like driving at night."

"You're not one of these guys who thinks he can drive with a flask on the seat next to him, are you?"

"No, sir."

"Another thing, I may need you on my bag on occasion."

"I'm not sure I follow you…"

"Golf. I may need you to be my caddie."

"Sure."

"Welcome, then."

We come to terms back in his office and I agree to start work the following evening. He gives me $5 and tells me to fill her up. I'm going to be covering a lot of ground.

"And keep the change," he says. "Did you have trouble getting out of the elevator?"

"Yes, I did."

"Sorry about that. I need to have that looked at. If you don't hit L when you get to the lobby, you may never emerge. I had a poor cleaning lady get stuck in there. I gave her a big tip and she still never came back."

"I think I better invest in some new tires, too. Just to be on the safe side."

"Okay, okay, here's another $20. Make sure they're quality. What I'm looking for is a safe driver and a dependable vehicle."

"New tires will help."

"I'll see you tomorrow night, and make sure you're on time."

The next day I take care of a few odds-and-ends, fill

up the tank, drop off some clothes at a Chinese laundry, grab a bite at a little restaurant down the street, and look around for the first time with more curiosity and less desperation. And I get some new erasers—whitewalls. The L.A. sunshine is a problem. My eyes are attuned to twilight, even midnight, but the noonday sun is painful. I can't venture out without sunglasses.

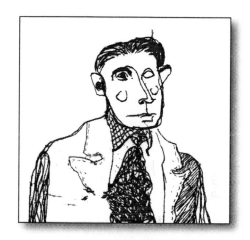

PART TWO
EAST OF HOLLYWOOD

The sea is calm to-night,
The tide is full, the moon lies fair
Upon the Straits;—on the French coast, the light
Gleams, and is gone; the cliffs of England stand,
Glimmering and vast, out in the tranquil bay.
Come to the window, sweet is the night air!
Only, from the long line of spray
Where the ebb meets the moon-blanch'd sand,
Listen! You hear the grating roar
Of pebbles which the waves suck back, and fling,
At their return, up the high strand,
Begin, and cease, and then again begin,
With tremulous cadence slow....
—Matthew Arnold, "Dover Beach" (1867)

CHAPTER 18

GRANYER

The sun is setting when I pull up to the international headquarters of Granyer Productions, Ltd. Granyer is originally from England, but he cut his teeth in the Far East—Shanghai—some place I've never been and I'll surely never go.

He had a dream when he went to the Far East—to pocket the keys to the vault of some modest little banking establishment. He was hoping to fill a war chest and if a bank teetered on the verge of bankruptcy, he would swoop in and "save" it. Then, he thought, licking his chops, the fun would begin. In Shanghai, a lot of banks put up a flimsier façade than sets on the back lots of Hollywood. Granyer thought banking had all sorts of swell possibilities. I only learned this later, of course. And why it hadn't worked out quite as he'd hoped.

He'd fallen for a Japanese woman, the daughter of a

powerful Japanese nightclub owner, and the Brits yanked him out of there, to try and forestall any serious scandal, such as their actually getting married and having children. It didn't matter how pretty or handsome or intelligent or educated or graceful or cultivated the children were, no one would accept them, not the Japanese and certainly not the Brits. The bank, which wasn't interested in losing the tycoon's business, ordered Granyer back to the home office in London. His family was dutifully informed and they were simply mortified.

'The tycoon wasted no time sending his daughter back to Tokyo and when Granyer realized there was nothing he could do, he sloughed off any romantic despondency he may have felt and fell back in the arms of a courtesan he used to know. He bought a boat and stocked it with Chinese bric-a-brac. Then one night he set out with his sing-song girl and they managed to make the crossing to San Francisco. He had no interest whatsoever in going back to Old Blighty. He stayed in America. A painting disappeared from the bank's boardroom at the time but they didn't press charges. A real entrepreneur. He'd made some connections outside of the bank and was able to keep himself going by selling his cargo in San Francisco.

He must have greased the wrong palms, though, because somehow he came to the attention of the local cops and was encouraged to keep on traveling. His sing-song girl slipped free in San Francisco, maybe scared by all the underhanded stuff he was engaged in. He slid south in quest of other opportunities. On his own when he left town, he was somewhat embittered. But one thing about Granyer, he was resourceful. Movies were being made in L.A. and people were packing the theaters to watch them. Why shouldn't he try his hand at it?

When I meet him he just seems like a prickly guy with bad teeth and rotten breath who wants to pay me. I'm an experienced night driver and I own a dark maroon limousine. *Et en plus, je parle français.* I learn that Granyer speaks passable French also. He enjoys being able to *pratiquer son français*, leaning back, smoking a cigar, me easing him around town in the Hudson. Like taking a Sunday drive in a bathtub. I insist he keep the window down. The smoke and the exhaust are too much like a double dose of L.A.

Granyer is an impatient guy. Once he climbs in the Hudson, other drivers become an endless source of discontent. As soon as someone slows us down the slightest bit, he starts making caustic remarks or even shouting. He waxes sarcastic about younger drivers, saying things like: "Okay, beautiful," or "Okay, gorgeous." But older drivers seem particularly galling. His running commentary features the heavy use of "Okay, grandma," and "Okay, gramps." To his credit, he becomes positively philosophical when we're stuck in traffic or getting dinged by a traffic cop.

It doesn't take long to get an idea of the kind of driving he needs. For one thing, he owns no car of his own, so we glide here and there running errands, hitting the pharmacy, buying groceries. I drop him at speakeasies, where he meets financiers he hopes to rope into backing his projects or to break bread with actresses he promises to turn into stars. The Hudson and I guarantee he makes a grand entrance.

While he's inside conferring, I cool my heels in the car. It isn't too terrible. I get paid by the hour and at the end of the night I have more folding money than when I set out. Hours later he comes out of the club, at times laughing uproariously and slapping guys on the back or whirling gals off their feet. After a parting joke or promise, he swaggers over to the car where I hold the door for him, and we drive off trailing what he hopes is a winning amalgam of style, panache, and success.

Sometimes things don't go as well and he comes back in a tense and foul mood. He has a temper, so I stick to driving and try to stay out of the line of fire.

When his sodden meetings do go according to plan, he follows up the next day, having me hand-deliver manuscripts for the project he's promoting. I enjoy touring the city on my own. I visit some swanky parts of Beverly Hills and deliver countless beautifully wrapped books to a swell group of maids and butlers. I get to know servants in Chinatown and Little Tokio, too.

I enjoy making these rounds later in the evening, when the air cools off and traffic thins out. People seem happy to see me, too. I'm not just another deliveryman interrupting them when they could be escaping the heat in the pool. I'm more of an event: special delivery from the Hollywood dream factory. I come bearing the possibility they'll one day see their name on a marquee.

Granyer and I develop a decent working relationship, a *modus vivendi*, and after a couple of weeks, he asks me if I want to move into one of the bungalows in his backyard rent-free, if I'll agree to chauffeur him around whenever he needs me, night or day. Considering he lives in Beverly Hills in a beautiful house on a huge lot, I figure *pourquoi pas?* It's pretty much our arrangement anyway. I go back to my creaky hotel, pack my bags, grab Vince, and motor over to Granyer's.

With few earthly encumbrances, it takes me the time to cross the threshold to move into Granyer's backyard bungalow. It's a cross between a shed and a cabin, pretty ramshackle, but the nicer of his two outbuildings. The yard is secluded, with a number of tall trees, and is surrounded by thick hedges. The cabin has a bed and dresser and a couple other sticks of furniture. Vince likes having a yard to explore and trees to climb, so he makes himself at home, too (after taking refuge in a tree for the first day and a half, casing the joint, seeing who his new neighbors are). Chauffeuring isn't half bad as a vocation. I just hope I don't get awakened at 3 a.m. too often, now that I'm really at Granyer's beck-and-call.

CHAPTER 19

A NEW ASSIGNMENT

Granyer invites me into his mansion for supper a couple days later, after I've done a lot of running around. He wants to talk to me, he says. We settle down at the table in his dining room and a maid brings us glasses of orange juice with champagne. Granyer has a buzzer installed under the table that he can step on to signal his kitchen staff. Next she brings us grapefruit on china. Each section of the grapefruit has been carefully incised, a maraschino cherry sits in the middle, and the whole thing's swimming in brandy.

As I finish squeezing the last drops of grapefruit into my spoon, a bevy of servants brings out the main course: new potatoes in rosemary, a fruit salad, and a huge platter of fish throwing off billows of steam. A cloud of steaming vinegar hits me, and tears burst from my eyes. "My God," I think, "What's this?"

My host looked at me benignly and smiles: "You're in

for a treat, Johnny. A Korean delicacy—fermented fish! It probably runs counter to the spirit of Prohibition, but…" His sommelier places a bottle of saké on the table. I quickly and as discreetly as possible drain a dram of the rice wine, hoping it will make it easier to stomach this abomination.

"Go easy on that stuff. I need you to make a run down to the coast later tonight. I have a shipment coming in and your land yacht will be perfect. We've picked out a very quiet cove. There shouldn't be any problem."

After dinner, one of his stevedores joins me. He's a quiet Asian guy who knows the way. We head north on the coast highway and eventually turn down a narrow, rocky road. He tells me to kill the lights. My car is complaining pretty noisily by the time we get to where my companion tells me to pull over. We step out of the car and quietly listen. Other than the surf, nothing. He has a flashlight and leads the way along a goat track that falls off down to a beach the size of a sandbox.

When we have sand underfoot, my companion turns his flashlight on and off several times. A rowboat approaches, riding low in the water. Two guys land the dinghy, and after a word of acknowledgment, begin lifting a dozen small wooden barrels onto the beach. Then they clamber back in their boat and pull away hard. We haul the casks up the winding path, load them in the car, and throw a blanket over them. Then we bump slowly back over the rocks to the coast highway and head home.

My companion is impressed: "Good car. Hold a lot." At Granyer's, more hands arrive to unload the cargo and Granyer oversees the operation, practically hopping with excitement. All the *tonneaux* are hauled down into his cellar and placed under lock and key, except one that he wants taken straight to the kitchen.

"Tap this and let's toast a job well done." They pour out glasses of saké all around and hoist them. "To next year's rice crop!"

The next day, runners from the best Japanese restaurants come and pay top dollar for a barrel of saké. Apparently this saké stuff is hard to bootleg well, making the real item rare and prized. And let's face it, Japan is a lot farther away than Canada or Cuba. Canadian whiskey and Cuban rum are plentiful in comparison. I'm an old hand at this kind of work and Granyer gives me a decent raise. I can't say I was overly surprised when he finally broached the subject.

A month later, the quiet guy and I pick up another shipment. After the barrels are unloaded, Granyer taps one of the kegs to celebrate. Everyone takes a nip and Granyer starts coughing and swearing.

"What's this?! It tastes like piss!"

"Not piss, boss. Tequila."

"Maybe the Mexicans have our saké."

"Can't even keep our orders straight."

"If I don't get my merchandise, someone's gonna pay."

In East L.A., some other smugglers are also perturbed. "*¿Qué es eso?*"

"*¿Urina?*"

"*¡Alguien va a pagar!*"

"*Cálmate, cálmate, eso es saké. Es posible que los asiáticos tengan nuestra tequila.*"

"*¡Espero que sí! ¡No puedo beber eso!*"

CHAPTER 20

GOLF ETIQUETTE

Talking through a mouth full of catfish, Granyer warms to one of his favorite topics. He's seeing to my education. "Golf is a noble game. A game of honor. A form of recreation played among gentlemen." (Let the pontificating begin.) "In the game of golf, one must follow the rules. A lot of rules. In fact, it is far more important to play according to the rules than it is to win. Every golfer who is a true gentleman follows the rules and will even call penalties on himself. In fact, one *must* call infractions on oneself. Otherwise, whatever one is doing cannot be considered golf and one is neither a golfer nor a gentleman."

I have to laugh. I sort of enjoy it when Granyer trots around on his high horse. Here he's a dyed-in-the-wool scoundrel 95% of the time and yet he clings to a few random principles that he thinks should be universal.

(His attitude about most principles is that they are imperative for others and voluntary for himself.)

For example, the old saw about "do unto others" gets squelched much of the time. He expects waiters and waitresses to act according to his idea of social standing. If the wait staff doesn't hop to and defer just the way he thinks they should, he gets haughty. Or dismissive. Immediately. He lays on the British accent and refuses to look at them, just quietly breaks off orders and waits for the help to disappear. When they return, he sits motionless and waits for his food to be deposited in front of him as if he's one of the royals, and then without a glance, he waves them off. Since I'm usually relegated to the car, I don't have to see him act like this too often.

On one rare occasion I join him for lunch in a speakeasy with a crowd of would-be actresses. Things are going well and he decides to order a second bottle of champagne. The waitress makes the mistake of starting with the girl to his left and continues around the table until she finally arrives at Granyer. There's only half a glass of champagne left for him. He dresses her down, telling her that she should have started with him, the person who ordered the bottle, and then he demands another bottle and announces that he is refusing to pay for it. The manager comes over and Granyer lets him have it, *sotto voce*, and then the extra bottle arrives, his glass is topped off, and he begins to calm down. Soon he's laughing and joking. He clearly enjoys getting exercised. The waitress serves us for two hours and he leaves her no tip whatsoever.

Another endeavor requiring correct conduct is the

game of golf. Not to mention caddying. Etiquette means a lot to Granyer and playing by the rules. That cheating is wrong is of course not unique to golf. Cheating is cheating, for God's sake. Name one game where cheating is considered acceptable. It's funny to hear him go on like this. He hates guys who improve their lie with their club or the toe of their golf shoe.

But what he really hates is losing a ball. That is a principle of a different order. The principle of objective reality. Material objects do actually exist. They can't just vanish. If he hits an errant shot and has no idea where he shanked it, it should still be found. It's got to be somewhere.

He tells me with satisfaction that once he was playing golf by himself and lost a ball. He was sure he saw it roll into a clump of bushes on the fourth hole. But search as he might (and he searched with all his might), his ball remained hidden. The next day, he couldn't stop thinking about it, so he hired a taxi to drive him back to the course, which was over an hour away. "I went back to that fourth hole and looked for my ball," he said, "and you know what? I found it." It was as if he'd won the British Open.

L.A. FRAGMENTS

One afternoon I'm driving down Hollywood Boulevard and there's a truck rattling along ahead of me transporting wooden crates filled with empties. Empty soda bottles. As I pull alongside it, I notice a couple guys riding in back. One shifts around suddenly and right in the intersection of Hollywood and Vine he upsets one of the crates. Coke bottles start sliding off the back of the truck and smashing in the road. The guy grabs for the empty crate and hauls it back upright, laughing. I'm having trouble figuring out the native Los Angeleno.

L.A. is an ambitious town. Everyone I meet seems to have artistic aspirations or a business scheme that they think is going to make them famous or at least land them deep in the gravy—acting, singing, playing music, making movies, taking over a bank, striking oil in their backyard, etc., etc., etc. The place is lousy with people drunk on dreams of grandeur, or hung over from them, now just trying to hang on.

It's also full of hard, clear-eyed people willing to exploit them. They know the dreamers will do practically anything, for free, if they think it will perhaps help them land in the big-time easy money down the road. A lot of the work that seems like an entrée to the good life gets done by saps for free. Only in Hollywood do you see prostitutes work for nothing. At least on the street, on Sunset Boulevard and Santa Monica Boulevard, the prostitutes actually get paid real money. The rest get fiddler's pay or monkey money, thanks and vague promises. People believe the hot air and keep holding onto this idea that they're going to make it big, that they'll become stars, superstars, super-duper-stars, not that they will create something great but that they themselves will become great, that everything will work out, until it hits them square in the face that it hasn't and it won't ever.

Like the painter, a fine arts graduate, who's eking out a living painting billboards.

Or the songwriter who's sure he'll be recognized as the next Gershwin. Except that the promoter he hooks up with confiscates his master recordings and won't give them back unless the rube pays him some sum that he doesn't have. Oh, yeah, and the singer doesn't have the rent and it's due in two weeks. But he does have some coke on a tray, and his works, which he keeps hidden within reach under his low-slung couch. He'll be right back and tell me more about how it will all work out, he's confident it will, somehow. I beat it out of there while he's holed up in the bathroom.

Or the would-be actress who keeps sleeping with producers *before* they give her the role. Before they ever give it to her.

Or the pianist, trained at Juilliard, who composes advertising jingles.

Or the classical guitarist who plays in the evening every other week in some French restaurant and moves furniture all the livelong day. And who has to listen to the waiters complain about why he doesn't come up with new material, who have no idea how difficult it is to master a single piece, who couldn't play a penny whistle if you held a gun to their head.

The guys with small rackets and no illusions seem more content. Like the bottle collectors who spill a crate on the road now and then and get paid for their services by the tire salesmen down the street.

Or the dope peddler who asks me if I can tell him what the best thing in the world is? Because he's figured it out. "Cash."

Or the guy from Kashmir who tells me that in L.A. the only relationship that matters is you and your money.

New York has its own version of these aphorisms, don't get me wrong. Here's one of my favorites: "When a dollar hits the sidewalk, three guys are there to dive on it."

The basic tenet is this: When things reach the point where actual money is liable to be made, people go nuts.

This is where Granyer is different. His philosophy is: scrape together a pile of money, then dream.

CHAPTER 22

GRANYER STUDIOS

The next day Granyer says we should go for a little drive. He wants to show me his film studio. We drive up into the hills until we come to two buildings in the middle of nowhere. The place is fenced in and the gate's padlocked.

"Welcome to Granyer Studios," he says, unlocking the gate and letting us in. He leads the way to a medium-sized round building, unlocks the door and flips on the lights. It's a big round barn of a room with a jumble of divans and rugs and lamps and glasses lying around. It gives off the unfortunate impression that someone neglected to clean up after the last party. Granyer looks nonplussed.

"Used much?"

"All the time," he says. "Go ahead and look around. You know why my movie studio is special? I can rotate and adjust the ceiling to get the light just right."

I look up and sure enough, the roof is composed of a dozen triangular leaves that resemble pieces of a pie. He explains to me that they can be opened separately or slid together to expose more or less of the sky and to track the sun. He can let in as much natural light as he wants. Conversely, the leaves can be slid shut to block out the sun or the occasional rain, depending on the weather and the scene being filmed.

Granyer admits he borrowed the design for his film studio from Thomas Edison's studio-in-the-round in New Jersey. In an adjacent building he's added a kitchen, a laundry, a tailor, and a sort of flophouse. When he's filming, he can take care of his crew right there and not have to waste time or money bringing anyone else in on his dealings.

A mural is painted on the underside of the adjustable ceiling in silver and black, red and white. It frankly depicts a raucous feast (or is it an orgy?) above a waterfall in the moonlight in some private, celestial garden with kimonos and bodies and trees and flowers and birds and starlight all entwined. The full moon and a raging river are both complicit. I want to lie down on one of the couches and spend a couple of hours dreaming on it, a pretty common feeling, I imagine.

Standing against the far wall are stacks of painted screens—a much more various collection of images—landscapes, sitting rooms, erotica, a couple of paintings that are clearly unfinished. The studio smells of fresh paint. His set painter will be there later, he says, I'll meet her some other time. Along another wall are racks of kimonos. Costumes. His is a movie studio writ small. Self-contained and self-sufficient.

"Looks like you have everything you need here. And some."

"In this line, one never has everything one needs. One can always use more of everything, especially money. Amateurs think you need taste and genius." Granyer laughs softly. "You know what real creativity is? Finding the wherewithal. Those who can do that, and I can, are real geniuses!"

As I feel the change in my pocket, I concede him the point.

"One of these days I'll let you visit the set when we're shooting. It's time to bring you along."

As we're about to head out, the door opens and a slender Asian woman peers in. "It is only I, Shoko," says Granyer. "Come in, my dear, come in."

"Good morning, Mr. Granyer!"

"Shoko, this is my chauffeur, Jean-Yves. And, Johnny, this is the artist responsible for painting my movie sets."

"Nice to meet you."

"You, too. These are your paintings?"

"Yes."

"They're fabulous. Especially the mural on the ceiling."

"Thank you."

"Truly."

"You're kind. But don't let me hold you up. I've work to do. If you stay, I might be tempted to add your likeness to one of my paintings. You want me to?"

"No, no, no. No portraits, Shoko. Ideal likenesses only."

"Not to worry, Mr. Granyer. I was only kidding. But you run along now. I'm busy, busy, busy. And please leave the door open when you head out. I need fresh air to work."

We cross the dusty ground outside the studio and pass a dented black Ford parked outside that I assume is Shoko's. After we're seated in the Hudson, I ask Granyer how he came to hire her.

"She's lovely, isn't she? This town is full of talent. It's a buyer's market. People respond in droves to every little ad in the *Times*. She's been working for me for about a year now. Not only does Shoko paint exquisitely, she's one of my more daring actresses."

"Her paintings are certainly daring."

"Believe me, so is her acting."

It's lunchtime when we return to Granyer's place, and he invites me in. "Let's see what's cooking, shall we?" As far as I can tell, the chef is up to no good. The house is filled with greasy steam. It smells more like rotting than cooking. The last time I smelled something like this was when I happened to pass a tannery in New York's meat packing district.

We sit down for lunch and Granyer looks positively gleeful. I, on the other hand, am afraid I'm awaiting my last meal and summary execution. Granyer offers me the usual, a drink that's clear and hot and strong.

"Saké?"

"Why not."

The seconds tick by and Granyer stops looking anticipatory and starts looking peevish. None too soon, the cook pushes through the swinging door from the kitchen bearing another enormous, steaming fish on a silver platter.

"Hmm," I say, "well, well," hoping against hope that it will taste better than it smells. Stalling for time, I swig some saké and make with the small talk.

"So, what kind of fish is this?"

"It's carp."

"Hmm." My fork wavers. It's gray and kind of slimy looking. It doesn't even seem completely cooked. "So," I ask, still stalling for time, "where do carp come from?"

"Stagnant waters," grunts Granyer with his mouth full, shoveling in a forkful of the wretched stuff. "How's the saké?"

"Just fine!" Fortunately for me, the saké is perfectly drinkable.

"It's from Japan. A certain amount gets smuggled into the country simply labeled as 'vinegar.' I prefer to consume it before it comes to that, of course. For the initiated, saké is one of life's little necessities."

"It warms you up."

"It was Oscar Wilde, wasn't it, who said that if he had life's luxuries, he could do without the necessities?"

"I think it was."

"Funny line. But 999 times out of 1,000, it works the other way around. The first to fall by the wayside is the unnecessary."

"Understandably."

"Take the White Russians in Shanghai. They fled the Bolsheviks with only what they could carry. They survive as outcasts in China, selling family heirlooms, their amber and jewelry and furs, until finally they're threadbare and penniless, dying to work at something.

The British, French, Americans, Japanese, and Chinese won't let them in economically or socially. It's a completely closed off city in all five directions. These Russians were once aristocrats and many end up having to work as pack animals and really the lowest of prostitutes. Most become opium addicts."

"Sounds awful."

"Terrible when the tables turn. How do you like the fish?"

"Mmm. Unusual."

"You know why I've managed to make a go of film-making? I know how to control costs, which is one of the main stumbling blocks to piecing together a movie—one of these cinematic *machines infernales.*"

"Hm."

"I use other people's money and other people's ideas. And what I hope to create is what all producers aim for—a perpetual-profit machine."

"Where do you show your movies?"

"I have a small theater in Little Tokio where I screen my films. I have a niche market, the city's Asian immigrants—the Chinese and Japanese. They're hungry for stories of the Far East, images of home, and saké."

All the while, the carp is giving us the fish face, eyes glazed over, as if reprimanding us for doing him in. I can practically hear his dying words: "Go ahead and taste me and admit it. You made a mistake. You caught the wrong guy."

CHAPTER 23

CADDYING ONE LATE AFTERNOON

"LeFouet," Granyer announces one morning, "I've a golf game this afternoon and I need a caddie. Ever done any caddying?"

"Never. What's a caddie do?"

"As my caddie you'll carry my clubs and refrain from talking when I address the ball."

"You're going to talk to your ball?"

"No! I'm saying I don't want you talking when I'm preparing to hit the ball!"

"You want me to be quiet."

"Exactly. And for your information, we may do some talking to our balls, but we usually wait until after we hit them. For instance, you may hear people yell strange things at their ball in flight, like 'Get up there, you bitch!' Golfers tend to improvise. Not phrases to repeat off the course. And this is especially important, I'll want you to watch my ball and help me find it, in case I foozle it."

"Do caddies make more than chauffeurs?"

"In your case, no. Caddies and chauffeurs earn the same generous salary. However, if I don't lose any balls and I win, I'll give you a big tip at the end of the round."

"How long will this take?"

"Eighteen holes usually takes four or five hours."

"What happened to your old caddie, Lester the Blister?"

"I got tired of his antics."

"For example?"

"Like rattling the clubs when I was trying to concentrate. Not paying attention to where my ball went. Misreading my line."

"Well, I like to read. I'll give it a go."

Granyer has a mid-afternoon tee time, and the sun is beginning its downward arc when I ease the Hudson up to the golf club. The place looks pretty swanky. His opponent is sitting under an umbrella on the porch nursing something with ice in it. Stuart Blanchard, Granyer's accountant, is the picture of dissolute gentility. Granyer introduces me as his driver and Blanchie makes a lame joke asking him how far he can tee off with me. Granyer says if I don't do a decent job caddying, he'll get plenty teed off, indeed. Hahaha. This isn't like Granyer, who's usually in no great hurry to speak. He's trying to make this guy comfortable, I guess. One bad joke deserves another. I give a little snort to let them know that I can recognize an attempt at humor when I hear it, and I leave it at that. Today my goal is to watch and learn. Granyer excuses himself and heads into the clubhouse.

As I go to sit down, his friend says: "Caddies aren't allowed on the verandah. Be a good fellow. Wait for us around the corner. You'll find the other caddies there." I'm used to waiting in the car for Granyer but I don't like this guy's attitude. I hope Granyer cleans his clock.

Turning the corner, I find a stooped old man who seems to be propping himself up on a set of clubs. Could he be the other caddie? I put Granyer's clubs down a few paces off and nod to him. I have no idea what the protocol around here is. He nods ever so slightly and then goes back to sleeping standing up. A few minutes later, I hear Blanchard's name announced. "The Blanchard party of two, on the first tee..." Granyer and his friend come hurrying up to us. Blanchard looks downright lopsided, as if he's spent his whole life lifting weights with one arm. Or playing too much golf.

"Oh, there you are," Granyer says to me, impatiently. "Let's not waste time now. We're up on the first tee." As if it were my idea to wander off. These guys are getting on my nerves. The old fellow and I shoulder the clubs. I'm wondering if there's some way for Granyer and his friend both to lose this match. After hitting his first shot, Blanchard pulls out a hipflask and takes a nip.

Caddying is tougher than it sounds. The tendency toward greater randomness is a constant problem. Clubs, when not handled just so, like to dump themselves all over the place, which makes a helluva racket. And they're surprisingly heavy. I get the hang of it eventually and I learn some new words, especially for bad shots—shanked, duckhooked, hoseled, skulled. I hear these expressions a lot. As the afternoon wears on, I begin to wonder if it should be called golf at all. Maybe this game should be called drinking and swearing. It's a bad sign that there's such a rich vocabulary for lousy shots.

To rankle his adversary, Granyer trots out some choice French golf expressions that he learned playing in the French concession in Shanghai. When Blanchard hits his ball forty yards over one of the greens, Granyer says to me pretending to be impressed, "*Il a bouffé du lion aujourd'hui!*" "What's that supposed to mean?" Blanchard wants to know. "I was just saying that you must have eaten lion today, Blanchie." When Blanchard dumps his ball in the middle of a pond, Granyer says in a mock whisper "*J'ai entendu une petite éclaboussure.*" "Now what?" Blanchie squawks. "I simply said that I thought I heard a tiny little splash..."

After he himself hits a string of terrible shots, Granyer practically moans, "*C'est la Berezina,*" referring to Napoleon's debacle fleeing Russia in winter. According to the metaphor, every time you think you might make it out alive, some Cossack gallops by and picks off another of your men. It's handy for describing a round of golf that's nothing but carnage, one casualty after another.

Late in the round, toward twilight, I understand why Granyer wants me on his bag. The two golfers are having trouble seeing where they've hit their balls. Granyer tells me quietly to keep an eye out for his ball. And that I should watch his friend like a hawk. He doesn't trust him and he wants to make sure he doesn't get away with any dirty play. They have a $100 bet riding on the outcome and he's hoping his opponent is going to lose a ball and he'll emerge triumphant. Losing a ball costs you a stroke penalty, I'm told. And, Granyer says, under no circumstances am I to find his friend's lost ball. Unless he tells me to. This is where I earn my keep.

Night is creeping up on us and I can see fine.

We get to the fateful 18th hole, the match all square, and sure enough, Blanchard hooks his ball off the tee. I see it disappear into the left rough between two trees. He has no idea where it's gone and he starts swearing like a tripe wife. In plus fours. Very hard on the ears.

Granyer looks at me steadily, giving me the eye, and pretends that he's going to do all he can to help.

"I'm sure you'll find it, Blanchie. We'll all just have a little look around. I'm sure it'll turn up."

The lopsided guy keeps ranting. "Where'd that damn ball go?" he shouts at his elderly caddie.

"We'll find it, if it's to be found…" the caddie begins.

"Dammit! How are we supposed to find our balls? It's the God-damn-middle-of-the-night!"

"You're playing a Spalding 2, no?" asks Granyer, knowing full well that's the ball the guy's chasing.

"Of course I am, God damn it. My initials are on the damn thing."

We march forth into the darkness and I lead my boss to his ball, while Blanchie spirals around in circles like a titanic drunk getting washed down a drain. Which, at this point in the round, he is. He's been drinking all afternoon and evening. I realize he's not so much lopsided as completely unbalanced.

Suddenly he pipes up, "Found it!" He's standing over on the right side of the fairway with a ball at his feet and I know he hasn't found his ball because I saw it clearly go sharp left into the rough. But the lopsided guy wastes no time and he hits his next shot straight and the ball trickles on to the front of the green. That one will be easy to find. Granyer makes a par, but Blanchie miraculously holes his long putt for a birdie and wins the match. He does a lot of gloating.

Granyer invites me to join them for a drink in the clubhouse. We don't even have to repair to a speakeasy. As we slake our thirst, Granyer asks to see his adversary's ball. Blanchard produces a Spalding with his initials on it.

"This is a Spalding 3, Blanchie. I thought you said you were playing a 2."

"It was pitch dark out there. I could barely see a thing on the back nine. I was playing this ball, that's all I know. If it's a 3, I was playing a 3."

"All right, Blanchie. If that's your story. But if I come back here tomorrow when it's light and I find a Spalding 2 with your initials on it, I'm going to claim the win and the $100. Until then, no money's changing hands."

"You're such a prick."

"Face it. 2's don't turn into 3's."

"Fuck you."

"You can come along, Blanchie, in case you think I'm going to manufacture a Spalding 2 with your initials on it."

"Fuck that. If you're really going to pull this kind of bullshit, take my caddie along. His eyesight's pretty good during the day. He'll keep you honest."

"I've got a better idea. You come with me. If we find a Spalding 2 with your initials on it on the 18th hole, you can play it from where it lies and if you still make a birdie, you win. Make a par, we tie. Make a bogey, I win. Can't be more sporting than that."

"And if you don't find a ball, which you won't, because it doesn't exist, you pay me double for calling me a cheater."

"And if I do find your ball, then you are a cheater, and you pay me quadruple for losing and cheating and bitching. Cheers, then, Blanchie. This round's on me."

"Okay. You're on. But the next round's on you, too, Chilblain. You lost. And tomorrow you'll owe me two C-notes. I'll take a Manhattan."

CHAPTER 24

MORNING AFTER GOLF

The morning after Blanchie loses his ball on the 18th hole, Granyer knocks on my door before dawn and a little bleary-eyed we head back out to the golf course. He wants to get there before anyone has a chance to find Blanchie's ball and spoil his coup.

En route, we pick up a disheveled, tight-lipped Stuart Blanchard. We load him and his clubs in and I put the pedal to the metal. Granyer is in a jovial mood. Blanchie looks like he'd like to clip him with one of his long irons. When we pull into the club's parking lot, Granyer suggests that Blanchard bring his clubs with him.

"Are you kidding? These are just for show."

"Suit yourself. It's going to be a bit of a hike back, though."

We hustle through the clubhouse, telling the sleepy guy behind the counter that we lost a club on the 18th hole and would like to retrieve it. He recognizes the two combatants as members and waves us through like a solemn, somnolent traffic cop.

Granyer and I spread out, with him walking up the left side of the fairway and me hugging the right, acting as if we have no definite idea about where the ball might be, just making a guess where Blanchie's tee shot might have landed. I've described to Granyer in detail where I saw the ball headed. He wants to do the honors of proving his friend is a liar and a cheat. He's convinced it will be hugely entertaining.

The sun has come up but it's still a bit chilly. The grass is wet with dew. Granyer hopes he will find the ball nestled at the base of a tree with no shot at all. The cheat will be stymied and that will be that. Match over. Of course, it wouldn't be over absolutely. He could chip out on to the fairway and then hole his approach shot. He could make a birdie like that. But it's exceedingly unlikely. Or he could make par and they would tie.

There's something weird about the 18th hole, though, and it's more than a little disconcerting. Small footprints in the dew, roaming all over. One of the grounds keepers might have been up and about before we got there.

Granyer looks and looks and after a while he starts getting agitated, whacking at clumps of grass with his club. Blanchie on the other hand starts to relax and then he goes back to being a smart aleck, telling Granyer that not only does he owe him $200, but he owes him an apology. I try to come to Granyer's rescue, looking among the trees where I saw the ball disappear. There's no ball there. I dread what the boss is going to say to me after we drop Blanchie back home.

Finally, we give up the hunt and stalk back to the car. Granyer is livid. His face is the color of lutefisk. Blanchie climbs in front next to me, having no interest in sitting next to Granyer.

As I turn out of the driveway of the club, I see a young Asian boy standing against a fence. He has a newspaper in front of him with a dozen golf balls on display. I pull up and stop.

"How much are the balls, sonny?"

"Five cents."

"That's a pretty good deal. Tell me, did you find any Spaldings this morning?"

He looks down at the balls on the ground and picks up three and brings them over to the car. One of them is a Spalding 2 and it has the initials SB stamped on it.

Blanchie howls. "I lost two balls yesterday. He could have found that anywhere."

"Where'd you find these, son?"

"On 18. People always lose ball on 18 after dark."

"Are you sure?"

"Yes." He smiles. "They hard to find at night. Easy to find in the morning."

"I've played this course hundreds of times. I've lost my ball on 18 before. He just found a ball from some other round."

"That's bullshit, Blanchie, and you know it."

"I don't know anything. Besides, say it was my ball. He moved it. How am I supposed to finish the hole?"

"Do you know where you found this ball, young fellow?"

"No. They all look alike. White."

"All right, Blanchie. Here's my offer—you get to replay 18 and if you get a birdie, you win, a par, we tie, and a bogie, I win. What do you say?"

He thinks about it for a few seconds and then to my great surprise, he agrees. So I turn the car around and we walk in silence back to the par-four 18th tee box, and this time Blanchie's carrying his clubs. He's a good golfer but inconsistent. To boot, it's still early in the morning, he's got an excruciating hangover, and we've already put him through a lot of rigmarole. The odds are tilting decidedly in Granyer's favor.

Blanchie takes his time, does a fair amount of stretching and swinging of his driver. Finally he tees up the #2 Spalding, waggles his club a few more times for good measure, and takes a rip. His ball goes crashing into the trees on the left of the fairway and this time we all get a good look where it's gone.

As he stomps off after his ball, he lets loose a string of pained and colorful epithets. It doesn't take long to locate his ball, though, and sure enough it's completely blocked by the trunk of a big oak tree.

From the tenor of his yelling, you might have thought he was some wounded Saxon opera singer.

Faced with no other choices, Blanchie plays his next shot left-handed using a putter and manages to jam it back onto the edge of the fairway. To win the match with a birdie, he would have to hole this next shot from 200 yards away.

And then he does something magical. He hits a magnificent shot that flies straight for the pin and actually hits it, but it caroms off and rolls about ten feet below the hole. He almost pulled off the impossible. When we get to the green, we can see the trail left by his ball in what's left of the morning dew.

"Make this and we're all square, Blanchie."

He pulls out his putter. He looks at the line from below the hole. He looks at the line from above the hole. He gets set to putt. He steadies himself. But then he freezes, as if he's turned to marble.

Years go by.

Finally he pulls his club back and takes a stab at it. The ball rolls to a halt a foot short of the hole.

He bellows as if he's just been speared.

Matter-of-factly my boss says: "Never up, never in, Blanchie. Never up, never in."

Blanchard grabs his ball and tosses it in the air as if he's going to fungo it to the other side of the solar system. He obviously thinks he's Babe Ruth. Granyer and I turn away to try to protect ourselves. He takes a tremendous cut at his ball in mid-air, but he whiffs, and the ball plops harmlessly, quietly at his feet.

We can hear the gnashing of teeth.

"I thought you were playing statue-maker back there, Blanchie." Granyer can't help rubbing it in.

The lopsided golfer doesn't say anything more, not that he's said much up till now, except the same four-letter words. Instead he roars something unintelligible and flings his putter in the air. It flies remarkably high, returns to earth, glances off his head, and knocks him out cold. He's lucky he didn't kill himself. That's what the doctor at the hospital tells us, anyway. What a nightmare.

My dear neighbor, Aunt Simone, was a large woman

and not at all athletic. A consummate intellectual. She played golf in her youth, though, and one day she made a hole-in-one. Finding it a perfectly delightful moment to leave golf and golfing to those who would have it, she put down her clubs and never played again.

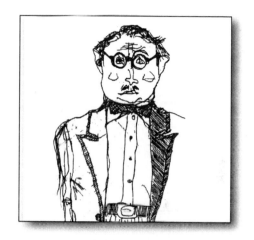

PART THREE
LITTLE TOKIO

Major Counsellor Kinto poked his head in.
"Excuse me," he said. "Would our little Murasaki be in
attendance by any chance?"
"I cannot see the likes of Genji here, so how could she
be present?" I replied.
—*The Diary of the Lady Murasaki* (11th century A.D.)

CHAPTER 25

MY STORY ADVANCES IMMEASURABLY

The next day Granyer tips me $20 for my fine caddying and tells me he has a new assignment for me. He directs me to a bookshop in Little Tokio, The Dragon and The Lotus, with instructions to pick up some books and deliver them to a dozen actors and actresses.

The Dragon and The Lotus is a small shop with books piled high in the windows and two blackboards on either side of the front door. The blackboards are filled with Chinese characters. Next to it is a florist. On the other side is a laundry belching steam, which makes me wonder if that's where they keep their dragon. Inside the front door is a heavy curtain that I push through. It's soothingly dark inside, a welcome break for my eyes from the L.A. sun. I take off my sunglasses and find a shop crammed with display tables and full bookshelves. It smells of incense. Dust motes are floating in the air.

The sunlight that would come through a front window is screened by flowers in flowerpots. I can't identify them, but they add a clean, happy, subtle fragrance to the place. What could be better than the smell of incense and flowers and books?

Behind the counter is a young Asian woman with her hair cut in a bob. She has a bright, intelligent expression on her face. There's a book open in front of her, but she isn't reading. She's cutting a page with what looks like a light-green jade letter opener. She gives me an open, inquiring look, holding the letter opener still for moment. Then she deftly cuts free two pages in her book. She sees I'm watching what she's doing and smiles.

"French publishers make you cut the pages yourself. You have to free them up one by one."

"Aha."

"It must save them money not cutting the pages themselves."

"Interesting."

"Or maybe they figure this way you have to buy the book to read it."

"It would make it hard to read for free in a bookshop."

"It would indeed. The good thing is I never lose my page. I always know where I left off." She sounds vaguely French.

"Unless you cut all the pages at once. I would imagine some people are like that. Overly efficient."

"I would never do that," she says. "I let the book divulge its secrets as it's meant to. From beginning to end. I don't believe in peeking at the end."

"I don't either. Though, I admit, I have to fight the

urge sometimes."

"Of course you do, when a book's really good."

"You know what I do sometimes? I cover the last page with my hand so I don't accidentally see anything that's meant to come later."

"I hope you won't think I'm jumping ahead if I ask what I can do for you?"

I tell her I'm there to pick up an order for Mr. Granyer and she nods quickly several times. She recognizes him, is expecting him, in fact. His books arrived yesterday afternoon from Shanghai.

"And you are, Mr...?" she trails off.

"*Monsieur*," I reply.

She gives me a charming smile and says, "*Monsieur, alors...?*"

"LeFouet."

"*Ah, oui, bon, M. LeFouet. Un instant.*"

She turns and goes to get the books. Quick, light steps take her behind a folding three-panel screen that portrays women in kimonos painting and writing. The painting is done in black ink with some red highlights and the frame is black and silver lacquer. The frame itself is elaborately carved, but it's too far away for me to make out distinctly. It looks like an antique. Nothing like the paintings in Granyer's studio.

As the bookseller doesn't return at once, I scan the bookshelves and start browsing. The books are almost all hard covers in Chinese. Or is it Japanese?

One small shelf in a far corner has a few books in English. I think to myself, maybe they'll have some rare find they don't care about because it's in English. Or they don't recognize, because it's lost its luster. Maybe they'll have some nice old books with leather covers like the ones my Aunt Simone had, Pepys or Matthew Arnold or Dickens. But, alas, no such luck. All they have are some dog-eared paperbacks. Forgettable stuff. And dust. This shop could use an experienced book duster.

I hear a door slide shut. Someone is returning and I smell a slight hint of perfume wafting my way. The girl with the bright expression reappears from the recesses of the shop. She's carrying a stack of books that's threatening to spill.

She just manages to deposit the books on the counter and proceeds to wrap each of them in light green paper, almost as if she were practicing origami. I have to smile. It's not perfume I smelled. It's Juicy Fruit gum. She positions each book diagonally on a sheet of paper and then folds the paper neatly several times before securing it with a single piece of tape. I watch and admire. Then she writes me up a bill.

"Twelve copies of *The Tale of Genji*. Mr. Granyer is a good customer. When he gets interested in a book, he doesn't buy just one copy. He buys a dozen."

"Maybe I should read it, if he thinks it's so interesting. Are these *en chinois?*"

"*Non.* They're not in Chinese."

"That's lucky. I wouldn't understand the first character..."

"If anything, they would be written in Medieval Japanese."

"*Oh, là!* Better yet."

"*Genji* is one of the world's first novels. Maybe the

137

first. It was written by a Japanese woman a thousand years ago. And it's a thousand pages long. This is in English, though. You could read it. You can read, can't you?"

"*Ça, alors!* That would be quite an undertaking!"

"Where did you learn French?"

"*Au Canada, mademoiselle. Et vous?*"

"*Moi?* Shanghai. I grew up in the French quarter in Shanghai. My mother is French."

"Have you read *The Tale of Genji?*"

"No. I wish I had the time to consecrate to it."

"I wish I had more time, too. What do I owe you?"

"Mr. Granyer has an account with us."

I pull out a check. "He told me to settle his account for him."

The young woman pulls out a ledger and quickly scans it. "In that case, $131 will settle our affairs. Between you and me, he's a good customer but very hard on books."

Granyer gave me the signed check this morning. I just fill in the amount and gather up the stack of books. After glancing at the check, she looks back up at me and smiles.

"*Alors, merci,*" I say. "*Et à la prochaine fois.*" She's awfully cute. I hope there is a next time.

"*Au revoir!*"

"*Au revoir!*"

She holds the curtain open for me and then the door. The heat outside is intense. I pile the books next to me in the Hudson. I reread the list of addresses Granyer gave me and plot my route. All of the addresses belong to actors and actresses living in Beverly Hills, stars Granyer hopes will consider playing roles in his next production, an adaptation of *The Tale of Genji*. It takes me a couple hours to deliver the load of them. Granyer is generally in the business of producing some pretty low-budget talkies, but he keeps probing, seeing if he can't interest a big name to act in one of his films. Maybe they will and he'll parlay it into a smash hit and a fortune. If he makes enough money, maybe it won't matter that his breath stinks and his teeth look like burnt corn on the cob. Then who knows what he'll set his sights on? Maybe he'll run for governor of California.

When I get back to the office, I still have a copy left, which I proffer Granyer.

"One extra…"

"Lay it on the table there. Such a famous book—and so fat—there's got to be a lot of great stuff in there. Enough material to make ten films. And it's all up for grabs. No copyright in force. No author to wine and dine. No royalties to pay."

"Do you mind if I borrow it? I'd like to read it."

"Read it? Are you kidding? You've got more important things to do than read. I've got people for that. We're in the business of making moving pictures."

"Words can be moving."

"You want moving words? That's what the stock ticker is for!" He picks up the book, puts it in his desk drawer, and actually locks it up. "Look, maybe you're right. Maybe you can work for me as a reader. I'll think about it but not now. We've got to pick them up and lay them down, Johnny. I've a meeting in 30 minutes." He snatches his coat off the back of a chair and wheels toward the door. I'll talk to him about it another time, at a quieter moment. I'd be good at it. I've read enough books to know a good story when I see it.

CHAPTER 26

LULU

You might wonder if I've met other stars in Hollywood than the faintly twinkling ones Granyer is sweet talking. Only in my dreams. Still, one day I pass a little hole-in-the-wall bookstore called Lulu's and decide to veer inside. Two older German men are talking with an elegant, younger dark-haired woman. They are speaking German and strangely I feel as if I understand what they are saying, even though normally all I know how to say is *Gesundheit*.

The men are famous, the playwright, Bertolt Brecht, and the filmmaker, Fritz Lang. Louise Brooks, the American silent film siren, is the bookstore's proprietor. A few years previous, she starred in the film "Pandora's Box," playing a *femme fatale* named Lulu. I recognize her right away.

I hear her say she's given up acting entirely to put her

energy into reading and writing film criticism. She's happy her bookstore is a haven for expatriate artists. From what I gather, Lang is trying to persuade her to take up acting again.

"I'm terribly busy at the moment, writing a theoretical critique of your film 'M,' Fritz, which I continue to find fascinating."

"I'm flattered but you're breaking my heart."

"There is no shortage of starlets in this town," she replies. "Coming to Hollywood has something fatal about it. It's like a cliff for the lovely stream that discovers too late it's a waterfall."

"Or babbling brooks."

"Bertolt, don't be silly."

"A real *nightmerikanisch*, this Hollywood," says Brecht, making a little joke.

"Maybe I will write something for you, Fritz, if the inspiration strikes me," she says.

"I would be delighted to read anything you write for me, Louise, you know that. Then he asks her, more seriously: "Why do you stay in Los Angeles, since you're no longer interested in film acting?"

"Most of what I did wasn't acting. It was posing."

"New York might suit you better. You could act in the theatre."

"I'm thinking about it, but I have friends here and my bookstore."

"Women with big books," says Brecht. "*Wunderbar!*"

"Ah, you! Stop! Anyway, I don't have the courage to uproot again. Here I have an endless stream of movies to watch and critique. Most don't deserve a second thought, but yours, Fritz, are different. They're works of art."

"Why did you come to Hollywood, Herr Lang," I ask, "if you have such misgivings about it?"

"Hitler asked me to become the Nazi Party's official filmmaker."

"Oh."

"I went straight home and packed. I left Germany the next day!"

Brecht smiles, unsmiling. "I was not welcome at all."

"We made the right decision."

"The sun's pleasant here."

"But everyday?"

"It's like vacationing in Spain."

"I prefer it here inside with Louise."

"You might want to audition a Japanese bookseller I know. She looks a little like Miss Brooks."

"She loves books and is quite beautiful, is that what you're saying?" asks Lang.

"Yes."

The door to the bookstore bangs open and who come in but the German novelist, Thomas Mann, and the German composer, Arnold Schoenberg. They're talking animatedly.

"I've spent the entire week at Venice Beach. It's a sweeping, golden expanse and the ocean is immense. It's always playing itself. I dip my feet in the water and feel as if I'm cooling my toes on the hem of some infinite indigo kimono."

"I'm glad you've come in out of the sun, Thomas," says Louise. "You've overdone it this time. You look horrific! Like hot pastrami!"

"I should have been an ancient Egyptian. I worship the sun."

"We had pastrami for lunch at Canter's the other day," Schoenberg chimes in. "It was fine. Delicious rye bread and the pickles were marvelous. We saw several movie stars there, but I can't for the life of me remember whom."

"I've been giving this some thought," says Mann. "What makes movie stars qualitatively different beings? I think it's that they're a constellation of all their roles and they're adorned and overlaid by all those bright lights. In one lifetime, they are reincarnated repeatedly before our eyes. When we happen to see them 'in real life,' they look ordinary but they come trailing clouds of their many previous existences. They remind me of Shiva, that blurred, many-limbed Hindu goddess of everything and its opposite."

"They don't seem like gods to me, Thomas," says Lang. "Delightful, certainly, but not otherworldly."

"Thomas has been picking my brain for a novel he's writing," says Schoenberg, "about a composer who sells his soul to the highest bidder."

"The devil is always the highest bidder," says Mann, "and everyone has his price. There was a squall yesterday afternoon at the beach and a full rainbow. I thought, 'That's it. We're not just matter. But we're clearly not just spirit, either. We're both. We're like the rainbow on the waterfall.'"

"That's what I resented about acting. Being hired for my body. A body that none of my producers seemed to understand I wanted to keep clad. The filmmakers wanted to make me beautiful, but beautiful like a body of water. It was so limited. How much acting does it take to run naked over the hills? I might as well have been a clown getting shot out of a cannon."

"I would happily pay to see you do that," says Brecht. "Even in a clown suit."

"Well," says Schoenberg, "if you've really given up acting for good, I'm going to give up composing. Thomas may like the sun and the heat, but it sucks the life out of me. It's giving me brain fever. I'm as dry as a mummy. This morning I looked at a score I'm writing and I couldn't tell whether I had my notebook right side up or upside down. I might as well have been trying to read Chinese. Besides, it's terribly difficult to raise my music to the level of the everyday—the clash of car horns in a city of traffic jams."

"You need a cold drink and so do I," Mann says. "I know of a speakeasy that makes the most refreshing drinks. It's splendid and dark. Just around the corner."

"We were there yesterday."

"Exactly. And in two minutes, happily, we'll be there today."

"Adorno is already there. He's expecting us."

As they leave, Lang turns to me and says: "Your friend looks a little like Louise?"

"She has something of her. I hope you don't find me impertinent saying so."

Louise Brooks just smiles and raises the fingers of her right hand, which were resting on a big book on the counter.

"But I'm prejudiced," I continue.

"Well, I'd like to meet her. Please give her my number and tell her to give me a call."

"Gladly."

"What's her name?"

"I must admit, I really must ask." They both laugh.

"Where's she from? Or don't you know that either?"

"No, I know that. She's from Shanghai."

"Accordion to whom?"

When I hear that, I get a little dizzy and hear myself saying: "Accordion to the song of the sing-song girl."

Then I throw in a few witty German asides and I even find myself saying *"Uberfooper"* and *"Donner"* and *"Blitzen."* Lang raises an eyebrow quizzically. He takes off his monocle and polishes it. Then Louise Brooks opens her mouth and he places the monocle on her tongue as if they are performing communion at a Catholic mass. We all raise brimming glasses of red wine (I have no idea where they came from), and toast each other, and I take several sizable gulps, suddenly overpowered with thirst.

We laugh and laugh until the actress raps the counter lightly, as if calling an end to this nonsense. She turns and practically floats over to the door of her bookstore and opens it wide. I hear the lapping of waves and smell creosote. The water in the harbor is sparkling and a black Chinese junk is anchored there and people are being tossed overboard and sinking like stones.

"I won't take 'No' for an answer, Louise. We'll talk again soon, yes?"

"Soon, Fritz. Shall we say 1941?"

Out of nowhere I feel The Dragon and The Lotus bookseller gently pressing up to me. She's smiling, wearing an emerald green gown. It's an embroidered silk kimono. It makes a crinkling sound that is almost musical. A dizzying, thrumming, drumming sound. I wake up with a sneeze as Vince is preparing to settle in for a long, comfortable nap draped across the top of my head.

CHAPTER 27

A DAYTIME RUN

It seems like I've been working for Granyer for eons when one day his junk comes in. It's February 1932. The phone rings and I pick up the party line as Granyer gets on. Even after a raspy voice asks for him and Granyer answers, I don't hang up.

"Granyer?"

"Speaking."

"That fruitcake you ordered is going to be delivered today in San Pedro. The fruit's a little undercooked, but you'll like it."

"I better."

"You will. It's delicious."

"The Department will hear from me if I don't like it, I hope you understand."

"I'd mosey on down there if I was you," is all the voice says, and then the line goes dead. I wait for Granyer to hang up before I do. Sure enough, he sends for me a couple minutes later.

"Bring the Hudson around by the garage, Johnny. We're going to put a boat haul on it. My yacht's arrived from Shanghai. It's waiting for us in San Pedro." For once he wants me to drive during the day. We go down to the marina and he signs all the necessary paperwork to take possession of a huge, handsome sailboat. A rail-thin, impassive Irish sailor is the one who's delivered it from China.

"How was the trip? Did she give you any trouble?"

"Not a bit," he says with a heavy Irish brogue. "A wee bumpy. A mite noisy. Otherwise, it was clear sailing. All the goods have dried out quite nicely. You'll see."

"Splendid."

"The port authorities like your boat."

"I'm glad. What did we say... $500? Here, take this, something extra for your trouble."

The sailor takes the cash, nods in our direction, and slowly walks away. One of the marina hands helps us winch the boat onto the boat haul. It actually dwarfs the Hudson. We look like a colossal escargot out for a Sunday drive. I start maneuvering it through traffic, back to Granyer's mansion and have several close scrapes, first with some blind guy in a jalopy and then with a telephone pole as I'm trying to turn north on La Cienaga. I've misplaced my sunglasses, which isn't helping matters at all. I try squinting.

Granyer lets me hear it. Every other block he's yelling. The yacht almost topples us over climbing one curvy road but I right us just in time. I pull over to catch my breath and try to regain my composure.

I take it *doucement* after that, nice and slow.

After a few false starts and back-and-forth maneuvering, I back the sailboat in behind Granyer's place, the way he wants it, out of sight. He has room back there. It isn't that tight a squeeze and I manage finally. We're both ready to snap by the time I kill the engine.

"I could use a drink," I blurt.

"I'll say. Next time less drama, eh?"

"Of course. Next time I won't lose my shades." The Hudson needs a drink, too. The radiator is boiling over.

When the sun goes down, and the California darkness descends, Granyer puts in a call to some Chinese movers he knows. They lean a couple ladders up against the boat and start unloading it. Why I had so much trouble pulling the yacht is no longer a mystery. It's loaded to the gills. Out come fifty cases of "vinegar" and a bunch of other trunks and boxes. I was handling a storm surge at every turn.

As the cargo is all being hustled inside a storage shed, a wicker trunk starts making noise. I unlatch it and inside is the rattiest, smelliest little old Chinaman I've ever seen. He looks as if he's been boxed up for most of the last century. We try to lift him up out of the crate and set him on his feet but he falls on the ground, moaning and groaning. Very, very gingerly he unbends his arms and tries to straighten his legs.

The elderly Chinaman starts coughing and clearing his throat and hacking and hacking. And then he starts talking. One of Granyer's Chinese workers speaks to him in Chinese but says he can't understand the stowaway. They pick him up, and he winces as he tries limping, and then he just lies down on his back. He gives us all a long, hard stare.

"You are Granyer?" he finally asks. He sounds like a British aristocrat who never learned English.

"I am."

"The Department sends regards."

"I was expecting a younger man."

"Change of plans. We talk later. I practically dead."

Some of the goons start laughing at the guy's accent, but Granyer cuts them short. "Quit acting like imbeciles. Help him up and take him inside where he can lie down. And get him some water. Easy now, gentle with him. And run him a bath."

Two guys help him up and the old man slowly limps toward the house, Granyer following close behind. "Finish unloading and lock up. Make it snappy."

After we haul the last crate into the shed and stash the last steamer trunk, we padlock it and start to walk toward Granyer's house.

"Where you going?" one of the movers asks me.

"I was going to see if Granyer needed me for anything else."

"Boss is busy. You call it a night."

That's fine with me. As I head to my bungalow in the backyard, I pass the side of the house, glance in a curtain that's open a crack and see the elderly stowaway sipping a glass of water and waving off Granyer, shaking his head. I stay and watch for a second. Granyer seems to be pressing him about something. The old stowaway looks up and suddenly gets quite agitated. Then he looks down again, drinks more water, and waves his hand in front of his face. Not now, he's clearly saying.

The next morning the old guy comes out to the storage shed with Granyer. He looks haggard but cleaned up, a far cry from the first impression he made. In a quiet voice, he points out various items that he wants moved inside. Granyer hails his stevedores and they pick up the suitcases, trunks, and crates he specifies. Some they muscle up the back stairs and into the house. The rest they shove in a free closet in my bungalow, of all places.

CHAPTER 28

THE STOWAWAY'S STORY

Granyer and the old man climb in the back seat of the limo and I drive them around town and listen to their conversation.

"I was expecting a different visitor," says Granyer. "A Japanese chemist recommended by a friend in Shanghai. By the name of Akihiro Michinaga. A Jack-of-all-trades, I'm told."

"Akihiro can't come. Sorry. Shanghai is bad. Japanese bombing. Chinese fighting, killing Japanese who live in Shanghai. Akihiro is too afraid to come out of hiding. He give me his spot on boat. Dangerous for everyone there."

"Too bad."

"Very bad. Worse than very bad," says the old man. After a long pause, he goes on. "Akihiro is very good chemist but he cross the wrong people—the Green

Gang, the Chinese, the Japanese army. They all looking for him."

"Pity."

"I am chemist. We work together."

"Really?" Granyer asks, encouraged.

"Yes. Call me Joe. I help you. You make films? Akihiro and I run film lab in Shanghai. He my apprentice. I develop lots of movie film."

"The Department surprises me. I'll say that."

"He don't know Akihiro stay in Shanghai."

"He assured me only a few days ago."

"Where is Big Department?"

"In New York."

"I help you, Granyer, but I need lab. I have many interesting projects. I think a lot crossing the Pacific."

"We'll see. First things first, Joe."

"A lab is first. Lend me your driver so I can get things I need." The elderly Chinaman leans forward and taps me on the shoulder. "Who are you?"

"Jean-Yves. John."

"Okay, John. You call me Joe, too. If Mr. Granyer say yes, you drive and help me with lab?"

"You can borrow Johnny. Just drop me at my place first."

After I deposit Granyer, Joe climbs in the passenger seat and we make the rounds. We hit a hardware store, where we buy beakers and washbasins and fans. Joe pays cash, peeling the necessary off a wad he has. Next we visit a toy store and buy a chemistry set for budding chemists.

"These very good," Joe explains. "They have what we

need." Later Joe goes into a pharmacy and comes out with some other active ingredients.

"This won't all explode, by any chance, if I hit a pothole?"

"A what?"

"A bump in the road?"

"No worry. I know what I do."

Next we head to Little Tokio and look for a place to rent. A little old Japanese woman with a cane takes us to an empty store that's available. It's a low brick building among other two- and three-story brick buildings. It's off a busy street filled with grocery stores and restaurants and shops. The area is busy with people following *leur petit train-train*. The daily hurly-burly. It's in the same neighborhood as The Dragon and The Lotus.

The woman unlocks the door and flips on a light. It's spacious inside. Joe nods his head as he explores it. It has a big front room with tall windows high up on the wall facing the street, and we manage to pry one open. The ventilation could be okay. It has a bathroom in back. When she turns on the faucet it kind of hiccoughs and bangs before rusty water sloshes out but soon the water runs clear. There are two other rooms toward the back. One's a bedroom. The other has no windows at all but has a big sink and running water. Speaking in Japanese, Joe and the proprietor come to an understanding. Later, as we're driving back to Granyer's, I ask him about Shanghai.

"So many opium shops in Shanghai. Thousands. On every corner. Hard to avoid. I leave to break the habit."

"Hm."

"In a shack on a bridge over Shanghai River, Japanese army is killing people and torturing people. They torture my friend. Hold him upside down and fill him with water. Then they stomp on him. So bad. How he survive, I don't know."

"Is that what they call the 'Chinese Water Torture?'"

"It is Japanese invention. 'Japanese Water Treatment.'"

"Good time to get away, I'd say."

"I get drunk the night we sail, for courage. Practically fall off gangplank. Devils chase me. Onboard I sleep like dead. Only wake up in middle of ocean."

"That must have been a relief."

"Not much. The Irish skipper, he good man. But I... He put up with me. I go through withdrawal. Sleep a week. Then I drink saké. It help, except when I get seasick. Finally, the drug sickness stop. Then I just watch sea rise, sea fall, sea rise, sea fall, and think about nothing. And how to win Go. We play Go, many games. Long trip. One day, I have to get in rattan basket and skipper hide me with blankets. So stuffy! Port workers not very curious. So here I am—sore, sober, philosophic. Some story, eh?"

"Welcome to L.A., Joe."

"You know Charles Granyer well?"

"I've been driving for him for awhile."

"I tell you secret. He in bad business in Shanghai. British ban cathouses in British Shanghai. Granyer make lot of money in French sector, where they don't mind."

"Hm."

"His club also opium den. He put on shows, singing,

dancing, music. Big crowd. British, French, Japanese, even Chinese. Respectable businessmen, family men, spend evenings there with little sing-song girls, eat like pigs, get drunk, smoke their pipes. Granyer get rich."

"How do you know?"

"He pretty infamous. He don't remember me. No reason he should."

He holds out his hand and I go to shake it. He pulls it away. He isn't offering to shake hands. He wants to show me something. "You notice?" he says, holding out the blackened thumb and forefinger of his right hand. "Opium does that."

"Hm."

"When I kick habit on boat, these fingers help me. I smell these fingers. Take deep breath. One day I suck these fingers, all day, hoping."

"I'm glad you're feeling better."

"Me, too! I make Granyer an offer, develop dailies cheap. He save money. Good for me, too. Steady work."

"Excellent."

"You know what Chinese call movies? They have perfect, poetic name for them."

"What?"

"Electric shadows."

CHAPTER 29

LAB WORK

Over the next days, Joe and I motor around town, buying more lab equipment, various chemicals, and a vacuum cleaner.

Joe doesn't waste any time. He assembles a fairly simple lab for developing film in the windowless room. The chemicals reek. We hang black curtains over the door to keep light out. And we install dim red lights so we can see and work without exposing the film. With my night vision, I almost told him not to bother.

"You smart guy, John. You want, you become my assistant. I need one."

"I studied some chemistry in college." (I don't tell him what I know about the distillation process. He may feel like sharing his life story but that doesn't mean I have to spill my guts, too. I think of Aldo's lesson about maintaining a presidential demeanor.)

"Why spend all your time driving? It boring, right?"

"Fairly." (Speeding in the middle of the night with cops shooting at you is plenty exciting, but I don't see any reason to argue with him.) "A string of red lights is a bore, that's for sure."

"All right then. You be my assistant. Remember, light is enemy. And dust. Now we have vacuum cleaner. But no worry, that not all you do. I bring you along. I teach you things."

Once again, I find myself in mortal combat with dust. "I'll talk to Granyer."

Granyer okays the idea of my becoming Joe's lab assistant as long as I'm available to chauffeur (and carry his golf clubs) when he needs me. I come to like the Japanese chemist. The ill effects of his trip wear off and he's energetic, full of ideas, funny. And he's clearly happy to have escaped from Shanghai. As for me, movie stills pose fewer professional hazards than the stills I tended in Canada.

I hear Joe tell Granyer that he's going to branch out, that he doesn't want to just keep doing the same old thing. Granyer seems to get pretty frosty with him, but what's he going to do? He's no chemist. When Joe's not around, Granyer takes me aside and tells me to keep an eye on him. He doesn't like his attitude.

"He owes me for bankrolling that lab of his. I don't want him getting sidetracked. Or taking a powder."

"He seems happy developing film and working on his experiments. He can't exactly run off with his lab."

"Just let me know if he starts packing."

"I don't think you have anything to worry about. He likes his work. And to do it, he needs a lab. He's not going anywhere."

159

CHAPTER 30

A HAIKU
ABOUT THE PAST

One day, when I have a break from work in Joe's lab, I can't fight the temptation to return to The Dragon and The Lotus bookshop. It's not too long a walk. It's the late afternoon of another baking L.A. day and the streets are bustling. As I come to the bookstore, I see that the blackboards flanking the doorway have something written on them in chalk. The one on the right is filled with Chinese characters. At least they are, as best I can tell, knowing as much Chinese as you can gather ordering *moo goo gai pan* and green tea. The other blackboard has some sort of short poem in English that reads:

Which overcasts what?
Rain, memories, fog, or night?
Then, now, then, now, then?

I think about what can only be called the misuse of the word "overcasts." I've certainly heard of overcast skies, but overcasts as a verb? It sounds as if something is throwing down or throwing over something else. Which is okay, in that sense it works. Which overthrows what? Does the past overthrow the present or does the present overthrow the past?

My heart leaps when I push aside the entryway curtains, peer into the bookshop and see the young bookseller, dressed in a green, pink, and silver kimono, straightening one of the rows of books at the back of the crowded bookshop.

"*Hallo,*" I call. "*Bonjour.*"

She smiles in my direction, "*Bonjour, encore!*"

She comes over to the counter, wearing that bright, open, friendly expression. She's a regular symphony in silver. She's wearing silver eye shadow, silver fingernail polish, and silver lipstick.

"*Mais vous êtes toute en argent! Pourquoi?*"

"I'm going to a party later. Do you think I'll make a splash?"

"*Tout à fait. C'est frappant, comme effet.*"

"*Merci. Alors, qu'est-ce que je peux faire pour vous aujourd'hui?*"

"*Ah, oui, ah, oui.* I'd like to buy a copy of *The Tale of Genji,* if you have one. For myself."

"We may have a copy. Let me check the shelves…"

She goes over to one of the walls and runs a silver fingertip down a long line of books, as if her eyesight is a little off, as if maybe she's a little far-sighted. She bends backwards slightly and the kimono tightens around her.

It's almost as if she wants me to see what a beautiful figure she has. She is beautiful, whether she's showing off or simply looking to find the book for me. She has a genuineness that puts the lie to the idea that she's being coy. She takes her time, leaning, looking, but finally she swings back toward me and gives me what the French call a *moue*, pursing her lips as if she's a bit thoughtful and a bit apologetic. "No *Genji* here."

She raises a finger. "Let me look in one more place. We do have some rare books. We might have a copy there. She goes to a far corner of the shop and moments later, beaming, returns with a big book in hand. "You're in luck. This is quite old, a bilingual edition of *The Tale of Genji*—English and Japanese. It's expensive—ten dollars—but a real treasure," she says, giving me a questioning, encouraging smile. "Do you want it?"

Ten dollars is a fortune to pay for a book, but it is certainly a huge book and in both languages. I would be getting two books for the price of one. And it has a beautiful leather cover that will shine later when I apply a little oil and give it a good polishing.

I take it from her and carefully open it. "This is quite a book. The Japanese is striking, even if I can't make head or tail of it."

"That's what the English is for."

"I'll take it."

As I dig in my pocket for my wallet, I try more or less discreetly to drink in the presence of this marvelous creature. She's pale, probably from spending her days indoors. She has short dark straight bangs, long eyelashes, and eyes filled with happy enthusiasm. She's fetching. Fetching me, anyway.

"I'm excited to start this," I venture. "Maybe you could 'consecrate' some of your time to reading *Genji* yourself. We could compare notes. I'm going to need help understanding it."

"Oh, I couldn't possibly. I'm reading stacks of other writers at the moment."

However, she surprises me by not being in a hurry to end our conversation. She wants to talk about *Genji* herself. "From what I understand, *Genji*'s author had a very deep feeling for people, their thoughts, as well as Japanese art and rituals, music and poetry. The author was a woman named Murasaki Shikibu. She's known as the Lady Murasaki. I believe she became tutor to the children of the Emperor. She wrote *Genji* during Japan's Heian Period, the 'peaceful period' at the turn of the first Millennium. It was a high point for Japanese culture, one of history's most sophisticated cultures ever."

"Sounds like you've already consecrated quite a bit of time to...!"

"Yes, yes. I admit I've read some. My grandmother is close to finishing a French translation of it. She's been working on it for a number of years."

"Hm!"

"It's full of beautiful, melancholy poetry. But it's a long book, as you can see. I haven't found the time to finish it."

"Is that where you get the poems you write outside?"

"Yes, sometimes. Sometimes they're earlier Chinese poems. They're haiku, which are seventeen-syllable poems. Sometimes they're mine. Sometimes they're my grandmother's. Though it's almost blasphemy. Haiku are supposed to be private thoughts. That was more in ancient times. It seems to make our customers want to come back. The idea with haiku is that it's incumbent upon you, if someone sends you a haiku, to respond right away with one of your own. Otherwise you're thought of as *gauche* or slow-witted or both."

"Who wrote today's poem?"

"My grandmother."

"It sounds quite sad."

"It's her birthday. That's why she's depressed. We're having a party later to cheer her up."

"Oh. Please wish her a happy birthday and many happy returns."

"I will."

"Thank you for *Genji*."

"I'll be interested to hear what you think."

"*Bien sûr.*"

"And take good care of it. It's a rarity you have there."

"I'll cherish it. *Au revoir.*"

"*Au revoir, monsieur. Et bonne lecture.*"

I shoulder my way back out through the curtains and into the harsh sunlight. I pass a hardware store and go inside and buy some oil and a chamois. When I get to my bungalow that night, all I can think about is the bookseller and how I'm going to find any excuse to spend more time in her company. Her bookshop reminds me of my Aunt Simone. And Manon. Under lamplight, I wipe the dust off my treasure. Then I put a few drops of leather oil on a cloth and I rub it into the cover, which takes on a deep brown color. It already looks happier. Then I polish the leather with the chamois. After a bit of rubbing, the book slips and slides pleasantly under the cloth and shines in the light. I open the book and admire the marbled paper on the inside of the cover. Very carefully, I turn the first few pages. It was published in 1867 in Kyoto, Japan.

And just like that, I begin to read *The Tale of Genji*. "In a certain reign there was a lady not of the first rank whom the Emperor loved more than any of the others...."

CHAPTER 31

THE TALE OF GENJI

Over the next days and weeks and months, I drink in *The Tale of Genji*, steeping myself in the Japan of 1,000 years ago, quietly turning the stiff pages of my increasingly beloved leather-bound book. When Granyer is embroiled in some movie deal and talking over dinner for hours with investors, I eat by myself and read about Genji and how he falls in love with the Emperor's mistress. (The Emperor, his father.) And she with him. And how they can't help themselves. And as time passes, she gives birth to a son who grows up to look uncomfortably like Genji, not like the Emperor. There is no mistaking his true father. It's the story of a terrible secret that cannot be kept.

It's also the tale of a highly cultivated civilization with simple pleasures, like moon-watching parties, where the Emperor, his family, and hangers-on spend the entire night watching the full moon shifting overhead, inventing poetry, drinking saké, and listening to musicians play the Japanese mandolin. The author, the Lady Murasaki, doesn't go out of her way to be complimentary. When she isn't impressed, she's honest about it. For instance, she write about one long night: "It isn't worth preserving the poems recited toward the end of the party, when the moon was finally disappearing. People had drunk too much saké. Their efforts were all mediocre, not in the least memorable."

Sometimes I read *Genji* late at night. More often I read it at daybreak. Morning is a beautiful time to read *Genji*, when it's quiet. Reading a page or two gives me the feeling I'm gliding along in a perfectly maintained 1,000 year old junk.

Who was this woman? The Lady Murasaki. The woman who invented the novel. Who was she really? She wrote a short autobiography, the way Gibbon did, after completing his own big, fat, square book. In her autobiography, she shows contempt for Sei Shonagon, a younger woman poet, the author of *The Pillow Book*, who is also part of the imperial court, slighting her for her conceit and her thin accomplishment.

I come to marvel at this about Murasaki Shikibu: Her characters experience much of the life she describes with mixed emotions, conflicting and nuanced and counterbalancing. She's a watercolorist painting with shades of emotion. She describes a culture that is conscious of tragedy and resignation, pleasure and melancholy, fatalism and poetry, joy and folly. Her characters are acutely and yet believably aware of their own thoughts and reactions and associations and assessments. I vow to try to be more aware myself.

Much of my time I spend with Joe working in the film lab. Or visiting the bookseller during my breaks, looking at books she recommends, adding them to my library. What's left of my time is spent chauffeuring Granyer and his friends around or delivering copies of *Genji*.

L.A. is vast. Getting from here to there eats up a lot of time. When Granyer starts filming scenes for his production of *Genji*, I really start careening around. I deliver the exposed film to Joe to be developed. Later I deliver the rushes to Granyer so he can see how the day's work went. The dailies alert Granyer to problems so that he can reshoot scenes if he has to, before he's had a set dismantled or released an actor. The lag in time between the shooting, developing, and screening gets on people's nerves. At the end of movies, they roll the credits. But what about the discredits? You never see them scrolling by. They'd probably be twice as long as the credits. Word gets around, though.

Joe is cheerful about the work. As long as he does his job, he's impervious to the problems of the filmmaking itself. He's a lot calmer than the other high-strung characters I meet making motion pictures. If the film is underexposed or overexposed or out of focus, it's not his fault, it's the cinematographer's. He has his part of the process down to a science. And he has no real stake in the outcome; it's all the same to him whether the film makes a mint or gets jeered. He probably wouldn't mind being associated with a movie that people like. But that's secondary. He gets paid upfront, like the brokers on

Wall Street. Glamorous it is not. The odor of acrid chemical baths permeates the place.

Joe decorates his lab one day by slapping up some still photographs, glamour shots of Asian film stars, including some he says were legends in Shanghai. He points to a handsome bit player in one photo and says it's him when he was younger and working as an actor.

Granyer says he wants to turn the 1,000-year-old, 1,000 page classic into an epic. He wants it to be the longest movie ever created, which is all well and good for the lab. With the production of *Genji* under way, Joe's going to have steady work, maybe for years.

CHAPTER 32

RETRIEVING THE BOOKS

Granyer tells me he needs to visit all the actors and actresses he's given a copy of *Genji* to. "That's enough time. I have other talent that wants in. Those are our scripts, Jean-Yves. I've called them. They know I'll be coming round. You can give them a copy of *The Iliad* later. Or *The Decline and Fall*. That'll keep them occupied."

He calls these his *Genji* meetings. I drive him to see all his unknown, struggling actors and he has a long drunken dinner at their place. Eventually he comes banging back into the car and throws their copy of *Genji* in the back seat. Most of the books look like they've been kicked around instead of read. I hate to see a book's binding crack; it pains me to see the state they're in.

"What do they do with these? Throw them at you?"

"You know how some actors are. They have less

reverence for books than they do for the theatre."

"Sad to see."

"The bookstore knows a place that fixes books. They'll know how to bind their wounds."

"I should have them fixed?"

"Definitely. We need these. It's not an easy book to come by. And in the future, tell them to handle them with care. I'm still looking for the right chemistry. Some of the players I visited are interested but, frankly, *je m'en fous*. I'm not ready to make a decision, yet."

CHAPTER 33

BOOK REPAIR

When I return to The Dragon and The Lotus book-shop, I bring a piece of chalk with me. Before I go inside with my battered books, I jot my first haiku on one of the blackboards outside. It came to me as I was half-asleep the night before. I wrote it down so I wouldn't forget. Carefully I copy:

Smiling, reading, bright.
You don't talk about money
as so many do.

Satisfied, heart pounding, I pocket the chalk, pick up my battered books and go inside to face the music, wondering when she'll see my poem. I know it's a bit direct for a haiku, but I don't care.

"I'm so sorry about these books."

"Don't worry. It's not your fault. Some publishers use very brittle glue. The French are especially hopeless.

Some of their books split the first time you open them. Or the whole cover just comes unstuck and falls off."

"Best not read them."

She laughs. "Truly. Better to admire them on the shelf. On your own shelf at home."

"One of these wasn't translated. It's in Chinese. Or Japanese."

She takes the battered book and peers at a page. "Japanese. Is one of your would-be actresses Japanese?"

"I'm not sure. I don't think so."

"Maybe that's why it's so mangled. She threw a tantrum when she couldn't read it."

"It would be frustrating."

"Childish, though."

She takes a piece of paper and pencil and quickly writes down an address. "This bookbinder does a good job repairing books. I've used him a number of times. It's just a block over from here."

"Okay, thanks. He's got his work cut out for him this time." She shakes her head a little.

"Do you have the dozen copies of *The Iliad* we ordered?"

"Yes, we do. I'll get them."

While she's gone, I look around the shop. When I return to the counter, I can't help but glance at the book she was reading when I came in. It's a book on art. I spin it around so I can make it out better. It turns out to be a book of erotic Japanese woodblock prints from the 19th century. I leaf through it, admittedly a bit furtively. It contains amazing images of men with phalluses that would look less alarming on a horse than a man. Women in deep distress. Couples in the throes of lovemaking. Everyone looking exceedingly bothered.

I hear the bookseller returning and spin her book back the way I found it. This does not escape her. She smiles, puts down a half dozen books wrapped in butcher paper. As she turns to get the rest, she calls over her shoulder. "Don't let me interrupt your reading."

"Can I give you a hand?"

"You enjoy yourself."

When she returns and has them all stacked in front of her, I ask her about the book of Japanese prints on the counter.

"That's a rare book that we just got in," she says. "They're woodblock prints by a famous Japanese artist, one of the most famous. Hokusai. They're shocking, and shockingly modern, considering he created them over 100 years ago."

"Is it for sale?"

"Yes, it is."

"In that case, I'd like it, also."

She looks at me a little nonchalantly, friendly. "I'll be curious to hear what you think of them the next time you come in."

"*Volontiers.* Oh, by the way, I wasn't going to tell you, but I wrote a haiku on your blackboard outside."

"*C'est vrai?* I can't wait to see it."

"*J'espère que ça te plaira.*"

"*A bientôt.*"

CHAPTER 34

FILMING JAPANESE WOODBLOCK PRINTS

When I finish my deliveries, I go back to my place and spread out the book of Japanese prints. It gives me a bright idea. Why not reenact these scenes on film? Start the film with a man and a woman. Film their romantic *tête à-tête* as it takes its course. And when they reach the pitch of excitement depicted in one of Hokusai's prints, freeze on their image and fade to the original work of art. Leave the audience gaping at the artistry and daring of Hokusai. Leave the rest to the imagination.

The next day I bring up the idea with Granyer and he likes it.

"Let's see the book. We can film some and let Joe develop them. I'll let him start with something small, something I can't have a commercial lab develop anyway."

"Okay."

"How old did you say they were?"

"Over 100 years old."

"Good. No copyright worries. And they're fine art. High-brow. Titillating and practically respectable, all at the same time."

"I'll bring in the book and you can see for yourself. To call them respectable might be a stretch."

The next day we spend a couple of hours at Granyer's studio with the book of Japanese prints. We go through the book and Granyer's cinematographer shoots a roll of film of the images. In some, the kimonos are hitched up, sliding off, and so tangled that they look like the lovers are drowning in a silk whirlpool, and instead of being carried away with lust and pleasure, drenched in sweat, they are being dashed in the sea, dying in a typhoon. The difference between the "little death" and death, between *la petite mort* and *la mort, tout simple*, seems pretty small.

"Do you have actors in mind for these mad lovers?"

"Of course. But the chemistry must be right. Without it, these vignettes would be worthless. With the right couple, we might pack the house. I'll need a small theater for discreet, private screenings. We could advertise them as 'C Movies.' You have to see them to believe them."

"Maybe you could use them as scenes in *Genji*."

"That's an idea. In the version we offer only to a select clientele."

"When we start filming *The Decline and Fall of the Roman Empire*, we can do something similar with the wall paintings from the bathhouses of Pompeii. They're something to behold, too."

"Keep this to yourself, Johnny."

"Of course."

There are many important female characters in *Genji*. Most only become noteworthy when *Genji*, the Shining Prince, seduces them. They cannot say "No" when he sees them silhouetted behind their drapes, and he decides to come inside their bedroom and stay the night. He's a sovereign. His licentious "romanticism" is a divine right of the royalty of the Heian Period. He might be Emperor one day. The women he conquers are accomplished, refined, erudite, but also insignificant and powerless. Once he's forced himself into their bed, though, he and they are forever linked. He doesn't completely forget them. They remain lovers or former lovers and he acts with some responsibility toward them. At least five women become his lover, consort, and dependent. It's as if in Japan 1,000 years ago a woman needed to be completely and securely hidden away. If a member of the royal family catches a glimpse of her or sees her face, he might conclude that this revelation, her having appeared to him, was intended, an overture that he now has the freedom to act upon.

CHAPTER 35

A SOMETIME ACTRESS

The next time I visit The Dragon and The Lotus, I write a second haiku on the blackboard in chalk. I wrote it this morning after I saw some flowers strewn on the sidewalk:

Some sumptuous lei—
unlaced overnight in the
rain's dark dalliance.

When I go inside, the bookseller is mouthing words to herself, talking quietly, as if rehearsing lines.

"I must look a little odd today, muttering to myself."

"Not at all. A lot of people move their lips when they read."

"I don't think I told you but besides selling books, I'm also a 'sometime actress.' I've played some simple roles for Monsieur Granyer."

"*Ça alors.*"

"Granyer wants me to play one of the female characters in his *Genji*. You might laugh, but I was just imagining myself playing a mad woman."

"Incredible."

"Why is that so incredible?"

"I never thought of you that way."

"What way?"

"As a starlet."

"Don't be silly. It isn't certain. Your employer is a real promoter."

"Tireless."

"He called yesterday and offered me a role. So, how about that? Now I'm reading *Genji*, too."

"Nice of him."

"He wants me to play a married woman, who's touched in the head."

"I haven't gotten to that part yet. Why is she mad?"

"Her husband is an important general and he cheats on her. Openly."

"People have gone mad for slighter reasons."

"Indeed. I wouldn't have liked to have been a woman then."

"May I come watch your performance?"

"Oh, let me think about that. I'm an amateur. I'll be terribly self-conscious."

"I understand. Think about it."

"Okay."

"When is the shoot?"

"I'm not sure."

"I don't know if Granyer even lets people watch while

he's filming. If he says it's all right with him, what would you say?"

"I might allow you. You'll have to tell me how marvelous I am, though. I mean how marvelous my acting is. You have to promise."

"I promise I will. I'm sure you'll be spectacular."

"I enjoyed your haiku, by the way."

"I hope you like my latest."

"You!"

CHAPTER 36

SHOOTING GENJI

When I get back to Granyer's, I mention that I'd like to visit his studio when a shoot is taking place, if possible when the bookseller is acting. He says that won't be for a couple of weeks but that I can come if I like. He says I can even come the next morning if I work hard and keep quiet. I can't make a sound when the camera is running and I can't tell anyone what I see on the set. I readily agree. At the same time, in the back of my mind I'm brooding, thinking he better not use the bookseller, my sometime actress, for his Hokusai experiments...

I've never been on a movie set before, even on the set of a small production like Granyer's, so I feel self-conscious the next morning when I step into his studio, the round building with adjustable skylights.

A few people are already there. There's the cine-matographer, who is arranging the lights and reading a light meter. There's the soundman, who's hanging a microphone. There's one of Granyer's stevedores, who helps with the lifting and shifting. There's a cherubic-faced Asian actor, who must be playing Genji, the Shining Prince. And there's a pretty Asian woman just emerging from behind a painted screen, dressed in a red kimono. No one takes particular notice of me and Granyer doesn't bother to make any introductions.

The day begins early and seeing that I'm eager to witness the magic of moviemaking, he offers to put me to work immediately "dressing the set." This sounds vaguely exotic and interesting until he hands me a broom and tells me to start sweeping. The place needs it. The set is a jumble of cushions, rugs, and folding screens, not as bad as the first time I visited, but still pretty much a mess.

Once the set is deemed sufficiently dust-free, the scene-shifter and I prop up and secure what's ostensibly a palace. It's just a facade with a door and a window with blue-and-white curtains. Behind this wall, we position a three-paneled screen that depicts a lion overpowering a gazelle, sinking its fangs and claws into its back. The gazelle's legs are buckling and its eyes are wide and wild. The screen serves as palace décor visible through the window.

The set firmly in place, Granyer hands me a notebook that he describes as the day's script and tells me to get ready to follow along. There's no dialogue noted. This is going to be a scene of action. They're shooting Genji forcing himself on a woman he sees one night getting ready for bed.

The script describes it bloodlessly, somewhat like a camera does, without acknowledging the horror and violation. That's for the actors to bring out.

The set establishes three spaces—outside the palace, inside a bedroom divided by a screen, and the bed behind the screen. The screen in the bedroom hides the bed.

When the filming begins, Granyer quietly utters the word "Action." Sometimes he simply says: "When you're ready." I do my best to position myself behind the camera so I can see what the lens sees.

Scene 1: (medium shot) Genji walks by the window and stops abruptly to look inside.

Scene 2: (extreme close-up) Genji staring, spying a beautiful woman who has left her blinds slightly open. He is mesmerized by the sight. He finds himself overcome with desire.

Scene 3: (medium shot) Genji plucks a flower and slips through the door into the house.

Scene 4: (Genji's point-of-view). A beautiful woman inside the house, walking by the window, passing in and out of view. She takes off her kimono, unpins and shakes out her hair, puts on some light bedclothes.

Scene 5: (medium shot) Genji appears in the girl's bedroom, flower in hand, surprising the girl, holding the flower out to her. He catches her by the wrist. She struggles and pulls hard to get away but he's strong. And he's the Emperor's son. With one hand he begins untying his own kimono. He continues to hold her with the other. He pulls her behind the screen.

Scene 6: (medium shot) What ensues is filmed in

silhouette through the three-panel screen. The shadows appear to be cast by candlelight.

Scene 7: (medium shot) Genji emerges from behind the screen, retying his kimono.

Scene 8: (close-up of the actress' face and her reaction when Genji unexpectedly appears in her bedroom) She's scared to death but she recognizes the prince. She accepts the flower but jumps when he grabs her wrist. She struggles. He is implacable. She is all alone. He is almost a god. She strains to free herself, unsuccessfully.

Scene 9: (close-up) She beseeches him. If he is going to force his way into her bed, let him then love her and protect her. She has heard that this is how the prince has treated other women, and hopes she will fare no worse.

Scene 10: (medium shot, behind the screen, the woman on the bed) Her kimono is open, the sheets barely cover her legs. She is crying. She is at the mercy of Genji but may yet benefit from his perverse sense of chivalry. She pulls the sheets up around her.

Scene 11: (medium shot) The actress gets up and puts her kimono back on.

Scene 12: (close-up shot of the sleeve of the actress's kimono) The actor grabs her by the wrist. She fights to free herself from his grip but he succeeds in drawing her, steadily, with him, step by step, out of sight behind the screen.

I tell Granyer that in the earlier scene, Genji grabbed the actress by her right wrist and now he's holding her by the left. Am I sure? I tell him I am and he thanks me. He has the actors switch arms and they reshoot that shot.

I realize where I've seen the actress before. It's Shoko,

Granyer's set painter. She is a daring actress. I didn't recognize her in costume.

This was a fairly simple scene—two actors, one setting—but it took six hours to film. The cameraman was methodical, shooting extreme close-ups, close-ups, medium shots, long shots. To be honest, there were no real long shots. Granyer's studio is too small for that. He would have had to film from outside, through the door or through one of the retractable windows. The studio was actually designed with that eventuality in mind, but we didn't do it today. This is truly a scene of intrusion and claustrophobia. There was nothing to be gained filming it from a long way off.

When Granyer says "Action," the atmosphere changes completely. Those of us who aren't acting practically stop breathing.

At the end of the afternoon, when everyone agrees that the scenes have been well played and shot from every angle and distance (to make the editor's life easier), there's a surge of relief and everyone starts laughing and chatting and bustling around, hurrying to change out of their costumes and into evening attire. The cameraman carefully secures the exposed film, taping the film canisters shut. I'll deliver them to Joe to develop. All told, we shot five rolls of film. Only tomorrow will we know how it went. Granyer tells us to leave the set as it is, until he sees the footage and is sure he's happy with it. That's easy enough to do.

I drop Granyer and the two actors off at Slapsy Maxie Rosenbloom's Café, where they are meeting up with the cameraman and soundman. I drop the film at Joe's.

Granyer tells me to join them afterwards, if I want, which I do. It's the first time I've been around people really making movies.

The cameraman commands everyone's respect. Ultimately, he's the one capturing the electric shadows. Setting up the lights, measuring the exposure, loading the film, running the camera, framing the images, keeping things in focus. He clearly can use an assistant. If I keep collecting part-time jobs, someday I'll be a complete something or another. I volunteer to help him. He says if Granyer wants to spring for an assistant cameraman, he'll think about it.

CHAPTER 37

FACHSI REAPPEARS

In the movies, time's divided into 24 frames per second, but I measure out my days and weeks watching the numbers tick by at the gas pump. Franklin D. Roosevelt gets elected President, Prohibition is repealed on December 5, 1933, and everyone bellies up to the bar. From one day to the next, Granyer's saké smuggling business goes bust. Everyone's back to being legit.

One evening, I'm sitting in my car on Sunset Boulevard and a monstrous midnight blue Bentley comes gliding by, and who do I see laughing her head off in the back seat with some old fogey? Fachsi. And as I'm staring and their Bentley is carving a beautiful arc around my car, she looks in my direction and she sees me and she sees that I see her, and her laugh freezes solid in midair as she looks at me, wide-eyed, and then they're past, free to continue on with their hilarity.

That Bentley had running boards the size of the Yankees dugout, headlights the size of manhole covers, and horns the size of trombones. *Grandiose, quoi.*

Staring after them, I try to start the Hudson, but it balks. I try again. A thin plume of smoke starts to seep from under the hood. I leap out and sure enough smoke keeps coming out of both sides of the hood. When I open it up, flames shoot out. I cast one last look after the blue Bentley disappearing down the street. I'm planted there for two seconds, holding the hood up, staring at the fire, when three sailors jog over asking if they can help me, a civilian in distress.

"I've got a fire extinguisher in the car…"

"We'll hold the hood."

The sailors take the hood from me and calmly prop it up. Are we going to get blown up? I dive into the back seat, find the extinguisher, and dart back to douse the flames. The engine's already covered in foam and the fire is out.

"Stan here's a leader of men. He poured his beer on it and we did, too. Put it right out."

"Thanks a lot."

"No problem."

"That was a three-beer fire."

"Refills are on me."

"Now you're talking."

"I know a place. A lot more comfortable than swigging beer on the street, begging for trouble from the LAPD."

I'm still reeling. That was close. I need my car.

Then I remember Fachsi. What a rotten moment that was to see her looking so happy with someone else. But even as bad as I feel, knowing she's in L.A. is slightly encouraging. She can't seriously be interested in that fossil, a livewire like her. He may be bankrolling her high jinks, which I'm sure she finds nice and easy, but nice and easy aren't the same as love and happiness. Those are completely different rings of paradise.

I lead the troops to the Parisee Inn, a place that used to be a speakeasy, where I go when I'm feeling restless. I'm not much of a drinker, but one cannot live on the classics alone. I like the Californians' idea of French *ambiance* and the waitresses keep the place alive between acts, taking drink orders in their crisp white aprons and skimpy black dresses. I'm sure the sailors will approve and I'm hoping a drink or two will take the edge off that queasy feeling that carburetor fire and Fachsi have given me.

They recognize me at the door, give us the nod, and in we go. The place is noisy and all the tables are taken. We have to do a fair amount of shoving to get to the bar. I order beers for my new friends, but personally I'm there to meet John Daniels or one of his hillbilly cousins. When I ask for a whiskey, the barkeep brings out a bottle with a Canadian Club label on it.

That takes me back, gets me thinking about dark nights shuttling shipments up and down the Eastern seaboard. I think about the time the Mounties and G-Men thought they had us in their sights and only managed to shoot one another. My driving saved us and 50 cases of Canadian whiskey, which ended up in some of the finest cellars on the Upper East Side.

I raise my glass: "Douse the flames, boys!" and that's

our battle cry for the rest of the evening. After we go around and around buying rounds, I'm dead sure I don't give a damn about Fachsi having a goddamn great time with someone else. She can do what she damn well pleases.

A jazz band settles in and starts heating the place up. An accordionist starts working himself into such a frenzy, he could be stoking a locomotive. We keep shouting "Put out the flames! Put 'em out!"

People are clapping enthusiastically when a delicate woman in a white wrap-around gown steps up to the microphone and starts singing:

It's lovely to be liked,
and it's likely we could love.
The difference between liked and loved
is a question of degree,
a simple question
of phenomenology.
I'd love you to like me,
and I'd like to love you,
but it isn't like me,
though it could be lovely.
The difference between liked and loved
is a question of degree,
a simple question
of phenomenology.
It would be lovely,
but it's quite unlikely.
It's too lovely to be likely.
A bit too lovely, most unlikely.

I have trouble not seeing double, but when I close one eye and concentrate, I see that the *chanteuse* is the bookseller I'm so crazy about from The Dragon and The Lotus. Now I'm sorry I've overdone it. If I can pull myself together, I'll tell her how much I'm enjoying her performance. She's the cat's meow! I get the barman to pour me a pitcher of H_2O and I start doing the best I can to dilute the effects of my long evening's unquenchable thirst. She finishes with a flourish and I clap as if my hands are on fire.

She moves around and sits down at the drum set and begins laying down the rhythm for the next set of numbers. When she finishes tearing it up, making the whole joint crackle with thunder and lightning, she throws away her drumsticks and the place goes wild. I leap up and bumble forward until I reach her. I whisper to her in French. "*Génial! Tu étais géniale!*"

A lot of other guys are crowding up to her, telling her how wonderful she was, but she recognizes me, gives me a conspiratorial smile, and slips her hand under my arm. They try to slow us down but we just keep snaking our way through the crowd toward her dressing room. That's what I'm thinking. Call it an intuition.

Then from behind us, a woman yells after us: "Go fuck yourselves to death!" I look over my shoulder and there's Fachsi with the King of Sweden. It figures she'd end up with one of her countrymen. Her face is so flushed she looks like she's about to explode. "Go ahead and fuck yourselves to death!" she screams again at the top of her lungs. Horrible. It really isn't like Fachsi to act like that. Crazed. Maybe her new life isn't so nice and easy after all. And besides, who said anything about fucking ourselves to death?

I look at the bookseller and she looks at me and she grabs my hand and keeps pulling me away with her to the safety of her inner sanctum. She has rough hands for a woman, but not for a drummer.

CHAPTER 38

THE JADE DAGGER

We duck through a curtained doorway. We're in a sort of labyrinth of rooms divided by oriental screens and embroidered curtains. Any pursuers would find themselves hopelessly lost. "Here we are," she says as she parts one last curtain and leads the way into her dressing room. Or maybe it's her bedroom. There's a bed, I know that, because she pulls me down onto it. And as she leans forward to meet my kiss, her gown slowly falls open, she lets it fall open, and I plummet into her arms.

In time, I encounter a hard bump under her left breast, a sharp point that I can't prevent myself from lingering over, feeling with my fingertip. I gently cover it with the tip of my forefinger.

"You've found one of my secrets. You must be careful," she says. "The point of that sliver of jade almost touches my heart. You don't want to actually love me to death, do you?"

"I think I already do love you to death."

"A tycoon in Shanghai wanted me and I refused him. He lashed out at me with an antique jade knife." At this she laughs a little. "And now it's mine."

I kiss her again and cup my hand over the shattered jade. The rest is a dream of black and white and red all over. Vows—A's (eh's)… and E's (ease)… and I's (eyes)… and O's (oh's)… and U (you)—and consonance, and hair and hands and you, lives and loves and me and you, rushing on and non, and non anon. "*La petite mort.*" A French euphemism. A Little Death.

We no longer care whether we're headed toward bliss and sleep or Death with a D. Waves of heat crash. *On s'en fout* whether we're chasing *l'oubli de la petite mort* or the real, total annihilation. We pitch forward and back and her hair falls over my eyes and she bites me on the cheek hard and on the nose and digs her nails into my chest as if she wants to be sure to take me with her. Waves of pleasure turn to pain. I'm jolted back to my senses, my waking senses, the ones that let me know I'm in pain, and I struggle to defend myself. I open my eyes wide, scared for her and particularly for me, and I see my cat, Vince, on top of me, clawing me, biting my face.

The room is on fire.

I jump up, trip and fall. Vince scampers off me and I stagger through thick black smoke to the door, throw it open, and he and I stumble out over each other. As we bolt, it's night, and I fall and roll and jump up again and run, coughing and coughing. Both of us sprinting barefoot. The grass is cold and damp. My little house is burning. I hear sirens in the distance. They won't arrive in time. Granyer runs toward me, bathrobe flapping, swearing a blue streak, though he does tell me later he's glad I got out. I'm lucky I had so little to lose.

CHAPTER 39

PICKING THROUGH THE FIRE'S REMAINS

The next morning, I wake up in my new domicile, the tool shed, and it takes me a few seconds to realize where I am. And why I'm moving down in the world. I start to get up and my head reverberates as if someone's banging it like a big brass gong. And they keep banging it and it keeps ringing. I have a world-class hangover on top of everything else. Drink is definitely not for me.

I limp outside and survey the scene through my puffy, half-closed eyes. It's some soggy sight, smelling of burnt cedar. A wall and a half are still standing. That's it. There's a huge burnt patch in the middle of the lawn. My bed is scorched and soaked, my clothes ruined, my books a pile of blackened covers. It's too depressing to begin to turn things over to see if anything has survived the conflagration. I add to this idyllic scene by retching in the bushes. I sit and survey the ruins from across the yard. My memory of Fachsi is also a bit nauseating, a smoldering ruin. Vince cautiously approaches the debris, but he doesn't venture into the charcoal either. He seems more than a little puzzled by his bungalow disappearing one day to the next. "What's all this sky doing overhead?" he seems to be asking.

Granyer and Joe come out of the mansion and join me. They stand looking grimly at the wreckage. Then Joe begins to pick his way over the fallen boards and piles of wet, burnt, unrecognizable stuff. When he reaches the part of the bungalow that had been a closet, he begins bending down searching for something. He has work gloves on and is shifting two-by-fours and various odds and ends until he hauls out something I didn't remember having—an alligator skin suitcase. Granyer had stuff stored in the bungalow. I guess Joe did, too. In the good old days, when I'd called this smoldering ruin "home," I hadn't paid much attention.

Joe looks almost despondent as he tramps back across the boards and out of the sooty mess, lugging the alligator skin suitcase with him.

Granyer asks him, "Find what you were looking for?"

"Yes. Some old experiments. Important to me, though. I forget we store them here. Until I hear about the fire. Glad you okay, John. Maybe time to get rid of cat."

"That beastly thing cost me a lot, I'm afraid, knocking over that candle. Promise me you're done keeping pets, that's one thing I insist on."

"That would be pretty ungrateful on my part. Vince saved my life. He bit me until I woke up. I'm the one to blame."

"Maybe we should keep Vince and take you to the pound."

"I'm sorry. I'm glad I'm alive to tell you so."

"You found your experiments, right, Joe?"

"Yes, I find them. John, you give me lift back to lab?"

"Of course."

"I called my insurance company. They're coming by later to inspect the bungalow, to make sure I didn't burn it down on purpose. Vince might be a hero but he's still taking the fall on this one. And no more candles."

"Definitely not. Candles are out."

I guess I fell asleep with my clothes on and my wallet and keys still in my pocket. That was lucky. But the car's not where I normally park it. Joe and I go out toward the street and there's the Hudson, all right. I don't know why I thought I should park on the sidewalk when I came home last night, but it seems I did.

I give the Hudson a walk-around. No dents. No blood. That's a relief. I have no recollection whatsoever of coming home. After the carburetor got its three-beer dousing, why did the car even start? Did I drive? Did someone drop me off? What a nightmare. My copy of *Genji* is on the passenger seat, though, spared.

I try to act nonchalant but can't. Joe gives me a look and shakes his head. We climb in and when I turn the key, the car starts right up. Might as well put it in gear. "Some party," Joe says. I have nothing to add to that.

When we get to the lab, Joe hefts his alligator suitcase onto a table and tries to open it. The latches are melted, though the skin itself hasn't burnt up entirely. Still, it's pretty well trashed. He finds a tiny key in a desk and tries to unlock the case, but it just gets bent. The lock doesn't budge.

He sighs and looks thoughtful and furious for a second. Then he rummages around in a drawer and pulls out a knife and a big pair of scissors and tries hacking away at the alligator hide. Very thick-skinned. He can barely nick it. Finally he pulls out a hammer and chisel and bashes at the lock and clasps. It works. He breaks them off one by one with some well-aimed blows. He puts down his tools and peels open the lid.

Inside are the remains of a dozen large glass bottles. Most have cracked in the heat and their contents have overflowed and burned. Joe picks up the knife and pokes at one blue-black mass. Next he wedges the prongs of the hammer under it to try and free it. Really exerting himself, he slowly rips it loose. The suitcase's lining tears out with it.

"Great," says Joe.

"I'm really sorry..."

"I mean it. This is great," and he chuckles to himself.

CHAPTER 40

GIVE HIM A CALL

The next time I stop by The Dragon and The Lotus to pick up books for Granyer, I write another haiku on the bookshop's blackboard:

> Hopes rise quick as gulls
> riding a sudden updraft,
> gathering like smoke.

"*Bonjour, monsieur.*"

"*Bonjour, mademoiselle.* I don't know if I should admit this…"

"Admit what?"

"I've been dreaming about you lately."

"Really."

"I dreamt that Fritz Lang wanted to talk to you." I don't tell the bookseller I dreamt she almost died in my arms. Or about burning down my house.

"*Pourquoi?*"

"So he could talk to you about a role."

She laughs.

"But I didn't know your name."

"It's Ariane."

"*Enchanté.*"

"*Et vous? Comment vous appellez-vous?*"

"Jean-Yves."

"*C'est un plaisir.*"

"*C'est moi. Est-ce que ça vous dérange si on se tutoie?*"

"*Pas du tout.*"

"*J'ai ce numéro de téléphone pour toi. Tiens. Le voilà.* It's Fritz Lang's number. Granyer gave it to me. He's met him."

"I'm not really an actress, you know. It'd feel absurd calling him."

"Think about it."

"What can I do for your today?"

"I'd like to pick up a book order. A dozen copies of *The Iliad.*"

"I'll get them."

When she returns with the books, I don't tear myself away.

"I'm enjoying *Genji,*" I say. "I'm pretty far along."

"It is beautiful. *Mais, ce prince, il prend pas mal de libertés.* Such a refined culture and yet the Shining Prince is practically a rapist. Really. No woman could say 'No' to the Emperor. Or his son."

"Some Hollywood producers also take liberties, I hear."

"What's that 'joke' they make? 'The casting couch?'"

"Pretty shameless."

"Do you need a hand?"

"No, thanks. I've got them."

Carrying the stack of books as if they were cordwood, I go to leave. Ariane holds the door for me, and as I pass back out into the flat, dry L.A. heat, she says: "*A bientôt,* Jean-Yves. We can discuss *Genji* again soon. And those Japanese prints. Hokusai is one of my favorites."

"Good luck with Fritz Lang!"

"We'll see. And thank you for the haiku."

"I wrote another."

I hoist the stack of books onto the hood of the Hudson before placing them carefully in the back seat. To what end? The actors Granyer knows won't care. They read as if they werewolves under a full moon. As I drive off, Ariane is studying my haiku. She turns and waves.

I spend the rest of the day and evening retrieving copies of *Genji* and dropping off copies of the *Iliad*. It's getting late but the thespians seem to expect me. I park outside the mansion of some actor who enjoyed his heyday before the talkies piped up. The place is huge and rundown, the grass is brown, the flowerbeds chock full of weeds. I knock and wait and the door finally draws open. The great man himself is standing there in his bathrobe. He seems to be coming out of a sound sleep. "I hope I'm not disturbing you. Here's the book that Charles Granyer promised to send round for the next movie he's casting—*The Iliad.*"

"I've been waiting all night for you."

"I'm sorry about that. Some other people are reading for parts, too."

"Swell."

"I need to pick up your copy of *The Tale of Genji*, if you don't mind."

"I haven't cracked a book that size in years. Now here's another one. *The Iliad*, huh? That's Greek to me."

"Indeed. By Homer."

"Homer who?"

"Homer. That's his whole name. Homer. The epic poet. From ancient Greece."

"Ancient, huh? If you say so. I'll be back."

He disappears for a few minutes, leaving me standing on his doorstep. He returns with a book with a broken spine and pages sliding out that apparently used to be a copy of *The Tale of Genji*. A few fall on the floor. I pick them up.

"Okay, sonny, here you go. You tell ol' lamebrain Grainy thanks for me."

"He told me to tell you that he'll call you soon to see if you're interested."

"I know the drill."

"And go easy on it, okay?"

"What?"

"Never mind."

At that, the actor bangs the door on me. Why should I lose sleep over the fate of an old book? A lifetime of habit, I guess. It was hard to believe he would read more than the first fifteen lines, if that. But he clearly was another book devourer. I would have thought he'd just say: "Tell him I read it and yes, I'd like the part. When's the gravy train swing by? When do we start rehearsing? How about an advance?" The pertinent questions.

CHAPTER 41

A HOLLYWOOD PARTY

After a successful week's work, Granyer throws a party for the cast and friends. Here's a dream come true— Louise Brooks and Fritz Lang arrive late. Granyer introduces me to them and I introduce them to Ariane. Lang comments on the resemblance between the bookseller and the film siren.

"I want Louise to write something for me," he explains. "Why won't you, my dear?"

"Most of what I write these days is critical of the movies. It would be quite paradoxical for me to fill pages disparaging film and the movie industry and then have you turn it into a film!"

"It might make an interesting film. Truth about illusion."

"Or delusion. Wouldn't it be horribly hypocritical?"

"Paradox is paramount anyway."

"Still photos moving."

"The depths of a flat projection screen."

"The diminutive become larger than life."

"Veronica Lake is tiny. She barely comes up to my shoulder. In studio publicity shots she looks as tall as the Chrysler Building."

"I think stars are diminished by their performances. In real life, they seem extraordinarily ordinary."

"You would enjoy talking to our friend, the writer, Thomas Mann. You know of him, don't you? He has some curious theories about movie stars."

"Books get made into movies because they're considered great or were wildly popular. Then they're 'improved.'"

"To their detriment."

"One of the virtues of what Granyer is doing with *Genji* is he isn't trying to improve it."

"Maybe he has the genius to leave well enough alone."

"There is a certain genius in being able to recognize another's greatness and to respect it and preserve it."

"I'll let you know when the premiere is."

"Do."

I glance over and see Granyer talking to Shoko, his set painter and most daring actress. He is clearly enjoying himself. He's in his cups and the veins in his cheeks are standing out like red cobwebs. In fact, he is at his most brazenly lascivious. He is literally licking his lips and leering. Embarrassing. She begins beseeching him about something and his expression darkens. His smile drops off and he's left with his natural expression, the frown of a fish with a hook caught in its mouth.

I hear her say: "Why are you holding out on me, Charlie?"

He shakes his head ever so slightly but definitively. She keeps whining until he interrupts her: "C'mon now Shoko. Now's not a good moment. I can't help you. Run along now and enjoy the party."

"Don't give me that. You're holding out on me!"

He starts to turn away but she latches onto his arm and detains him just long enough to throw her drink in his face. A couple of Granyer's goons hustle her toward the door as he wipes the champagne off his face with a silk handkerchief. She lets him hear it on the way out. As she's rushed past a tall blue urn in the entryway, she manages to swipe at it and topple it over, spilling sand and cigarette butts all over the floor. That gets people's attention.

When I drive Ariane home later that night, she tells me that the ashtray incident reminded her of something out of *Genji*. I ask her why, but she tells me I'll have to wait to find out. She brushes aside my offer to walk her to her door. She dismisses the idea with a laugh and just hops out of the car and disappears into her bookstore. I wait for her to shut the door behind her. When I see the lights come on inside, I ease away from the curb.

CHAPTER 42

UPTON SINCLAIR AND THE EPIC CAMPAIGN

One eventful July day in the summer of 1934 it's sweateringly hot and I imagine the citizenry working up a quenchable thirst. I'm delivering copies of *The Decline and Fall of the Roman Empire* to a host of actors and actresses, the usual voracious readers, when I come across a big gathering. Curiosity gets the better of me and I park and get out to see what gives. People are holding signs that read "EPIC," but it's hard to imagine all these down-on-their-luck characters are lovers of epic poetry. Most likely it's a soup kitchen.

It turns out the mob has come to hear Upton Sinclair explain why they should vote for him in November to be the next governor of California. Somewhat improbably, Sinclair, the author of *The Jungle*, is the front runner in the governor's race. He's running on the EPIC platform, whose goal is to End Poverty in California. Running as a

Democrat, he's leading in the polls.

Sinclair's wearing a hat and glasses and is a slight, unprepossessing man in his fifties. He has been traveling throughout the state for months, giving a stump speech so full of common sense and inspiring such hope during the economic crisis that it looks as if he actually has a chance to win the election. All of the powerful people whose livelihood depends on the *status quo*—business as usual, politics as usual—are taking him dead seriously. And when they discover that he is not interested in bribes and has no intention of selling his future political appointments for campaign contributions, they become his determined enemies.

A smear campaign financed by the haves and willingly promulgated by the major California newspapers is hammering him mercilessly, charging him with promoting Socialism, Communism, free love, white slavery, not to mention adultery, bigamy, venality, and un-Americanism. If the broadsheets are to be believed, Upton Sinclair is Joseph Stalin.

Sinclair is wearing a dark suit, in spite of the heat. He strides up to the podium and begins speaking into the microphone. As best I can recall, he says: "Friends, I've written many books in my working life and my opponents have been having a swell time taking my words out of context. As you are surely aware, they have been doing a hatchet job on the EPIC campaign, spreading lies about me all over California. I now realize that that's what you have to expect if you run for public office and try to change the way things are done, even in this great country, the United States of America.

"According to these propagandists, I'm some combination of Caligula, Attila the Hun, Don Juan, and Lenin. That I'm an American writer who cares deeply about his country and the fate of his fellow countrymen is getting buried in an avalanche of lies. One California newsman I know told me he couldn't remember the last time he wrote something he believed. That, I'm afraid, is what we're up against. One lurid lie after another. I almost felt sorry for him.

"My campaign for the governor of California has very little to do with me. It's not about the political ambitions of Upton Sinclair. The EPIC campaign and the EPIC platform are about one thing and one thing only: implementing a program of production-for-use in order to End Poverty In California. Friends, how many of you are currently unemployed? Let's have a show of hands. That looks about right. About a quarter of American adults are out of work these days, and that same 1-in-4 ratio is true here in California. And at a time when so many men and women can't find work, are starved for work, factories are sitting empty and idle and fields are lying fallow. The country's ability to manufacture and grow is running at a fraction of what it's capable of. People have lost their homes. Families have lost their farms. This economic Depression is grinding on with no end in sight. And Washington and the political establishment seem incapable of coming up with any new ideas to change the situation.

"Here in California, our groundswell EPIC movement has many good ideas. What we're asking is for the chance to put them into practice. The basic idea, and it is an epic idea, is to put all that unused productive capacity to work. The factories and the farms, and our human strength and potential. People need an opportunity to use their energy and skills. We have to think beyond an economy that depends solely and strictly on the use of money, the availability of money, and the exchange of money. That particular commodity is in woefully short supply these days. Does that mean no one should work? No one should grow food? No one should build houses? Of course it does not.

"Instead of the country going deeper in debt, producing nothing while spending money to support the unemployed, we are proposing that people go back to work immediately producing goods for use. Fallow fields can be planted with crops. Farmers can go back to raising food to feed themselves, their families, and their neighbors. Empty mills can be reopened and workers can go back to producing clothes for themselves and their neighbors. The extra clothes can be traded to farmers for food. And the extra crops can be traded for clothes. This kind of exchange can be expanded to include all people's basic needs. And this barter system could be implemented relatively easily and everyone would benefit. It could be used to put people back to work and to provide people with the things they need until the country truly emerges from the Depression. Until then, people can work to support themselves and their families. The government will not have to spend so much money to provide people with public assistance. And the country will harness all the energy and will power that has no outlet in the terrible plight that we find ourselves in.

"That, my friends, is the EPIC program in a nutshell. Our goal is to End Poverty in California. And after the rest of the country sees that this is a viable solution to our problems, other states can adopt the EPIC program to help their citizens. We are proposing that people be allowed to work and produce for their own and for other people's use. For a vibrant economy, we need economic activity. And not the kind of fictitious economic activity that consists in playing the markets. We know what happened when too many people got caught up speculating in stocks on Wall Street, London, Frankfurt, and Shanghai. We need to promote economic activity that creates food and clothing and housing, and builds schools and hospitals and fire stations. In November, if you vote for the EPIC candidates and get your friends and family to vote for us, come January, we'll begin to End Poverty in California. It can be done and with imagination and will power and common sense, we will all roll up our sleeves and start doing it."

Without my sunglasses on, he looks a lot like a pencil sketch of Don Quixote.

As Upton Sinclair finishes speaking, a black car speeds by with a Tommy gun poking out the window firing at the podium. He's shot. Two other people, too.

CHAPTER 43

STOP AT THE NEXT GREEN LIGHT

I run up and volunteer to take him to the hospital. I'm parked right there. I whip open the back seat and shove a pile of books on the floor. Several bystanders help ease the wounded men into my car and I gun it out of there. Upton Sinclair is doing his best to hold himself upright in the passenger seat. The other wounded men, both campaign workers, are lying in back.

They talk fitfully. "Since I wouldn't take their bribes, they're starting to play rough. Not used to being turned down."

"That guy from the Los Angeles Stock Exchange and all his talk about 'penny-ante stocks' wasn't very subtle. Talking about what would happen if we didn't listen to him and his colleagues."

"They don't like my idea of putting a tiny sales tax on stock trades."

They press handkerchiefs to their wounds, and I keep giving it the gas. Sinclair is calm and talking to his guys, trying to keep their spirits up. "We're going to make it. We're going to be there any minute now. Hang in there, boys." I'm speeding, honking, and swerving through traffic. It's like an oven in the car, sweat is pouring off me and practically sizzling when it hits the seat. My passengers are suffering.

Suddenly, up ahead I see something, broken wooden crates right in my path. Smashed green Coca Cola bottles are spilled across the road. I hit the brakes but it's too late. The limo barrels over the broken glass. It sounds like more shooting but it's the sound of tires blowing.

The car starts skidding. My mind's racing. Can I make it to some flat stretch? Where I can get the car to stop? If I can just make it over the rise up ahead and through the light at the foot of the hill, after that it bottoms out. We might be all right. We're almost to the top of the hill already and the gates smile upon us. The light is green! I take my foot off the brake and hit the accelerator. Got to make that green light.

As I crest the hill, I get my first good look at what's really up ahead, what the very crest of the hill had hidden. There's a truck blocking my lane, waiting to turn left at the green light! And a car is next to it, waiting to turn right! I slam on the brakes, again, frantic. The car skids, fishtails. I look farther right... What's this now?! The sidewalk's filled with school kids, skipping and laughing, heading home!

The car blocking the right lane slowly begins to turn

and the curbside lane, which is oh-so-narrow, actually opens up. I stop trying to jam the brake through the floor and we fly through the gap between the truck and the kids. I don't even have time to sound the horn or anything. I blow through the opening like water bursting through a dam. And then I let the car coast until I ease over to the side of the road and we come to a halt.

Sinclair and his two aides wonder why I'm driving so badly. "Why are we stopping? Are we at the hospital?"

"Not yet." I jump out and flag down a cabbie. "I've got the next governor of California in my car. He's been shot!" A minute later I watch as the cabbie roars off, hoping he gets them to Mt. Sinai before anybody expires.

CHAPTER 44

THE ROMAN AQUEDUCT RUNS RED

The next day a tire guy helps me replace all four tires. My old ones were no match for those Coke bottles. Afterwards I sit behind the wheel for a minute, thinking about Upton Sinclair and the sound of bullets. I thought I'd gotten away from speeding black cars and machine guns. I wonder if the shooting victims are going to pull through.

Sinclair said something in the car, what was it? Something about "penny ante stocks?" That's what the thugs who killed Aldo Pennebeck had said. And that's not what they're called. Nobody calls them that. They're penny stocks. What did he say? "The guy from the Los Angeles Stock Exchange?" Yeah, that's what he said. No guy who works on a stock exchange would make that mistake. They might accuse you of running a "penny-ante operation" or they might suggest playing some "penny-ante poker," though that's doubtful, but they're not going to call penny stocks "penny-ante stocks."

I feel sick thinking about it. Slowly it comes back to me that I have books to deliver. My list of addresses is crumpled on the floor under the passenger's seat. I retrieve it and smooth it out. Then I glance into the back seat. The books are gone. Then I remember they're on the floor back there. I shoved them off the seat to make room.

I open the back door and sure enough they're there, and I start gathering them up, arranging them as nicely as I can. But I was pretty rough with them yesterday in the heat of the moment. And they've been trampled. Some of the butcher paper wrappers are sticky with blood. No one wants a blood-soaked book to read. I'll have to rewrap them, start fresh.

I drive back home and take the stack of books inside. I start unwrapping first one, then another, inspecting them. Some look okay. Some have a little blood on them that seeped through the butcher paper. I try dabbing it off with a wet towel and that works pretty well. When I'm done it isn't noticeable. I put them aside to dry before I rewrap them.

I clean a half-dozen copies of Gibbon this way, but I still have piled before me several that got pretty badly mangled. When I was a teenager, working for my Aunt Simone dusting books, I also restored a few volumes with her. I unwrap one book that looks as if someone danced on it roughshod. The big fat square book practically pours out of the butcher paper.

It takes a second to realize what's happening. A pile of

white powder is pouring out of the butcher paper onto my black kitchen table. The cover and binding are cracked and the sands of time are pouring out.

I fill a bucket with water and grab a rag and go outside to look in the car. Sure enough. Blood and white powder, streaks of white and red, and white footprints. I wash it all off, as best I can. What is that white stuff anyway? Not powdered sugar.

What if the doctors notice some on the campaign workers' shoes and test it? How can they miss it? Jesus Christ. That would be the end of Upton Sinclair. He sat in front, though. The books were in back. Lucky I didn't go into the hospital. They took the taxi driver's photo instead. It's probably plastered on the front page of the *Los Angeles Times*. "Local cabbie saves Upton Sinclair's life." I hope he saved him. That was some speech he gave yesterday. Someone may have taken a photo of the Hudson as I sped away from the rally. Probably did. The press was out in numbers. They would have been tripping their shutters like telegraph operators.

CHAPTER 45

THE GUY IN THE DARK

I go back inside, lock the door, and pull the curtains. Maybe I should take a powder. No pun intended. Everyone I know seems to be in on this, including yours truly, though I really didn't know until now. I can see how this will shake out. I can't confront Granyer or the bookseller or the would-be actors or Joe or the bookbinder. The only way they tolerate me is as the simpleton. The guy in the dark.

And if the customers don't get their wares, I'm going to pay. They'll get this batch, just a little late, that's all. I continue the triage. Undamaged books go in a box, which I stash away. I let the bloodstained books that I washed off keep drying. Each book with a broken spine I put in a bowl or pan of its own, so it won't spill it guts too much. I sweep the powder on the table into a sugar bowl. Then I try to hide the whole disaster by carefully sliding the books under my bed and straightening the bedspread so that it reaches to the floor.

I have a lot to do and not much time. People waiting for these kinds of books tend to be on a pretty tight schedule. Impatient. Then again, they're probably used to waiting. I need supplies—more butcher paper, bookbinding paper, cardboard, glue. It only takes me about an hour to find an art supplies store and the clerk is even nice enough to explain some of the rudiments of bookbinding to me.

It takes me a while to figure out how the white stuff is packed in the book covers but I do. Then I begin repacking the bindings, cutting new paper and cardboard as needed, and using a paintbrush to glue it back in place. I dry them in front of the heater. When they're dry, no one will give them a second glance.

While the books are drying, I shave and change into fresh clothes. It's been a long couple of days. I carefully pack the rest of the books in a cardboard box. I mix up the undamaged ones with the ones that I cleaned and the ones that I repaired, somehow hoping that will reduce the chance that anyone will notice anything. Sort of bringing luck into play, the luck of the draw. I put the box in the back seat of the Hudson and cover it with a blanket.

Then I begin making the rounds. I obey all the traffic signs and other laws of the land. I stop scrupulously at stop signs. I slow down nice and smooth. I signal to give my fellow drivers a clear understanding of my every move. I see the LAPD everywhere.

I've ferried a lot of this stuff around town unwittingly,

but now that I know what I'm really doing, my palms are sweating and I feel sick to my stomach. I just want to get this stuff to its unlawful owners. Then I'll see about changing my line of work.

All the actresses and actors, and their butlers and maids, look quite different to me this time around. Understandably. I deliver the last volume to a haunted looking woman who clutches for the book and then vanishes back inside. I drive a few blocks away, turn a few corners, and then slow down and pull over. No one is around. I chuck the box into a dumpster in an alley. As I pull away, I finally begin to relax. It's late when I get home.

CHAPTER 46

ANOTHER DISCOVERY

The next day I pay Joe an early visit. He's in the lab, heating up some noxious concoction. When I get his attention, I tell him about Upton Sinclair getting shot but don't say anything about the books. It only captures his interest for a couple seconds.

"Johnny, I make a discovery. Very important."

"Really?"

"Remember when you burn down Granger's shack?"

"Unfortunately."

"One of my experiments is in your closet. Fire does something. Solves problem I work on long time."

"Happy something good came of it."

"Bring Granger here. Tell him I have interesting proposition for him."

"Sure."

"If he not busy, have him come today."

As I motor back to Granyer's, I wonder what Joe has in store and whether I should say anything to my boss about what I know about his choice of reading material. I find Granyer at home. He's curious to hear Joe's proposal, so we climb in the car and make our way through stop-and-go traffic back to Little Tokio. The chemist answers the door to the lab in high spirits.

"Come in, Charles, Johnny. Come in, come in. Smells bad in here, I know. Some good experiments stink. Come. We talk quietly in back." We follow Joe to his room.

"Sit down. You want tea? Yes?" Joe returns with all the necessaries on a tray. He pours us each a cup and after we've taken a sip of our constitutional, he begins.

"I tell Johnny your sad fire isn't all bad. Silver lining. You know I leave my suitcase in his shack? It contain important experiments. I never unpacked. Too busy working on your film, Charles. I completely forget."

"What experiments? Come out with it already."

"Please excuse me, but I can't tell you yet. Trust me. We make a huge fortune."

"Let me get this straight. You want me to come over here so you can tell me you have something to tell me that you can't tell me."

"Correct."

"Fine."

"So you invest?"

"Sight unseen?"

"Charles, you thank me later. For a nice drive," says Joe. "You use to work on Wall Street, Jean-Yves, right?"

"For a while."

"You still know people?"

"Maybe. But I haven't talked to them in a long time."

"Tell me this. If I invent something bad for companies, can we make money?"

"We could. By shorting their stock. Instead of 'buying low and selling high,' like you normally try to do, we would sell high, buy low, and pocket the difference."

"How much money we need?"

"Not that much."

"Well, that's good news," Granyer interrupts, "because I don't have much to throw at you, Joe."

"Are these public companies?" I ask. "Do they trade on the stock exchange?"

"Yes, I think so. I make a list of companies. All right?"

"In theory, it sounds fine," I say. "But it still takes money to make money. It takes capital to capitalize."

"What if the discovery doesn't turn out to be unfortunate for these companies after all?" Granyer asks.

"That would be bad. If their stock price goes up, instead of down. We could lose more than our investment."

"Sounds less than perfect," says Granyer. Then he pauses for quite a long time.

"What we need is a syndicate," I say, "a handful of investors who are willing to pool their money and make this play with conviction."

"Joe," Granyer says, finally, "you seem convinced you're onto something big. I'll see what I can scrape together."

I'm not close with J. P. Morgan's circle of friends, so I'm going with the people I know.

Time has passed, but have the wounds healed? Maybe I can make it up to the New York widows Aldo suckered into investing in his penny stock scams. I unearth Aldo's little black book and start making calls. It doesn't go well. The first number is disconnected. The second call goes through, but the guy on the other end is definitely not the woman I'm trying to reach. He doesn't know how to reach her but he's pretty sure she had a stroke and is in a hospital or a nursing home or Poughkeepsie. All he knows is the family sold her apartment and he lives there now.

I call a third number and the phone rings and rings. My mind wanders and I almost forget I'm making a phone call when someone answers. The receiver sounds as if it's dropped or knocked against several pieces of furniture and then finally a weak voice comes on the other end.

"Hello…"

"Is this Mrs. Van Willingden?"

"Who wants to know?"

"This is John Still. A broker named Aldo Pennebeck gave you some investment advice in 1929 and I'm calling to see if I can interest you in an investment that will turn out much, much more favorably?"

"That's a good one. I lost everything I had on that penny stock scheme that fellow pitched me. I should call the police. What are you trying to do, kill me?" The line goes dead. The good news is we didn't actually kill her.

I get another idea. I'll call the rest of these poor people and find out who's survived. If I make money on Joe's plan, I can send them a share. Of the 23 widows Aldo conned, 11 of them are where he found them. Rather than get their hopes up, I tell them I'm with the Census Bureau. I duly note the spelling of their names and their mailing addresses. Maybe I can make it up to them.

John Bull got slaughtered in 1929, but the stock exchange still exists, at least in name. I get on the horn and try tracking down some of the people I used to work with. The spectral Speckler may still be in Philadelphia. And Unterfisch may still be haunting the NYSE trading floor.

Speckler sounds genuinely shocked to get a call from me. Aldo's accounts were in a complete mess and with his "suicide" and my disappearance from one day to the next, the executor had a devil of a time sorting them out. Speckler listens politely, nevertheless, hears me out, which doesn't take long, and then quickly demurs when he realizes I don't have any particulars to offer up, that I want his money on faith.

Next I make a series of calls and actually speak to Unterfisch. I apologize for ditching him outside my apartment. I tell him my only excuse is that Annemie put me under some sort of spell. He admits he actually used my apartment for the next several weeks, on and off, laying low. I suggest that I can square things with him by bringing him into our syndicate, which, as I'm trying to make clear, is a sure thing. All he needs to do is place a bet and maybe find one or two other discreet investors to join us. He scoffs and tells me to go jump in a lake, and not in so many words. Why would I think he has money to invest? He's working for chump change. He says floor traders have nothing to do four days a week and are selling apples on the corners on Fridays. He doesn't know a soul. He'd appreciate it, in the future, if I'd spare him the prank calls.

After I hang up, I take a deep breath. This is bad. Poochie's people might have money to invest. But let's not forget there are risks and rewards. The reward is that I make everyone, including myself, a lot of money. The risk is that Poochie and his friends pay me a visit. We got along, way back when. I wasn't the one calling any shots. Why would they hold anything against me? I chauffeured them safely down a lot of dark roads. And I always picked up the tab.

In the little black book, in smudged, tiny script, I find a number for Poochie. I dial it and he picks up. He grunts into the phone and that's all it takes. I'm sure it's him. I tell him it's me and then keep right on rattling along, apologizing for falling off the edge of world like that. Without so much as a drink to say "So long." If anyone can hold up his end of a conversation in chips of monosyllables, he can. Even with dead silence coming from the other end of the line, I'm pretty sure he's still there. I lay out the basic idea for the syndicate and somehow I get the impression he's not averse to the proposition. At least he hasn't hung up. Then he actually formulates an entire sentence. He wants my number. He'll get back to me after he talks to Big Department.

CHAPTER 47

THE GENTLEMAN FROM SHANGHAI

About a week later, a gargantuan gentleman from the British banking industry in Shanghai arrives to see Granyer. The impassive Irish skipper, the fellow who delivered Granyer's yacht, is with him, and they have a blonde in tow. Granyer acts a bit thrown to see them but invites them in immediately, making all the requisite signs of respect. Bowing, scraping, practically genuflecting.

"Nice to see you Charles."

"And you, B.D. You and our friend, the skipper, and your lady friend."

"It wasn't too hard finding you. Eva, this is Charles Granyer, businessman *extraordinaire*."

"Welcome, welcome."

"It's always a pleasure to join you at table. Our impromptu visit won't inconvenience you too much, I hope?"

"Of course not." Granyer rings for his chef and gives him a number of instructions. The chef bustles away and a butler returns with a tray of glasses, ice, and bottles.

"Two pink gins, Rudy."

"Do you want those in or out, sir?"

"B.D., I forget how you take yours…"

"In."

"Make both of them with the bitters in, Rudy."

"Yessir."

"And what can we get your friends?"

"A glass of champagne for Eva, isn't that right? With a splash of orange juice. Do you have French champagne, Charles?"

"Happily, yes."

The young woman smiles broadly and smacks her lips. "Please, yes. Thank you."

"Finnbar, you prefer Irish whiskey, don't you?"

"If he's got any."

"Would you like that neat?"

"On ice."

"An Irish whiskey on ice for our guest."

"Yessir."

Drinks in hand, Granyer raises his: "To Shanghai."

"May it stay where it is," the gentleman from Shanghai replies.

"Here's mud in your eye."

"Skol."

"Do you have my sailboat securely moored, Charles?"

"Yes, of course. Everything's shipshape."

"And what about my dear friend? Is he making himself

useful?"

Granyer takes a sip of his drink before replying. "Your friend never made the trip, B.D."

"What?"

"He gave up his spot. The man who stepped off the boat wasn't the man you promised."

"Finnbar described the man to me. So this doesn't come as a complete surprise. But you disappoint me, only telling me now."

"I planned to tell you, of course, but things have been running smoothly. It didn't seem urgent. His stand-in has his own know-how. An able replacement."

"But does he feel the same sense of loyalty? For Akihiro to beg off like that shows an unseemly lack of gratitude on his part."

"Your arrangement with Akihiro is outside of my ken, obviously, but his replacement, Joe, is a man of many talents. He's practically an alchemist."

"After lunch I'd like to meet this fellow."

"Certainly."

"What are we having for our luncheon, anyway, Charles?"

"Blue marlin. I caught it myself."

"Hm."

"First some delicacies that you can't get in Shanghai. Rudy is a master in the kitchen."

"Fine."

"Another pink gin?"

"What kind of white wine do you have?"

"You name it."

"Chablis?"

"Rudy, a bottle of the Chablis, if you please."

"Yessir."

After a creamy potato soup and fruit salad, the chef wheels in the main course.

"Did you catch it from my skiff?"

"It took three of us to haul it in."

"Good show, Charles. One never gets to taste marlin in Shanghai."

"I'm having its head mounted."

Finnbar finally finds something worthy of comment. "Where'd you catch it?"

"Off Catalina Island."

"That's a fish tale," the sailor replies. "Blue marlin are Atlantic dwellers."

Granyer hesitates a few moments then laughs. "Okay, I admit that was a white lie. I purchased it. It's good, though, isn't it?" The colossus laughs and pounds the table. "You haven't changed, Charles. Still indulging in hyperbole. You're an inveterate fabulist."

"I prefer to think of myself as a purveyor of dreams."

Over the next three hours, Granyer's British guest proves he comes by his girth through honest and assiduous effort. He puts away what can only be described as an obscene quantity of food and liquor. It is of this, apparently, that the good life consists for British bankers in Shanghai—a daily overindulgence in gastronomy. Four square meals a day. The wiry sailor, Finnbar, acquits himself well, also, but he's not the type to savor each mouthful. He disports himself more like some starved barracuda.

The blonde shows little interest in the food after the

first taste, but she makes steady progress on the Chablis and chain-smokes. She amuses herself by breaking off bits of bread and rolling them into balls between her slender fingers. The conversation and the company clearly bore her.

"When can I meet the passenger who rode my yacht from Shanghai? Finnbar says he spent the trip kicking his habit and playing Go."

"Spent the first week sick as a dog. Don't know what made him sicker... kicking or drinking saké."

"He's something of a research scientist. He'll be pleased to meet you, I'm sure. He thinks he's on to something and he's looking for investors."

"He is, is he?"

"He thinks he's discovered something we can make a fortune on. In the stock market."

"Stop. You're giving me indigestion."

"We'll talk business later."

"Let's. This marlin deserves to be left in peace."

When the three men can eat no more, they push their chairs away from the table and Granyer rings for his butler.

"Cigars, Rudy."

"Very good, sir."

He returns with a box and offers them up.

"Straight from Havana."

"Splendid."

They sit pensively smoking. Their woman friend pulls another pack of cigarettes out of her purse, tears it open, and puts one in her mouth. She waits for one of the men to give her a light, which they do.

"Is it too late to pay a visit to Joseph?"

"What time is it? Five? He may still be at work. I'll hail my driver."

"We'll follow you in the Bentley. Lead the way."

CHAPTER 48

FURTHER DEVELOPMENTS

At the lab, I knock loudly until Joe comes to admit us. I follow Granyer, the Shanghai banker, the Irish skipper, and Eva inside. Joe is looking more and more like a mad scientist.

Granyer introduces Joe to his visitors and they pull up seats as best they can in Joe's cluttered laboratory. He and Finnbar already know one another, having crossed the Pacific together. When the gentleman from Shanghai asks him whatever happened to Akihiro, Joe explains that he's Akihiro's uncle on his father's side.

"Akihiro tell me he plan to leave Shanghai. I beg him let me go instead. I have a problem. Afraid I never shake it if I stay. Did Finnbar tell you about me?"

"A little."

"My nephew coming later. Any day now."

"How will he find you?"

"I write him when I get here. You know him?"

"A long time ago, he worked for colleagues of mine. They told me he's quite a scientist."

"Joe's done good work for me, I assure you," Granyer interjects. "Akihiro sent a capable man in his place."

"Thank you, Charles. What can I do for you gentlemen?"

"Keep Charles happy, that's all."

"I try. We have excellent partnership."

"You'll let him know when Akihiro comes to town?"

"Certainly. I introduce them. Maybe he hire Akihiro, too. Not easy to come to new city or new country and find work. Especially now."

"You have something you want to show our friends, Joe?"

"Yes, absolutely, I do. I make long story short. I have some luck recently. One of my experiments turn out better than I ever hope. I show you."

Joe gets up and comes back a minute later with a set of golf clubs. He unzips one of the pockets and pulls out a blue-black ball.

"I make this. I believe it make investors and me very wealthy. Watch." He drops the ball on the ground, it bounces quite high, and he catches it. "Very lively, yes?"

"May I?" The fat man reaches out his hand. Joe bounces it toward him and he catches it. He rolls it around in his hand, looking it over carefully.

"Catch," he says, and bounces it back to Joe, a bit too hard. It bounces all the way over Joe's head.

Joe steps back and snatches at the air to try and catch it. Instead he loses his balance tripping over the golf bag lying on the floor and rams into the shelf behind him. The ball caroms off some glass bottles and beakers on the shelf.

A brown bottle tips over and spills all over Joe before falling and breaking on the floor. The golf ball rolls back off the shelf and bounces and bounces and bounces across the lab until it comes to rest somewhere out of sight.

Joe gathers himself up off the floor and reaches for a towel. He mops at the chemical that spilled on him, quick to inspect the broken bottle. It's labeled $AgNO_3$. When he straightens back up, he's got a queer smile on his face.

"Some mess."

"Sorry, old man. That ball really bounces."

"Please, you excuse me. I wash this off right away."

As Joe is wiping his face with the towel and dabbing at his wet clothes, his hair begins to turn black. He catches sight of himself in a mirror on the wall, changing before our eyes. Makeup is running down his cheeks. The obese banker begins to stare.

"Very unhealthy. Excuse me," mutters Joe. "So clumsy."

"Are you okay," Eva asks.

"Yes. I think so."

She sticks a cigarette in her mouth and pulls out a pack of matches.

"No, don't do that," Joe says. "Don't smoke. Too many fumes."

She takes the cigarette out of her mouth. "I'll be outside." She gets up from her perch, gives me a look, and leaves.

"Okay, sorry," Joes says. "I be back."

Joe turns and heads quickly toward the back of the shop. From behind, he no longer looks like an old man. His hair is dark, his stride purposeful.

"Did you see his hair turn black?"

"Indeed. He looks thirty years younger. What was it that spilled?"

I decipher the chemical formula on the label of the broken brown bottle. "Silver nitrate."

"What's that?"

"It can be used for hair dye."

"Aha."

"Silver nitrate's the active ingredient in film stock, too," I add. "If you don't mind, I think I'll step outside for a smoke, too."

"Wait on that, Johnny. The spill's asphyxiating us. Open those windows and find something to clean this up with."

"Okay." I find some rags in a bin while Granyer, the banker, and Finnbar stand up and move away from where the chemical spilled.

"He must use silver nitrate for his film work," says Granyer. "I must say, he's been a great help developing the dailies for my latest film project."

"I understand he ran a very successful lab in Shanghai, when he wasn't acting," says the banker.

"I thought you didn't know him."

"We've never actually met. But, I believe that's Akihiro. He and I have some unfinished business to attend to. He's going to have to cut me a much sweeter deal on that golf ball of his. Finnbar, be ready when he comes back. We wouldn't want him to get the drop on us."

The Irish skipper gets up and positions himself toward the back of the shop, out of sight. I keep wiping the floor with the towels I find.

"There's no back door to this lab, is there?"

"I don't think so."

"Good. Johnny, see if you can't hurry him along a bit."

"Sure."

I go to the bathroom and knock. All I hear in response is a big nothing. I call Joe's name, but he doesn't answer. I try the door and it's locked.

"He's not answering and the door's locked."

"The snake."

The fat man springs to his feet with surprising, almost frightening rapidity and storms back to the bathroom. Finnbar follows him. "Joseph? Are you all right, man?" He rattles the doorknob a couple of times. Then he lowers his shoulder and cracks the door open.

We all crowd the doorway, almost afraid to look. All we see is an open window and no Joe. The fat man sticks his huge head out the window and discovers a narrow airshaft rising to the roof. He's ten times too big to follow Akihiro aloft.

"Not happy to meet me, apparently. You should have had him over for dinner more often, Charles, he wouldn't have been able to squeeze his way out. I'd heard he had a variety of talents. I didn't know he was an acrobat."

"He's definitely a contortionist," says Granyer. "You

237

should have seen him climb out of that rattan basket."

"That was painful to watch."

"I was impressed when he climbed in and I shut the lid," says Finnbar. "He hardly made a peep."

"Do we know where he lives, Charles?"

"As far as I know, he lives here. There's a bedroom off the hallway back there."

"Seemed like a nice old guy who happened to know chemistry," I say, tossing in my two cents.

"He's wanted on three continents," says the banker. "He's a lesser prince, from what I hear, the Emperor's nephew. He refined the purest heroin in Asia. The aristocrats of Shanghai loved his work. But he got hooked himself, started making poor decisions. It became uncomfortable for him to stay."

The blonde slowly opens the front door and steps back into the lab. Granyer raises his voice: "Why don't we discuss this over dinner, shall we? It's time for supper. These chemicals are giving me a headache. I'll get a ride with my friends, Jean-Yves. You stay and figure out what Joe's done with my film. I must have it developed. And if he comes back, tell him he has nothing to worry about. He has my word."

"Where did he go?" Eva asks. "I didn't see anyone leave."

"He's vanished on us, and he didn't even say so much as 'Cheerio.'"

"It's true I was a little startled to see him," says the gentleman from Shanghai, putting on his coat. "I'd only seen his photo, and not a good one at that. But tell him I'm all for letting bygones be bygones. I'm intrigued by

his extraordinary golf ball. I might invest. I'll look
forward to discussing it over a round of golf. We'll see
how it performs under fire."

"I'll tell him, if he shows."

"Call me with updates, Johnny."

"Okay."

"What's on the menu tonight, Charles?"

"Lutefisk."

"What, pray tell, is lutefisk?"

"A Norwegian delicacy—fish that's packed in lye for
six months before it's prepared."

"Sounds ghastly."

"Not at all. We'll wash it down with aquavit. A
shipment's just come in that went around Cape Horn, all
the way from Norway. They took it the long way to give
it a good jostling."

"Hey, listen," the blonde suddenly pipes up, "I'm
tired. And I'm not really hungry. This lab's making me
sleepy. I want to go back to my apartment. Maybe John
can give me a ride? It's not far."

"I can give you a lift. Then I'll find the dailies."

"Are you sure, Eva? I can't vouch for lutefisk but
aquavit is a rarity. A most heady elixir!"

"I need a nap."

"John has work to do. We'll give you a ride home,
sweetheart." I didn't say anything. I waited to see how
this would play out.

"Will we all fit?"

"You know the Bentley."

"But, Department, you're big... you're larger than
life."

"Ha! *Très drôle*. You'll see. We've plenty of room."

"Then let's go. I hate chemistry."

Eva stands by the door and is forced to wait a little longer. The banker walks ponderously across the lab and bends over slowly to pick up Akihiro's golf ball and pocket it. As he straightens up, he notices one of the photographs on the lab wall. The one of Joe acting. He gives it a long look.

"After you, Eva. Gentlemen," says the banker.

"We'll try out that ball on our next round," Granyer says, making small talk.

"What do you mean 'We'll' try it?" the massive guy shoots back. "I'll try it!"

"Of course you will!"

As the three men bang out the door with their blonde friend, Granyer calls back: "Keep me posted, Johnny, about my movie. And about Joe. Persuade him to stick around, if he has a change of heart and comes back." I nod and watch them depart. The blonde turns and catches my eye.

"See you, Eva," I say.

"You will?"

"Definitely."

"It's in the cards?"

"I hope so. It might depend on the game."

She looks unconvinced. After a last look, not unsympathetic, she shrugs and follows the crowd. Finnbar slides in behind the Bentley's huge, white steering wheel. It's roomy, that's for sure. Even so, the huge guy punishes the back seat climbing in. I'm afraid he'll capsize the thing. Eva climbs in next to him, from the other side. Granyer slips in the front seat. Engine purring, the Bentley pulls away, crunching some gravel, listing to starboard. My head is spinning, and my heart is peppering me with questions. So that's Big Department. That certainly was my old girlfriend, Eva-Maria Fachsi.

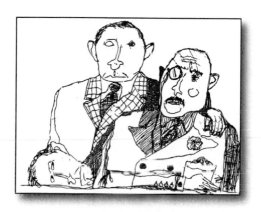

PART FOUR
THE DRAGON AND THE LOTUS

Ah, love, let us be true
To one another! for the world, which seems
To lie before us like a land of dreams,
So various, so beautiful, so new,
Hath really neither joy, nor love, nor light,
Nor certitude, nor peace, nor help for pain;
And we are here as on a darkling plain
Swept with confused alarms of struggle and flight,
Where ignorant armies clash by night.
—Matthew Arnold, "Dover Beach" (1867)

CHAPTER 49

IN COOL PURSUIT

Once they're gone and I find myself alone in the silence, I lock the front door, pocket the key, and toss a dry towel on the last of the spilled silver nitrate. I wipe it around with my shoe. That was a shock to see Fachsi. She looks tired. Some company she's fallen in with... Big Department. He's practically as big as my hopes once were. A gentleman from Shanghai. Last I heard he was in New York and Poochie was working for him.

I tell myself I'll find a private moment to talk to Fachsi. Then we'll see what's what. I pick up the black towel and drop it in a bucket. While I try to muster a thought or two, I slop the towel in the bathroom sink and turn on the faucet. Once it's exposed to light, silver nitrate turns black. That's how it works. It slowly washes out of the towel like some inky river in search of thoughts and paper. Joe is not coming back, I would bet.

He doesn't want to be reintroduced to Big Department, if he can help it.

I stick my head out the open bathroom window and inspect the airshaft. About twenty feet up is a square patch of sky. In the twilight, I can make out a metal ladder anchored to the wall opposite me.

I shove the bathroom window open as wide as I can. It's a bit tricky leaning out and grabbing onto the ladder, but I manage. I give it a shake to make sure it'll hold me. Then I pull myself the rest of the way out the window and clamber onto the ladder. Feet securely planted, I don't look down, and proceed to climb quickly to the roof.

I'm probably too late, but to have any chance of finding Joe, I figure I've got to go after him now. When I reach the roof, the sun is setting and the sky is stretching orange and pink for miles. This is a magical time of day in L.A. The houses are baking hot inside but the air on the rooftops is cooling off and the city is quiet and almost peaceful.

CHAPTER 50

THE ELUSIVE
INVENTOR

For half a second, the soft warm evening air almost persuades me to abandon my pursuit. It's delicious. I feel like sitting on the roof's ledge and just collecting my thoughts. But this is no time for daydreaming.

The buildings in Little Tokio are connected, some wooden, some brick. It's immediately apparent that when Joe fled to the roof, he had only one escape route. In three directions the adjoining buildings are either a story too tall or a story too low. And there aren't any ladders or fire escapes leading up or down. The rooftop to the building in front of me is the only one beckoning.

I swing myself over a four-foot high ledge and let myself down onto a tar rooftop. Night is falling and it's getting darker by the second. I can see fine. This roof also presents a single escape route. It has access to only one of the buildings connected to it. I slip over this next ledge and continue quietly exploring. Neither of these buildings has obvious entryways into the buildings themselves. No doorways or stairwells.

I creep along as quietly as I can, scale another ledge, and ease myself down onto the roof of what seems to be a pretty rickety wooden structure. The sun is down and what's left of the sunset is a dark purple gently bleeding into the black of night. The smell of jasmine fills the air.

Anything at all visible is visible to me and I have the feeling that I've found Joe's trail. The roof of this building has a small wooden-framed skylight that appears to be slightly ajar. The walls of the roof are lined with planter boxes and climbing jasmine. Their white blossoms are glowing in the twilight and their fragrance is heavy. I barely notice them. At best, any pleasing effect they have on me is subconscious.

I slip my fingertips under the edge of the dingy skylight and try lifting it up, as slowly and noiselessly as possible. It budges. Chains on either side hold it vertical when I get it open. A narrow ladder is visible, poking up out of the darkness. Where it leads is exceedingly dim.

I listen for sounds coming from inside. Nothing. I reach for the ladder and give it a shove to see how stable it is. It moves a little but seems fairly solid. I lower myself into the opening, feeling for a rung to rest my foot on. My right foot finds it and I begin my descent, rung by rung. I consider pulling the dirty skylight closed behind me but think better of it. What little light there is will help. And, anyway, who could possibly be after me? Fachsi? The Department? Not likely.

I keep descending cautiously. The air is musty. I

suspect I'm climbing into an abandoned building. I can't imagine that Joe has set up shop here, but I'm not turning back now. It might help me figure out where he's gone.

If I have the misfortune to run into anyone, I'll say I got trapped on the roof and this was the only way I could think to save myself.

A sudden gust of wind kicks up and the skylight overhead bangs shut! If anyone's here, they'll be coming to investigate any second now. I'm suspended in mid-air in utter darkness.

Seconds crawl by and my eyes adjust and I can see, or I think so anyway, a cluttered floor about twenty feet below me. I relax momentarily and take a deep breath. I take another step but there's no rung there. That's an unpleasant surprise. I slip and grab for the ladder with both hands but my left hand misses. I find myself clawing instead at a flat wall. My fingers find something solid to catch at and I try to steady myself by my fingertips. But it doesn't hold. Whatever it is tumbles out from under my hand and crashes in the shadows below.

My right hand has a death grip on one rung, though, and one of my feet has landed on a lot lower rung. A ladder missing the occasional rung is better navigated by day. I'm in a warehouse all right and I'm beginning to make it out. The walls are jammed from floor to ceiling with books.

CHAPTER 51

AN INNER SANCTUM

I climb the rest of the way down as quickly as I can while never taking either hand off the ladder. Once my toe finds the floor, I step off the ladder and heave a sigh of relief. Then I edge my way along a wall, making out some dark contours. I almost bang into another floor-to-ceiling ladder. I only see it when it's about six inches in front of my nose. Stepping around it, I make out a door. I try the doorknob. It turns and ever so slowly I push the door open.

Inside is a darkly glittering room, impossible to make out except for *quelques reflets*, a few reflections off some small golden lacquered boxes and a large three-paneled wooden screen. A candle seems to be lit somewhere back of it. I hear a rapid rustling sound and from behind the screen emerges a ghost-like cloud that floats straight toward me.

A candlestick appears and shadows climb the walls. I can see paintings and low chairs and a table with a scroll and pens and paintbrushes.

"Who's there?!" The white cloud coalesces into the powdered white face of a woman dressed in a dark kimono. It's Ariane. Dressed up. But only for a second do I think that it is she. In the candlelight, before my eyes, she ages fifty years.

This quite elderly woman barks at me in a hoarse voice: "What are you doing? Stay right there!" Her teeth are black. They make her look even paler, almost two-dimensional in the half-darkness. She's pointing a small gun at me.

"Excuse me. I'm sorry. I can explain. I got trapped on the roof. This was the only way I could get down."

"Put you hands up!"

"Of course, of course. I work at a film lab near here."

"Don't move, you."

"Is this the bookstore on Aliso Street? I'm a friend of the bookseller, Ariane."

"Ariane!" The old woman shouts weakly. We wait as she holds the gun on me. I hear someone running toward us and Ariane hurries in.

"Are you all right?" The two women confer rapidly in what I take to be Japanese.

Then the elderly woman in the kimono motions toward me. "He says he's a friend of yours... funny way to pay a visit!"

"Ariane, it's me, Jean-Yves. I'm sorry! I climbed up on the roof of the film lab to watch the sunset and the door locked behind me. I was stuck. The skylight was ajar. It was the only way I could get down. I had no idea it would bring me here."

"What a story! Put away your gun, Grandmother. I know Jean-Yves. He works for Charles Granyer."

"Hm."

"It's true. One of your loyal customers. Please forgive me for frightening you. What a crazy adventure, ending up in your bookshop like this. I thought I'd have to spend the night on the roof!"

"I'm glad you don't have to."

"Well, now that I'm back on *terra firma*, I certainly don't want to impose on you any more than I already have."

The grandmother says something else in Japanese to her niece.

"Come, Jean-Yves. Follow me."

"And don't try anything. I'm not putting down my gun until you're good and gone."

"Grandmother! That's really not necessary."

"Good riddance. The next character who tries coming in my rooms is going to get shot."

"A thousand apologies!"

"How am I supposed to get any work done?"

"Please forgive me. I am terribly sorry."

As we start to leave, Ariane's grandmother exclaims: "That skylight needs to be locked."

"Do you want me to do it?" I ask, trying in some way to make up for the disturbance.

"Yes I would!"

I slowly climb the ladder back up to the skylight, past the missing rungs, and slide a rusty bolt into place. I can see the bookshelves clearly now in the candlelight. From floor to ceiling shelves are lined with beautiful, leather bound books, many with gold filigree. The two women are waiting for me to make it down and go.

"Thank you, Jean-Yves."

"Of course. The least I could do."

"My advice? Stay off the roof. That route is shut for good."

"I'll take your advice, don't you worry. Thanks again for saving me from myself."

"That's up to you to do. In the future."

"Goodbye."

As I pass the elderly woman, she steps back to let me by and loses her balance. She quietly sits down on a carton of books.

"Oh, gad!"

"Are you all right?"

"It's just so frustrating."

"Here, I'll help you up, Grandmother."

"It's so embarrassing. People must think I'm drunk!"

"No, really. That's the last thing anyone would think."

"Let me help you to bed."

"Again, terribly sorry to have barged in on you like this."

"It's ridiculous. All I drink is tea!"

Ariane takes her grandmother by the arm and accompanies her off down a dark corridor. After a minute, she returns.

Ariane leads me out of her grandmother's drawing-room, past the wooden screen, through another large storage room lined with bookshelves and piled with boxes. Some of the boxes are sealed, some half-unpacked.

"My grandmother had a stroke a year ago. Since then she's become very unsteady on her feet. It's a shame."

"I'm sorry about that."

"She tips over. You just saw her. When she's around, I do my best to hover near her to try to catch her if she starts to fall. She's a brilliant writer. She writes marvelous poetry. I think I mentioned already, she's translating *Genji* into French. She's been working on it a long time. But her balance has completely deserted her."

"How is she with a pistol?"

"Probably pretty bad. I would hate to be an innocent bystander."

"How was I even able to get in through that skylight?"

"I have a roof garden. I must have forgotten to lock up after myself."

"That's what I smelled. What are you growing?"

"Tomatoes, for the most part. And jasmine. I enjoy the peacefulness of the evenings up there."

"I understand completely."

"I make corsages out of the flowers and sell them to the florist next door."

"I would never have guessed your bookstore was so enormous."

"It's not obvious from out front."

"Where do you buy your books?"

"We import most of them from Shanghai."

A heavy curtain hangs at the far end of this storeroom and when we pass through it we emerge into the bookstore and cross directly to the front door. The flowers in the window are also giving off a lovely perfume.

"*Merci, encore*," I say quietly.

"Okay, *salut*. You know where the entrance to the store is. I suggest you use it the next time you visit."

Ariane unlocks the door and I smile at her and leave. She doesn't try to make any more conversation and neither do I. Best to get, while the getting's good. I'm lucky the police aren't waiting for me.

I hear the lock turn in the door behind me and I look back and wave. She pauses in the window of the doorway for a second and then disappears through the curtains. Which way now? Left? Right? I try to orient myself, before deciding to turn right, which takes me toward the nearest corner. I circle back around a very long block to where Joe's lab and my car are. It gives me time to think.

Could they not know what's in the books they're selling me? They really seem much too nice to be drug smugglers. There must be some other explanation. I wonder if I should try to talk to Ariane about it. If she is in on it, it would just tip everyone off. They'd know I know too much. But if she doesn't know, maybe I can spare her some serious trouble. She might appreciate it. She probably would. And so might her grandmother, the tumbledown poet.

CHAPTER 52

A MAGIC SHOW

I unlock the door to Joe's lab and sleepwalk back inside. I flip a light on, slump down on a stool, and begin to think. Or rather, not to think. No one is going to be bothering me for a while, I can afford to close my eyes and rest the old cabbage. After a minute or maybe ten, I get up and start looking for Granyer's latest film shoot.

I'm scrutinizing some promising looking film canisters in the darkroom and thinking about Ariane and Fachsi and Joe's dramatic exit when I hear someone rapping at the front door. It's Joe, or should I say, Akihiro. He wants in pronto. I lock the door and kill the lights and we retreat to the lab in back, where we can talk bathed in the dim red light of the darkroom.

"While I'm still thinking about it, where is the footage from yesterday's shoot, Joe?"

"On those two reels. They come out fine, well

exposed."

"Granyer'll be happy to hear."

"I can't stay, John. Have to get some things. You understand. Big Department and I are no friends."

"They wanted me to tell you that all is forgiven. The Department said he might want to invest in your new golf ball."

"He say anything." Akihiro quickly begins shoving papers in an alligator suitcase.

"Where are you going?"

"Don't ask. Dangerous for you to know. I contact you. Our plan still on. You be my frontman, place orders, and we share profit after."

"I'm still in. Those guys were playing me for a patsy anyway. I don't appreciate it."

"Dishonest people. Stick with them and things turn out very, very bad."

"Just when we were about to make a fortune shorting Spalding and Wilson and Titleist."

"Golf ball just a magic show. The insides revolutionize more than golf. I think I discover man-made rubber. Synthetic rubber."

"Really?"

"Yes. I call it 'rubberish.' How that sound?"

"So-so. I'd keep working on that."

"Before only way to get rubber is from rubber trees. Now I make my own rubber. Fire is final step in process—intense heat."

"What do you make it out of?"

"Don't ask, Johnny. Trade secret."

"I understand."

"Once we make our short bets, we announce my invention. Bad news for all tire companies. Their shares pop and we make our fortune."

"Synthetic rubber."

"Yes, John. Cheap tires."

"We can short the spot market for rubber, too."

"We talk more in car. You give me lift, right? I lie in back seat and you drive."

"Sure. Do you have everything you need?"

"I think so. Go check out front. Let me know when coast is clear."

CHAPTER 53

DROPPING OFF THE DAILIES

I drop off Akihiro at a spot he directs me to, on the corner of a street I've never seen before, in the dark. We leave it that he'll contact me and let me know when to start putting our short bets in place. That he isn't actually an avuncular scientist is a surprise, I admit, but somehow I still trust him. If I never hear from him again, I guess that'll mean we just said *sayonara* rather than *au revoir*.

I swing back by the lab and grab the film for Granyer. I'm in no great hurry to get there, but until I figure out what my next move really is, I need to act as if everything is normal. When I get to Granyer's place, his lights are on and the front door is slightly ajar. Out painting the town red apparently. I wonder if Fachsi is with them. Damn their eyes! I turn off some lights and pull the door shut as Vince comes walking purposefully toward me over the lawn. He and I walk to our place in back, the tool shed. I climb into bed and pull the covers up over me. Vince jumps up and settles himself at the foot of the bed and begins purring. Soon he's whistling in his sleep.

I turn the light off and for some reason think of Manon, a long time ago, half-seen through the shower's frosted glass door. I don't know why I think of her all of a sudden. Our minds have a mind of a mind of a mind of a mind of a mind of their own. I turn the light back on and write a haiku in pencil:

> A wet girl, naked,
> toweling off. Rosy dawn,
> buffeted by clouds.

I won't write this one on the bookshop's blackboard.

CHAPTER 54

GRANYER'S DISAPPEARANCE EXPLAINED

The next day is a beautiful sunny day and there's no sign of life in Granyer's house. My phone rings. It's Granyer.

"I'm down at police headquarters, John. They've got me locked up. Damned inconvenient."

"What happened? Did Eva make a scene on the way home?"

"Who's Eva?"

"Big Department's blonde girlfriend."

"No, she had nothing to do with it. I threw a party to show my banker what fun L.A. can be. I invited a dozen sing-song girls, hired a band, and the whole thing got out of hand, too loud for the neighbors. It was a riot. The cops came and shut us down."

"They arrested you for disturbing the peace?"

"They arrested me for a number of preposterous things. They're not letting me out for a while. I don't know how long."

"Do you want me to come bail you out?"

"They're refusing me bail. They think my actresses are too young. I told them I could prove they were of age. They said they were going to make a big deal out of it in the newspapers. Smear me with making dirty movies. You know what I think? I think people don't like competition in this town."

"Could turn into a lot of free publicity."

"That's the spirit. I need you to finish filming *Genji* for me, Johnny, posthaste. While I'm getting all this press. I'll have my accountant send you funds."

"Wouldn't one of the other members of the crew be better suited...?"

"You're the only person I know who's read the book. You're practically the only person I know who reads books, period. The rest of us are devoted to the cinema."

"You should spend more time in bookstores."

"I don't have time for that. Now listen, we need one last scene. The one with the mad woman. You've got the book. Find it and put together a shooting script."

"Right."

"When you've got the script done, the cinematographer and the editor can take over. You know them. But first we need the script. I need you to find the scene and transcribe it."

"Won't the police raid us and confiscate the footage?"

"How will they know? Anyway, my lawyer's taken care of that."

"Yeah?"

"He argued in court that shutting down my film

would be added punishment exceeding the usual sentence for my peccadilloes. Cruel and unusual punishment. Or double jeopardy."

"Hm."

"The court agreed. The police have to let us continue, provided we stop filming people rolling around on top of each other naked. And, believe it or not, you have no choice, either. He checked on that, too. You'd be contributing to my uncalled-for financial ruin. The answer's yes, right, you'll do it?"

"Of course."

"Excellent. I knew I could count on you. We'll shoot that last scene, edit it in, and call it a movie. Hold a premiere. Start playing it non-stop in my theater. Sell buckets of tickets."

"The cast keeps its clothes on?"

"That would be wise."

"Which lab should I use, now that Joe's disappeared?"

"Any of them. This won't be the same sensitive material. You get me? Under no circumstances is it to be the same kind of material!"

"I'll work on the script tonight. We'll get started with the shooting when I hear from your accountant."

"Okay, Johnny, don't let me down. And turn off the lights in my house and lock up."

"Where's the gentleman from Shanghai?"

"I'm not sure. It was too hot at the party. When people started keeling over, he beat it. He got lucky."

"So did I."

"I wouldn't go looking for him, even to see that girl."

"Yeah, maybe." I'm not interested in seeing Big

Department. I would like to talk to Eva-Maria. For old times' sake.

Later that afternoon, Finnbar shows up at the door to my shed. He asks me if Akihiro ever came back. I level with him. I tell him that he did, but that frankly he's nervous. He throws a scare into me by suddenly reaching inside his coat. I think he's going for a gun. I recoil and start to dive for cover. He tells me not to be so jumpy. He pulls a check out of his coat pocket and hands it to me. It's made out to me, for $10,000. He says Big Department wants to invest in the golf ball and that this money is to show Joe he has no hard feelings. His one request is that we make him an outsized profit. I notice my hand trembling as I take the check from him. I wish I could make it stop.

The next day I get a call from Joe. He's still lying low. I tell him that Big Department is in to the tune of ten G's. We can start placing our short bets. We agree we should short the spot market for rubber, rubber futures, and the shares of all the major tire companies.

He's poised to go public with his discovery as soon as we have our short positions in place. I give him the news that Granyer's in jail. We agree that's one party we're lucky not to have been invited to. He tells me he'll be in touch and hangs up. I place our short bets with a broker at the Los Angeles Stock Exchange. For good measure, I short Spalding and Wilson and Titleist.

CHAPTER 55

RECRUITING ARIANE

That evening I open my beautiful old copy of *The Tale of Genji* and comb through it to find the story of the mad woman. It's a long novel but eventually I fall upon it. I draft a shooting script and use several sheets of carbon paper to make copies.

The next morning I drive over to Ariane's bookshop. It's cloudy out. On the blackboard is written another haiku:

In dead of winter,
jutting from blue and grave hills,
a bone-colored moon.

I read it a few times carefully. Inside I scan the shop for signs of the more obvious miscreants. No one's there. The air is fragrant with incense, though. As I approach the counter, I hear light footsteps and Ariane steps out from behind the painted screen that hides the passageway to the store's cavernous book repository.

"*Salut*, Ariane."

"*Salut*, Jean-Yves. You used the front door!"

"Indeed. Thank you again for the other night. Saving me from being taken for a second-story man."

"It was rather strange having you drop in on us like that."

"I had no idea where I was. That was lucky, really, for me anyway."

"It's all okay now. My grandmother was alarmed, understandably, but she got over it."

"I'm glad she didn't have a heart attack."

"Or shoot first and ask questions later!"

"Say, did you ever talk to Fritz Lang?"

"No. I never called him. He has so many actresses to choose from."

"You're still a 'sometime actress,' though, aren't you?"

"I find it amusing."

"We have one last scene in *Genji* to shoot. The one that Granyer mentioned to you. The one with the mad woman."

"Ah."

"Do you still want the role? We plan to shoot it soon, in the next few days."

"Why not? My grandmother can run the shop. I remember the scene from the book. It's not terribly complicated."

"No, but it's dramatic."

"Yes. It's quite memorable."

"I have a script for you then."

"Nice."

"Let me know what you think. Maybe you'll have some suggestions…"

"Sure."

"I'll be curious to know."

"This is exciting."

"I can give you a ride to the shoot, if you want."

"That would be convenient."

"We'll know soon which day we're shooting."

"Okay. You'll have costumes, everything I need?"

"Yes. We'll have everything for you there."

"*A bientôt, alors.*"

"*Oui, c'est ça.*"

"How did you like today's haiku?"

"I liked it and the wordplay on 'grave' and 'gray.' Quite somber."

"My Grandmother said she was thinking of a huge winter moon she saw once when she was a girl in Japan."

CHAPTER 56

A DAY OF RECKONING

I get a call later that day. It's Granyer's accountant, his apoplectic golf pal.

"John Still?"

"Yes?"

"Johnny Boy, this is Stuart Blanchard, Charles Granyer's accountant."

"I've been expecting your call."

"He tells me you're moving up in the world, that you're going to oversee the completion of his film."

"I'm willing."

"But you'll need the wherewithal to do so."

"Exactly."

"Come by my office and I'll give you some petty cash. For all other expenses, you're to have vendors send me the bill."

"That should work. What's my boss charged with?"

"They're accusing him of smuggling saké."

"Prohibition's been repealed."

"And heroin trafficking."

"Hm."

"And prostitution."

"Hm."

"And white slavery."

"At the moment, I believe they're screening a choice reel of *The Tale of Genji*. One that was meant for private parties. I think they're going to accuse him of being a pornographer, too, for good measure."

"*Zut.*"

"He told them it was art, and as the saying goes, they laughed mirthlessly."

"*Zut, alors.*"

"His real problem is they're going to charge him with attempted murder."

"Oh, là."

"But his lawyer's going to fight it. Someone brought some drug to his party and people went crazy. All hell broke loose."

"What was it?"

"The lab says it was a combination of cocaine, elephant tranquilizer, and Spanish fly."

"*Quelle honte.*"

"A young guy went berserk and started shooting up the place. He didn't clip anybody, just let in some starlight. But three girls overdosed and ended up in the hospital. When the police arrived, they came in swinging their billy clubs as if they worked for Pinkerton's and were breaking up a longshoremen's strike."

"Granyer wasn't hurt?"

"He only drank champagne that night. And when things got frantic, he told me he took cover behind his Chinese gong. Like a true gentleman. He's not going to be swindling his friends at golf anytime soon."

CHAPTER 57

SHOOTING GENJI AGAIN

Three days later, with a film crew lined up, I drive over to pick up the bookseller. I offer a haiku of my own, not wanting to disrupt our exchange. I quickly write on the blackboard outside The Dragon and The Lotus:

> Blue turns to black, but
> blazing and improbable
> sunsets intervene.

Ariane lets me in looking wide-awake. She's wearing a light-yellow silk dress. "Have a seat. I've a treat for you." She goes over to the white flowers growing in her window planter and carefully extracts a small packet from one of the flowers. The flower is just starting to open in the morning sun. She comes toward me smiling and holds a sachet up to my nose.

"Tea?"

"My special green tea. I let it steep in jasmine over-night..."

"...sleep in jasmine..."

"...and now I will brew some for you."

"*J'ai de la chance!*"

"Yes, you're in luck. A trick I learned from *The Memoirs of a Poor Chinese Scholar.*"

"Beautiful. I can't wait to try it."

She and the tea have an almost mystical effect on me. Instead of driving to the film studio, it seems as if we simply float there, except for the glaring and predictable stoplights that intervene. Ariane assures me that she's learned the role of the mad woman and that she's looking forward to the day's shoot.

When we open the studio, we're confronted with the cold debris of some previous debauchery. It's clear it was one of those classy soirées where people amused themselves spilling drinks, knocking things over, and taking a tumble. The place is a shambles. *Un vrai bordel.* I apologize and set Ariane up outside on a folding chair, until we're ready to do her makeup and hair and can let her change into costume. She takes the delay in good spirits, saying it will give her time to reread the script.

The crew and I open the doors, windows, and skylights to air the place out. An hour-and-a-half of cleaning and the place is in shape for filming.

This last scene takes place in the mad woman's bedroom. The soundman and I arrange the set, a living room big enough for the three Japanese actors—the mad woman, her husband, and his attendant. Light meter in

hand, the cinematographer adjusts the lighting and the
skylights. He confers with the three actors after they've
put on their costumes and makeup.

We're ready. Ariane takes a seat on a cushion on the
floor of the bedroom. Her hair is disheveled and her
makeup slightly smeared. Her eye shadow, lipstick, and
nails are all painted dark gray. Her silk kimono is a pale
blue. It almost appears to be carried aloft by the deep
blue cranes embroidered on it. After giving me a quick
glance and a blink of recognition, she falls into the
trance of an actress entering into her role. She sits stock-
still, half watching, half dreaming.

The cinematographer implores the actors to
concentrate. He would like to film the main action
without a cut. As he explains, he's hoping to capture the
most dramatic moment in a single take, as if the actors
were performing in the theater, letting the intensity of
the actors build. It isn't a scene that can be done again
and again. Having written the shooting script, I know
why. He has the actors rehearse the scene once, twice,
three times.

Then, satisfied, we begin in earnest. He cues the
lights, the camera begins whirring, and the actors begin.

The imposing fellow who plays the husband, a general
in the Japanese imperial army, is being helped on with a
fancy dress kimono by his manservant. He's going out
for the evening. The bookseller, who plays his unhappy
wife, accuses him of going to see his mistress. He doesn't
even pretend otherwise. Such arrogance is maddening.

Looking elegant and impossibly self-satisfied, he is
about to leave for the evening when his wife climbs to

her feet. She picks up the incense burner smoking in the corner of the room and dumps the burning cinders on his head. The embers trickle down his silk kimono and begin burning dozens of holes in the fabric. His attendant tries to brush off the burning incense. The general's hair and face are powdered with gray ash.

Ariane backs away, letting the incense burner fall on the floor, crouching and cowering in fear, smiling in hatred and triumph. The husband curses her but he restrains himself, knowing she's ill, convinced she's unhinged. The attendant wrestles her out of the bedroom, then returns to help the husband out of the ruined kimono, getting him another to wear. We succeed in filming her act of revenge in a single take, and Ariane is towering, magnificent, nothing like her usual self, nothing like a quiet, retiring scholar.

The next day we have the film processed. It's perfect, a triumph, and the editor can now add the final piece to Part 1 of the epic film version of *The Tale of Genji*.

CHAPTER 58

GOING SHORT

The next day Joe calls and tells me he's gotten involved in a stock car race to be run that afternoon. And that it might be an important development. The results are published in the newspaper. His car was the front runner from the start and won. When the reporter interviews the winning driver, he drops a bomb. He tells the reporter that his car won racing on a new kind of synthetic rubber tire.

The story gets picked up by the wire services. The next day it hits *The Wall Street Journal.* The day after that *The New York Times, The Financial Times,* and *The Times of London.* Investors can see the implications and the share prices of tire companies start to sag. Joe calls, beside himself with glee. How far down will the shares go, he wonders? When do we buy the shares back? How greedy can we be? Is it time to hold a press conference to explain his break-through discovery in more detail? To reveal himself as the man behind the tires? Not only will we drive the prices even lower, but some rubber company will certainly want to buy the rights to his invention. We'll make money coming and going.

Then something happens that we didn't anticipate. Word hits the news that Germany is rearming, violating the Treaty of Versailles. The price of rubber firms back up. Our short positions start throttling us. *Et là, naturellement, j'ai un moment de solitude.* I've become the master of my fate, the captain of a boatload of trouble.

CHAPTER 59

MORE SHOOTING

My phone rings and before I can even start in with any social niceties, there's someone braying in my ear. "You gotta put up more money on your short positions. That's the way it is, Still. The tire companies are up 20% today and their shares are soaring." It's Squidrow on the horn, my broker at the Los Angeles Stock Exchange.

"I'll call you back," I say and hang up.

I have to think. The Japanese are armed and forcing their way into China. Now the Germans are rearming. War devours natural resources. How long will it last? Probably longer than I can afford to be wrong. Someone has to cover these short positions. And if we do, at that point we'll take another huge loss.

The phone rings. It's the gentleman from Shanghai. He dives right in. "Okay, start talking, where is he?"

"Who?"

"Akihiro!"

"How should I know? Last I saw he was headed to the bathroom to wash himself off."

"Don't give me that. Finnbar told me you've been in touch with him. You're helping him put over that damn rubber deal. You must know how to reach him."

"I'll try."

"Akihiro's going to have to make me whole. He gave me a bum steer and now he has to take it off my hands. Our contact at the Los Angeles Stock Exchange is laughing at us. He says war is imminent and it's giving the rubber market a real boost. He's terribly obnoxious about it and we used to be quite friendly."

"He called me, too, threatening me."

"I don't like my friends getting cocky at my expense."

"War profiteering is fine by him, apparently."

"Going to war with me won't be. Okay, Still, this is what you're going to do. You're going to track down the chemist and we're all going to sit down with the stockjobber and come to an understanding."

"Maybe I can find him. I'll call you back."

I hang up and dial a number. After it rings a couple dozen times, Joe answers.

"Yes?"

"Joe, it's me. And I've got bad news. The short play is a bust. We've got to get out now. Where can I meet you? Every second counts. Okay. Okay. At the bookshop? Okay. See you there in 20 minutes."

I call the Department back and give him the address to The Dragon and The Lotus.

"And call the guy at the stock exchange, Squidrow.

What a name! Tell him to meet us there. Akihiro better be full of bright ideas."

I dial Squidrow's number and arrange for him to meet us. "We'll be there in a half-hour. We'll get this straightened out," I promise.

"That would be wise."

I head outside and climb into the Hudson. It's another hot, washed-out L.A. morning.

The Dragon and The Lotus is open for business, and the Department is already there. I must say, when he's around, one's a crowd. He's driven himself, the Irish skipper apparently having had other things to do. Ariane is behind the counter, looking on edge but happy to see me. I try to explain in French what's going on but the fat man cuts me off, letting us know that he can understand.

"If you don't mind, please lock the door." The Department is giving orders now. "I'm afraid we're going to have to deprive your customers of their literary diversions for the time being." A couple minutes later, Squidrow, the broker from the Los Angeles Stock Exchange, knocks. With the fat man's nod of approval, Ariane lets him in. It's getting stuffy inside.

"What kind of penny-ante operation is this?" Squidrow wants to know.

"Don't talk to me about penny-ante. I'm still gagging on those penny-ante stocks you force-fed me."

"I told you twelve-times-tomorrow, Department, they're penny stocks. Penny. Stocks."

"Regardless, you foisted them on me and you owe me."

"Okay, Department. But the way things stand, you

owe me more for the tire company shares you borrowed. I'd like them back. Besides, it's in your interest to cover the short positions. The market can smell war 1,000 miles off. The shares are going sky-high. The boys think they're worth a lot more than what you got for them. I'd like to sell them myself."

"You're feeling rather chipper about this, aren't you?"

"If your plan had panned out, you'd be plenty cheery yourself."

"It may still. That's the point of this meeting. We're going to persuade Akihiro, when he graces us with his presence, that it's in his best interests to give us a healthy share of the royalties from his invention. To help him to ease out from under his debt. Once his synthetic rubber's in production, we'll all make a small fortune. Especially if there's a real war."

"It's tempting. But it's too dicey to take care of today's more urgent matter. This is a margin call, Department. If you don't want to buy back the shares you borrowed and return them to me, you need to put another $20,000 down to keep your short positions where they are."

"Where's that blasted Akihiro? We're not going to resolve this without him."

"He's supposed to meet us here. This is the neutral ground he wanted."

"It looks like he's stood us up. As they say, time and the markets wait for no man. What'll it be, Department?"

"You're starting to get on my nerves, Squidrow."

"I've got to get back to the office. I did you a favor coming here. Time to settle up like gentlemen."

"Okay, Still, where in blazes is Joe? We're losing money as we speak."

"If I knew, I'd tell you."

From the back of the bookstore comes the sound of footsteps. The curtains behind the counter part and Ariane's grandmother comes shakily into the room. She addresses Ariane in a husky voice, speaking to her in Japanese. The two go back and forth, both clearly upset.

"I understand," Ariane says in English. "It should only be a few minutes." Her grandmother silently admonishes her with a last look before she retreats back into the recesses of her bookshop.

The Department cuts to the chase. "Okay, Squidrow. What'll it cost me to buy these shares back?"

"I'll call the Exchange."

Ariane passes the phone to the broker who dials the stock market. He checks the current prices with a colleague.

"As of this moment, it would cost $34,000 to close out your positions."

"Prices still rising?"

"That's the word."

"Okay. No use sitting on our hands. Buy them."

Squidrow says into the phone: "Buy them and put them back on our books. Yeah, that's right. They're covering their shorts."

"We're covering something."

"Correct. They're coming back home where they belong."

Department pulls out a checkbook, sits down heavily at the shop counter, and begins writing. I'm thinking

about my good fortune, not having had any money to invest. He tears out the check, looks at it a bit longingly, and hands it to the broker. Squidrow gives it a glance and slips it in his billfold.

"Thank you, Department, for your, uh... *largesse*. There'll be other opportunities. I'll see if I can't bring you in on a better deal, something sure-fire."

"Let me get the door," says Ariane.

"No need. I can find my way out."

Big Department just gives him a dull look. He's wheezing. Squidrow adopts a professional look of commiseration. He gives a nod of adieu, pushes through the curtains in front, and bangs the door. Big Department waits a moment before laughing without any humor at all.

"That check isn't worth the paper it's written on. I'm calling my bank and putting a stop on it. But meantime our bet isn't getting any worse. We stopped the bleeding."

"I'm not sure that's going to work," I can't help saying.

"If I ever get my hands on that inventor, I'm going to thank him personally for bringing me in on this deal."

"Go ahead and thank me."

We turn and there's Ariane's grandmother, pointing a gun at Big Department. Her feet are planted squarely on the ground.

"Granny, put the cap gun away. I wasn't talking about you."

"Oh, no?" And then it becomes obvious. The elderly woman wrapped in the green-and-silver kimono is Akihiro.

I try to intercede. "Department, you don't want to put a stop on that check. Sometimes, like right now, the best thing you can do is cut your losses."

"The hell I am. Akihiro over there is going to make me whole if it's the last thing he does."

"We can discuss that, of course."

"You're going to give me royalties from your invention. I might excuse your *maladresse* for a sizable percentage..."

"It's possible."

"It's definite. But first I'm calling the bank. Please allow me."

"Be my guest."

The Department pauses before he rises to his feet. His face is a splotchy red. He looks as if he's literally gnashing his teeth. As he lumbers across the room, Joe steps to one side of the counter to let him through. I follow and try to get between them to keep things from getting out of hand. The Department picks up the receiver and starts dialing. At the same time, he reaches behind him and takes hold of the beautiful, heavy, antique screen that hides the corridor to the rest of the bookshop. It depicts a group of young women painting and writing poetry. He rips it so hard forward, and so suddenly into Joe and me, that he succeeds in knocking us both over. For a disorienting moment or two, we find ourselves under the fallen screen's beautiful, serene young ladies. We could be actors in one of those turbulent Hokusai woodcuts, just minus all the fun. I'm lucky Joe doesn't accidentally shoot me.

The Department kicks the gun out of Joe's hand.

Then he reaches down and grabs Joe by the neck and starts squeezing. With his other hand he seizes me by the neck. He's so big and strong, he hauls us up off the floor easily. We get to see him enjoy his revenge as he strangles us. It's not a sight anyone can enjoy for long. As Joe's face turns dark red, I spy Ariane's jade letter opener on the counter and I struggle with everything I have left to reach it. The big man is too quick. Before I can close my hand around it, he dashes me flat on my back.

Somewhere behind us, a gun goes off. And it's from this lowliest of low angles that I see the Department's surprise at getting shot. He feels the back of his neck, then he buckles and falls squarely on Joe. They hit the deck and twenty books are bucked off their shelves.

I crawl over to where Joe is squawking the tune of someone asphyxiating. I pry the Department's hand from his throat. The way the Department is bleeding from the bullet wound in his neck, there's clearly nothing to do for him. He's finished his round. I try to roll the Department off Joe. In this wrestling match, the behemoth is determined to go out a dead winner and does nothing to cooperate. The guy must weigh a thousand pounds.

For a moment he gives me a vaguely dirty look and his arms and legs twitch. Then he takes on the appearance of someone lost in thought, as if he were trying to remember a point he wanted to make.

I turn away expecting to see Ariane holding a gun, but instead I see Squidrow standing there.

"I thought I better stick around. I figured the guy was going to try to stiff me."

"Lucky."

"I couldn't let him murder two of my best customers."

"Help me move him, would you?"

Squidrow and Ariane both help. She's crying what sounds like "*Tonton*" and quaking. We tug and shove and pull on the dead man, trying to tip him to one side without completely bulldozing Joe. We manage to create enough daylight for Joe to wriggle free.

The Department's face is turning gray. He bears a slight resemblance to Granyer's undercooked carp. Joe looks decidedly unwell himself, moaning on the floor, covered in blood. The wig he's worn has fallen off and his kimono is stained red. We are all quietly screaming in our own way. Very quietly, not wanting to rouse the neighbors. So far no one has come investigating the sound of that gunshot.

Ariane is the first to move. She gets up and goes to the counter and begins writing.

"What are you doing?"

"Cancelling the book club."

"Good idea."

She hurries to the front door, locks back up, and pastes the notice in the window to ward off the club members, who are scheduled to arrive any minute. She also closes the blinds.

Joe climbs to one knee, then gets unsteadily to his feet.

"Thank you for saving me."

"Don't mention it."

"That was a nice shot."

"He's as big as a barn. I practically missed."

"But not quite."

He holds the gun out to Joe. "Here. Wipe my prints off, eh?"

"Certainly."

"I mean right now."

"Okay." Joe takes a handkerchief and carefully wipes down his pistol.

"Dangerous business, finance," Squidrow observes.

"Clearly."

"Will you all be all right?"

"I hope."

"Now I'm really off. I'm going to bank his check while it's still warm."

"Don't worry about police," Joe says. "We all witnesses, you saved our lives."

"You're going to the police?"

"No. No police."

"If it can be avoided, it would be a lot less complicated," says Squidrow. "In any event, I was never here."

"Of course not."

"I mean it."

"Sure, sure."

Ariane unlocks the door and lets Squidrow out. Joe trails off and Ariane follows him, leaving me with the dead man's corpse. Ariane comes back with towels and blankets and tries to dam the pool of blood spreading across the bookshop floor. The Department is sprawled on a big Persian rug, which is soaking up a lot of blood. Ariane and I pick the screen back up and position it in front of the counter to hide the dead man. Joe returns eventually. He's washed himself off and changed clothes.

"How are we going to get rid of him? He's the size of a Greyhound bus."

"The three of us can't move him."

"Can you give me one of those blankets? I can't stand seeing him there."

Joe and I spread a horsehair blanket over his corpse. Then we take one edge of the rug he's fallen on and fold it up over him. At least he isn't just croaking there in broad daylight anymore.

"We wait till sundown. We have time," Joe says, thinking out loud. "No one's looking for him here."

"What about your grandmother, Ariane?"

"She's away."

"It was obviously self-defense. Or justifiable homicide."

"He went crazy."

"First he strangling us like kittens. Then he squash me like roach. I'm sore all over."

"No one's calling the police," I say. "They're probably on his payroll. For the police, we're nothing but a pay cut. We just did away with their meal ticket."

"That Squidrow was some cool customer," says Ariane.

"What if he'd actually left when he said he was leaving?"

"Or missed?"

"He better change before he goes to the bank. Blood money."

"When sun goes down, I make a call," Joe says.

Ariane goes into the back. Joe and I position a table over the corpse. We throw a blanket over the table and stack some books on it. I can't help thinking that it's some kind of crude metaphor for the world's "thin veneer of civilization" and all that.

"Let's find my niece."

So that's it. Joe's her uncle. Her *Tonton*. All one big happy family. As we wend our way back, Ariane is nowhere to be seen. I use the bathroom and wash as much gore off as I can. When I come out, no one is there. Almost ineluctably, I walk to the ladder at the back of the storage room, the one that leads to the roof garden. The skylight is open.

I climb the ladder, navigating the broken rungs, and hoist myself onto the roof. It smells like a funeral. Ariane is there among her jasmine, leaning against the wall, balancing on one leg. The other is pulled up and the sole of her foot is flush against the calf of the leg she's standing on. She looks like Shiva. Joe is sitting in a chair in the shade of the plants looking solemn. Who can blame him?

I come over and we all just breathe in the fragrance of the jasmine and hold our peace. We have time before the sun goes down. There will be time to talk of important matters. For now we'll simply meditate.

I eventually break the silence and begin asking Ariane and Akihiro some of the questions I have for them. "Do you really even have a grandmother, Ariane?"

"Of course I do."

"Well, where is she?"

"Out of town, visiting her sister in San Francisco. She won't be back for a few days."

"Was that really your grandmother, who met me when

I climbed down the ladder the other night?"

"Absolutely."

"Did your uncle come down the same ladder that night before me?"

"Yes, Jean-Yves, he did."

We lapse back into silence. Then Ariane says, "I have a question for you, too... Who's that dead man downstairs?"

"He was the head of the Green Gang in Shanghai," says Joe. "Big international crook."

"How did you know him, Jean-Yves?"

"From New York," I say. "I made the mistake of contacting one of his associates about your uncle's business proposition."

"Some mistake. Especially for him." We all invest some silence in thinking about that.

"How did you end up in L.A., Ariane?"

"Shanghai was poison. The French section was lawless. That's how I met Charles Granyer. He's the one who got me out. I crossed the Pacific with him."

"Were you his girlfriend?"

She shakes her head. "I was no sing-song girl. I was an actress. He owned the nightclub where I performed."

"*Il est un vrai mythomane.*"

"He does exaggerate, but he's got some good sides to him. Even so, I didn't trust him. I let him know I was armed. I was prepared to defend myself, if he'd tried to take advantage."

"What was his reaction?"

"He laughed a bit nastily. I'll give him this, though, I never had to remind him. It might have been unnecessary to warn him like that, but I didn't want to find out otherwise, when it was too late. He's not at all my type." She lets that sink in for a bit and I enjoy letting it.

"Joe, are you really Ariane's uncle?"

"I'm your father's younger brother, aren't I, Ariane?"

"Of course you are. My uncle was becoming a well known actor when Shanghai started to fall apart."

"When I fell apart," he says.

"The Department says you're actually the Emperor's nephew?"

"Hah! Very funny. I play him once in a theater in Kyoto."

"Maybe he saw the play and is confabulating."

"I don't know. Maybe. I know people who can help," Akihiro says. "We get through this."

"Should I perhaps go down and check on the gentleman?"

"Where's he going to go, John?"

"I have another question for you, Jean-Yves... It's a big question. Do you believe in God? Or karma?"

"Why do you ask?"

"*Comme ça.*"

"Do I believe in God? Goddesses, yes. Squidrow showing up when he did was providential, I'll say that."

"What I'm wondering is whether this is fated? Or just some terrible mistakes and accidents?"

"I'm sure I don't know. I'm going to wait and see."

"I don't want to wait to know God," says Ariane quietly. "I can't help but think about what the Heian Japanese believed: That our lives are as ephemeral as dew on the lotus."

"But what's that have to do with God?"

"It means our time here is fleeting. We shouldn't put off thinking about the important questions."

"What about you Joe?"

"Scientists explain things scientifically. But I believe in karma. No waiting for karma, either."

With Big Department downstairs dead and us on the roof in limbo, our conversation again evaporates. Or sublimes. I concentrate on the fragrance of Ariane's rooftop garden. She sits tilted over now, deep in her own thoughts. Her mouth looks like a hyphen. Joe looks like a cipher.

"What about those books I've been buying and handing out all over town? That was a mean trick to play on me."

Ariane looks surprised. "I thought you enjoyed *Genji?*"

"I'm talking about what was in the books."

"What do you mean? The story is in the books."

"There was more, though, wasn't there, Joe."

"We talk later, okay?"

"Heroin. In the covers."

"What?! I didn't know a thing!" Ariane protests.

"I'm sorry, Ariane. Hard to stop. I try. Big Department and Granyer make me do it."

"That was a pretty rotten way to use your niece and me."

"I make it up to you."

"Do I still have any of your special books in my bookshop?"

"Three or four boxes."

"Are others on the way?"
"I think so, but I'll cancel the rest, I promise."
"After the dead man, the books are next to go."
"Agreed."

CHAPTER 60

THE SANITATION DEPARTMENT

At 8:30 p.m., Akihiro makes his call, after disguising himself again as the old chemist. He looks completely different with gray hair and makeup.

"I have drain problem. Yes. Can you send me plumbers? At least four. Make it six, to be sure. Very big job."

He rings off and twenty minutes later we hear a discreet rat-a-tat-tat at the door. Joe tells Ariane and me to stay out of sight in back. He goes out and peers through a gap in the curtains. It's the company he's expecting. Acme Plumbing. He unlocks the door and six burly Asian guys wearing beat-up gray hats and carrying bulky bags come stalking in one after the other.

"Where's the clog?"

"Over here." Joe slowly walks over to the table covering the Department and pats it.

"Nice rug."

"Not any more. You can have it. I don't want it. Just want it removed and my drain running again."

"How'd it happen?"

"How does anything happen? It needs to unhappen."

"None of my business anyway."

"It's a distraction. Bad for business."

The guy lifts the blanket and looks under the table. "That's some load."

"I know."

"Five hundred and we flush it for you."

"I have something maybe you take instead."

"What?"

"That Bentley outside. Owner lost his license. Permanently."

The plumber goes over to the door and peers out. He takes a good look at the Department's limousine. "Deal. Let's see the keys."

"Should be on him."

After this deal's struck, these guys are the height of efficiency. They move the table out of the way and empty the Department's pockets. Then they roll him up as snug as a bug in a rug. Joe kills the lights and one of the guys cracks the front door to take a look around. It's late and the street's deserted. Another guy follows when he gives the signal. They duck into an alley and slide off a manhole cover. The other four beefy guys play pallbearers. They lug the deceased down the alley where they plan to dump him rug and all into the Los Angeles sewer system. Joe follows to make sure all goes as planned. The Department's so immense he gets stuck, but with six guys shoving, they succeed in thrusting him on through the opening and down. He makes quite a splash.

Joe comes back inside alone. "No more Department."

"Jeez."

"*Tonton*, can you please take your books, too? I really don't want them here."

"John, you help me? We drive them to my lab. No one around to see us."

"Sure."

The three of us go through the shop's back warehouse and find the books that have to go. There are four heavy boxes. We decide to forge ahead, since it's still dark out. Joe and I move the boxes to the front door, while Ariane works to wash away the last traces of the Department's demise. She's exhausted, as we all are, and impatient and exasperated and distressed. Understandably.

Sure no one's in sight, we fill the Hudson with the books and drive the short distance to Joe's lab. Some go in the trunk, some in the back seat. Maybe we should have just dumped them somewhere but Joe says he knows someone who'll take them off his hands. It can be tough to stop kicking the gong around, or resist making money selling the stuff.

We're about to unload our reading material when a man steps out of the shadows. It's Finnbar, the Irish sailor, and he's got a gun in his hand. Not another guy with a gat.

"Gents."

"What's the gag?"

"Where Big Department, Johnny?"

"Beats me. Must be in bed by now."

"He's not at his hotel."

"Well, what are you pointing that thing at me for?"

"I want your full attention."

"You've got it. Quit pointing that."

From the opposite direction, another man appears. A very large man. He's holding a gun, too, though it's more the size of a small cannon.

"How's you and me?" he asks.

"Poochie."

"Johnny."

"Who's the weed in the thousand-mile shirt?"

"A colleague of mine."

"The hell he is," says Finnbar. "That's the escape artist with the golf ball."

"Where were you this afternoon, Finnbar? You're kind of an escape artist yourself. The Department says you left him high and dry."

"When'd you see him?"

"I talked to him on the phone. Granyer had me call him about playing a round of golf."

"The screws collared me for a wrong bit," Finnbar says, incensed.

"What for?"

"Some highway mopery."

"A big deal around here. Jaywalking."

"I explained to the copper, 'I'm from New York,' I sez. 'Where I'm from, when it's green, we walk, and when it's red, we walk.' He said he didn't like smart guys from New York and that this wasn't New York. He was gonna have to teach me a lesson about walking in L.A."

"Had nothing better to do, I guess."

"Said I better think twice the next time I try to walk in his town. I tried to ring up the Department, but there was no answer. I'm lucky Poochie showed and put up the twenty clams. They said they might just keep me till kingdom come. Said I was a menace to the natural ebb and flow of traffic."

"They gave Finnbar a floater," says Poochie.

"Yeah, I got twenty-four hours to leave town."

"But I ain't no disappearing act, Johnny," Poochie says quietly. "I'm a balancing act. Finnbar thought we might find you here. You and your syndicate have some settling to do. You said it was gonna be duck soup."

I'm thinking things over when Akihiro speaks up. "We settle with you, no problem. We have some precious cargo in our car. You can have it."

"What is it?"

"Junk hidden in books from Shanghai. Valuable to right customer."

"How valuable?"

"Very."

"Let's see."

I open the door to the back seat and let Poochie peep in one of the boxes of books.

"Mooch. In the covers. They're brimming with the stuff."

"You're making progress. But it ain't enough. We lost a fortune on your penny-ante schemes."

Finnbar has an idea. "What about the sailboat? We could use that, too. This town is beat."

"Okay," I say. "I'll drive you to Granyer's and hitch the

yacht to the Hudson." The sailboat is actually Big Department's, but as Aldo might have said, the tough customer is always right, and anyway, at this point, the gentleman from Shanghai ain't gonna miss it.

"Yeah? Then what?"

"Then I chauffeur you to a cove I know and you'll be on the sail."

Finnbar quietly confers with the big galoot: "What say you, Poochie?"

"I say, okay."

"Okay," I say, "let's ramble."

Poochie sneers in Joe's direction. "What about him?"

"We've got too much cargo already," I say. "The hacks are gonna wonder why we're all jammed in my boiler. You know, like, 'What's the big party?'"

Poochie grabs Akihiro and raises his fist as if he's about to clock him, but he just shoves him instead.

"Okay, the golf ball stays."

"All right, then, let's scram."

I give Joe a hasty nod before jumping in the Hudson. Poochie and Finnbar wedge themselves into the back seat. Neither puts his gun away. The street's still deserted and I put the limo in gear.

"You know, we ran into an old friend of yours this afternoon. What's her name? Fachsi?"

"No kidding."

"Yeah, for a couple seconds. She said she was leaving for New York. Said she was sick to death of L.A."

"Did she say anything else?" I'm driving fast and for a second the wind seems to be blowing right through me.

"She said, 'With friends like these, I need an enemy.'

Then she just kind of sniffed at me and scattered."

"I guess things weren't panning out for her here," I say, acting as if this is a normal conversation. I keep driving and for a chilly moment I imagine Fachsi and Annemie back together, making Manhattan. Our New York days are long over. Nothing to do now but shake my head, which is what I do.

We find Granyer's place pitch dark and dead quiet. The gardener's apparently on vacation and it looks abandoned. I know where he stashes an extra key and let us in. The living room is a mess, glasses all over the place, stale smoke still curing the joint. It helps me picture the wild party going full tilt that bought him a bit. All that's missing is a couple hundred bacchants and a phonograph blaring "Minnie the Moocher." I look for the key to the sailboat while Poochie slips a bottle of whiskey in his pocket. I let them know I've found the key and that we can keep rolling.

"What's the hurry, Johnny? We could lay low here, right, Finnbar?"

"Granyer won't mind. He's got a new home."

"Food, booze, beds."

"The cops are coming back with a warrant," I say. "They're going to toss the joint. You know what they're like. I say we keep moving. But it's up to you."

"Of course it's up to us, you!"

Finnbar agrees with me. "This town ain't right. Let's grab some stuff and get out of here."

"So long as it's good stuff."

Poochie keeps me covered, while Finnbar grabs some bedding, throws some food in a bag, and empties

Granyer's liquor cabinet. Before we leave, Poochie pockets a silver ashtray. We carry the plunder out to the car and shove it in the passenger seat. We secure the sailboat. With my passengers kicking back training their guns on me, I head to one of the private beaches where we used to fish for barrels of saké.

It's risky, boating this time of night, but I take some roads less traveled to get out of town. Eventually the lights of the vast city fade and I carry us down darker and darker roads, hoping soon to be rid of my old friends. It's a cloudy, moonless night. The narrow path that leads down to the cove and the water is filled with bumps and humps. Finnbar gets out to help me navigate and I back slowly, bouncing and jouncing, to the water's edge. He has me stop just short, and we load it with Granyer's booze and boxes of fine literature from Shanghai. Then I back the car up until the sailboat is afloat. I get good and soaked unhitching it. It's damn cold in the middle of the night, even in Southern California. I'm so cold and nervous, I'm shivering, beside myself waiting for them to sail. Poochie comes over to me, to say goodbye, as big as the nighttime sky.

"You better hope you never see me again, Johnny."

"Poochie…"

"You still owe me a drink, and you always will."

I don't know what he cracks me with. It could be his gun, maybe a blackjack. Maybe he just cold cocks me. The darkness swells up and I don't know anything about anything. For a moment I feel as if I'm floating, warm and relaxed, then the night swallows me whole and I'm everywhere and nowhere, everything and its opposite.

Like Shiva or a dead man.

How long I'm out, who knows? It can't have been that long, because when I come to, it's still night. I'm on my lips, literally, facedown on the sand, as if I'm trying to give mouth-to-mouth resuscitation to the whole world. Something's throbbing. I think it's my head.

I roll over on my back. For the first time since I was a teenager, I can't see a thing. Not a thing. I blink and blink. I wipe my eyes with the back of my hand. Still nothing. I feel the top of my aching head and its sticky with blood. Better and better. Like some marooned pirate, I drag myself up the beach, away from the sound of the lapping waves. I don't crawl far before I scrape up against the boat hitch. Using it for support, I follow it to the car. I stretch out in the back seat, close my broken eyes, and dream.

The markets keep tumbling. The trading floor is mayhem. Guys are staring at the ticker with their mouths hanging open. They look like carp mouthing words of complaint in a fish tank in Chinatown. *The New York Times* on my desk is dated October 19, 1987.

I wake up with a lunge. It's pitch dark and I feel sick, woozy. The back seat is comfortable though. I try to let myself drift off again. Wall Street gyrates through my mind. It's a bit confusing, but I'm returning from lunch and hear a big commotion coming from the stock exchange as the steel doors bang open and guys start piling out. Some are bloody, some collapse on the sidewalk. Others manage to shove their way through the crowd gathering outside.

I see our old floor trader, Kyle Unterfisch. His white

shirt is bright red from the knot of his tie down. He grabs my arm to steady himself. I ease him onto his back on the sidewalk. He barely whispers, "Bye." Another bleeding trader, who's fallen a few feet away, opens his eyes wide and groans, "Sell, sell…"

A *Wall Street Journal* blows down the street and gets stuck to Fish's side. The date at the top of the page reads September 2008. Fish always was a contrarian. Eyes rolling back in his head, he whispers a few famous last words, "Buy. Buy. Bye…" This time I wake up for good. It's still 1934.

I lie in the dark, wondering what time it is. I'm rocking. Slowly I realize, I'm on a boat. I don't even like boats. I start to get up and immediately bump my head and bang my elbow. It dawns on me I've been Shanghaied. Doped and loaded on a boat like so much ballast. I start hammering for all I'm worth and yelling for help. "Hey!" I yell. "Hey! Help!"

The boat slows and the sea calms. My eyes are blurry but I seem to make out Fachsi floating above me. Then my eyes adjust and I see Ariane, looking at me, smiling hopefully, concerned. Then I open my eyes, for real this time, and the velvet headliner of the Hudson is hovering over me like the pricey lining of some fancy coffin, plain as day. I'm awake and alone and I can see. I hear waves lapping against the tires. The tide is coming in.

It takes me maybe a minute, I don't know how long, to get my bearings. The cove is empty. No sailboat to be seen. No beachcombers. I'm happy about all that. I feel wretched. Rather than get out and get wet, I climb over the front seat and move the car before the water rises any higher. I drive back to Granyer's, the empty boat haul rattling behind me.

For a change, the L.A. sunshine seems damped down. I don't need my sunglasses, even though the sky is clear. I pass a Rolls Royce with its hood open, broken down by the side of the road, two members of the monied class alongside. I almost hit the brakes but don't. In the past, when I was more devil-may-care, I might have laughed. But I check my baser instincts. Instead I offer them a moment of not particularly useful sympathy and drive on.

I park at Granyer's and take refuge in my shanty in the back yard. In the bathroom, I clean the wound on my head. As I look in the mirror, I see something funny. My pupils are no longer pooling out, as they have ever since I fell off that ladder so long ago. They're fairly small, in fact.

CHAPTER 61

THE PREMIERE OF THE TALE OF GENJI

Don't misunderstand. I'm grateful, truly, for my changed perspective. But having everyday, relatively normal eyesight takes getting used to, as does not being able to see at night. But that's what lights are for.

Poochie and Finnbar haven't returned to port, but I keep looking over my shoulder anyway. I suspect Poochie's on the lam. He must have gotten bunged up in some barrel of laughs in New York and has to keep sailing. Otherwise, I couldn't have kept him from taking up permanent residence at Granyer's, at least not so easily.

Under the circumstances, of which there are many, I think it's best I move. I leave my *pied à terre* and find an out-of-the-way apartment that no one I know has ever seen, a place no one can connect me to. Then, for the next few weeks, I hole up in a dim editing room with Granyer's film editor. Ariane comes and keeps us company one afternoon. I love seeing her but I have a crowd of awful thoughts intruding on me. Poochie and Finnbar, Big Department and Granyer, Akihiro and Fachsi are all plaguing me. My brain is filled to overflowing. Even so, the editor and I actually finish cutting *The Tale of Genji*. The lab pulls a print and I get the word out that we're having a screening.

Several dozen people attend the premiere, including Shoko, Ariane, and the other actors. Some potential investors that Granyer suggests are there. When the closing credits begin to roll, the applause is enthusiastic. Afterwards, we're all chatting when some well-tailored guy appears at my elbow and quietly insists we talk in private. I extricate myself reluctantly and he suggests we repair to the peace and quiet of the great outdoors. As we head out, I think I see Louise Brooks at the back of the room, standing apart, looking serious and terribly elegant. I didn't see her arrive. Maybe she'll write a review. That would be something. Once outside, the dapper guy starts talking in a low, calm voice.

"That was a great movie. A great picture. We'd like to buy the rights."

"Marvelous."

"But only because you didn't know better. We're doing you a big favor here. This is the last film you will ever make like this. Now that you know better."

"Huh?"

"We're the only ones making sex films in L.A. If you try to make another film like this, I assure you, you'll be very sorry."

"It isn't a sex film. If anything it's an art film, a literary

305

film. It certainly isn't pornographic."

"As far as I'm concerned, art is just failed porn. Art requires imagination. Even great art. Porn doesn't. Porn's better. People prefer it." There's no point in arguing with this guy. "Our audience doesn't like imagination. If they liked imagination, they'd stay home and use it. They like reality. Or maybe they don't have much imagination and all they can think is they could use a lot more exciting reality. They need our help. That's our business—cutting out imagination and dishing up reality."

"*Genji* cost a lot to make. A lot of time and work."

"We understand. Go ahead. Name your price."

"How about $50,000?"

"We'll give you $3,000. Take it or leave it. Either way, this is the last time you send light through that film."

"We'll take it."

"We know about the other scenes. We're putting them back in."

"The police confiscated them."

"We know that. We got them back."

"Hm."

"In this town you need connections."

"Clearly."

"Leave 16mm alone, sonny. It ain't no good for you. Now let's go up to the projection room and get the film. You'll write me up a nice sales receipt, and I'll cut you a check."

A couple of days later the check clears. These guys wanted the legal rights to *Genji*, apparently, to wrap around the experimental films we made of Hokusai's woodblock prints.

CHAPTER 62

THE FLOATING BRIDGE
OF DREAMS

I wake up and find my cat, Vince, sleeping next to me, breathing heavily. The phone is ringing. It's Ariane. She's the only one I gave my new phone number. She's calling to see if I can give her a ride somewhere with her grandmother.

"Of course," I say. "Where?"

"My grandmother wants to pick up three Buddhist monks from the Daisha Mission on Jackson and San Pedro."

"Okay."

"I told her what happened in the store. I had to. I couldn't keep it from her."

"And…"

"She says the only way to cleanse the spirit of her bookshop is to have priests perform an exorcism."

"When do you want me to come by?"

"Now, please, if possible."

"I'll come right over."

When I arrive at The Dragon and The Lotus, Ariane and her grandmother are dressed in black, waiting for me. I'm glad I put on a dark suit myself. The grandmother gives Ariane directions in Japanese and Ariane translates, relaying to me where I need to go to get to the Buddhist temple. It's only a few blocks away. We don't talk much during the drive.

Three monks are awaiting us. They are wearing yellow robes and carrying big satchels presumably with the *accoutrements* needed to perform an exorcism. They climb into the car, and two sit next to me in the front seat. Ariane and her grandmother ride in back with the third. Their tall red hats block my view in every direction.

"How does one perform an exorcism," I ask the one next to me, "if you don't mind my asking?"

"Certainly not. We chase away evil with prayer, chanting, drumming, and what is known as the incense of 100 paces."

"Hm."

"When we're done, if it goes as we hope it will, the home, which we understand also is a home for books— for knowledge and thought and learning—will be cleaned, freed from the karmic residue that always remains after a violent death."

From the back seat, the third priest says: "We will disperse the darkness before it settles in and becomes permanent."

"In that case," I say, "I would like to stay and lend my

moral support."

"You may. It's all right."

The ceremony of exorcism lasts the evening and much of the night. The priests only leave off chanting and drumming at dawn when they quietly pack up their tools. They tell us they're satisfied and the women should have nothing more to fear. The most senior priest instructs Ariane and her grandmother to continue to burn the 100-paces incense for the rest of day and he hands them several sticks. Then he blesses each of us in turn.

"And you, young man, though you're not as young as all that, my advice to you is to stay away from the men you've been associating with. These alchemists have beguiled you with impossibilities. You thought they were selling such exciting wares—golden libraries!—but as you've seen, their books are empty. They contain nothing but blank pages, numbered pages. Pages of mud and worse."

"And," says a second priest, "you should get a shave."

I drive the priests back to the Daisha Mission alone and then, exhausted and not sure what to do, I visit Akihiro's laboratory. The door is locked. A sign in the window says "Closed." I peer inside and it looks as if it's been cleaned out. Joe was able to move his lab, after all.

I have only one place to go now, but I'm afraid of the welcome I deserve. I go back to my apartment and feed Vince. He's happy to see me. I lie on my creaky bed and think and read. The next morning, I shower, shave, and put on my dark suit. I drive to Little Tokio.

On the blackboard outside The Dragon and The

Lotus, I write:

Even the strongest
bamboo bows. My bare hands sting,
shaking the snow free.

I knock and Ariane opens the door to her bookshop. She's wearing a celadon green kimono. She invites me in.

"*Bonjour, Ariane.*"

"*Bonjour, toi.*"

"I delivered the priests home safely."

"I'm glad. I was wondering about you."

"I checked on Akihiro. His lab is empty."

"Don't worry about him. He'll resurface, if and when he wants to."

"I liked him when he was an old man."

"My grandmother always said my uncle was a man of too many talents."

"Then I went home to sleep and think."

"We all have had a lot to think over."

"I have an idea."

"*Je t'écoute.*"

"Before our lives become too eventful, I was wondering if I could work here for you and your grandmother?"

"Doing what, Jean-Yves?"

"I'd like to make amends. I could be your duster of books. Books appreciate the attention. And it's a form of meditation. And therapeutic. I'd be happy to repair the rungs on your ladder to the roof, also."

"*C'est gentil de ta part.* I'll ask my grandmother. Maybe she'll say 'yes.'"

"I was thinking perhaps we could hold a reading here afterwards, too."

"That could be nice."

"You could read something. You have such a beautiful voice."

"*Comme quoi, par exemple?*"

"How about something from *Genji*. Maybe the last chapter?"

"You could read, too. *J'aime bien ta voix, aussi.*"

"*Avec mon accent canadien.*"

"*Et moi, avec mon accent franco-japonais.*"

After hearing my proposal, Ariane's grandmother actually offers to hire me to be a part-time book duster, but I tell her I don't want to be paid. In the string of mornings that follow, Ariane serves me her otherworldly jasmine tea and then I work my way methodically from ceiling to floor and floor to ceiling. I dust the shelves and books one by one with a whiskbroom and chamois cloth, oiling and burnishing the leather covers, just the way my neighbor Simone taught me to. Quickly and carefully.

When I break from dusting, Ariane and I take turns reading out loud from our book of choice. She reads in Medieval Japanese—I'm curious to hear what it sounds like—and I read in English.

"I asked my grandmother if she'd like to read from her French translation, but she said she's too worn out."

"Another time maybe."

When we're ready, we pick a date and schedule the bookshop performance. I hope the dusting and reading will help restore her resplendent bookshop.

The day of the event, Ariane writes our announcement in chalk on the blackboards outside, one in Japanese and the other in English. I enjoy seeing her swiftly and deftly writing the Japanese characters. The English reads:

Please come tonight at 7 p.m. to a public reading of the final chapter of *The Tale of Genji* by Murasaki Shikibu. Tea and cookies to be served afterwards.

She hangs three traditional festive decorations off the front of the store—billowing orange paper carp. There's some breeze and they stir from time to time and in a friendly way jostle one another.

A dozen people come that night to hear us—a tarnished knight errant and a scholarly princess. The text is beautiful and the audience quiet and attentive, except for one elderly man who sneezes twice and blows his nose. (I almost wrote: "blows his noise.")

After reading the last chapter, called "The Floating Bridge of Dreams," we serve tea and *gateaux secs*, and some of the listeners thank us and one or two offer their congratulations, and eventually the talkative stragglers depart. As we straighten up, and put away the chairs and dishes, Ariane and I agree that it went as well as we could have hoped.

"And now our audience can say something that not many can say—that they've *finished* the epic *Tale of Genji!*"

"*Précisément.*"

"In English and medieval Japanese!"

"*Exactement.*"

"*Et ça, c'est beaucoup-beaucoup.*"

"*Toi, t'es beaucoup.*"

"*Et toi, t'es trop. Et juste assez.* You're my *sine qua non.*"

Ariane surprises me by pulling out a bottle of champagne and two glasses and asks me to do the honors. It's cold and spills, foaming like sea surf, until our glasses overflow.

"To the pursuit of happiness."

"To happiness."

We touch glasses and take a sip.

"Let's toast to hearing from your uncle again, someday, in happier circumstances."

"*Ça, oui. Absolument.*"

"And to the world's first novelist, the Lady Murasaki."

"And her shining prince."

"To everything blowing over."

"To The Dragon and The Lotus."

"No one knows your uncle. Everyone thinks he's an elderly owner of a film lab who's closed his business. And no one's going to shed any tears over the Department."

"I hope you are right."

"Even Poochie won't miss him."

"Who's Poochie?"

"The pugilist who gave me my eyesight back."

"Nice of him."

"I don't think he meant to be nice. I think he's one of the gangsters who tried to kill Upton Sinclair."

"*Oh, là!*"

"And he definitely killed my boss in Manhattan."

"*C'est vrai?*"

"*J'en suis sûr.* Let's not think about it."

"*Toi, alors.*"

"I'll tell you about it some other time. More ancient

history." I take another sip of champagne.

"I'll say this for New York, I was happy to escape it in 1929."

"You said you liked New York."

"Oh, definitely. Lots of interesting people. Lots of bookstores. But I left there in a hurry, after my boss Aldo was killed. I think I was next on the list."

"Hm."

"People who read love New York."

"*C'est bien préferable.*"

"And it has seasons, more or less."

"Which season do you find more beautiful? Spring or Fall?" Ariane urges me to answer. "Don't give it a lot of thought,"

"In New York, *l'automne.* Spring only lasts a week, so it's hard to appreciate. There's so little to savor. The winter is long and snowy, and the skies are blue. Then spring comes and you have to jump over piles of slush. And then a week later summer hits, and it's broiling and muggy and truly malodorous for months. Fall in New York is crisp and wonderful," I say.

"Chinese scholars and poets debated this question back and forth and forward and back," says Ariane. "Those who prefer Autumn claim their preference is the subtler one, that the Spring's charms are too obvious. They say people who prefer Autumn tend to be a little melancholy."

"Hm."

"You always did strike me that way."

"Not anymore. *Tu m'as changé.*"

"I'm glad. *Comme la vie est belle.*"

"*Parfois.*"

I pour more champagne in each of our glasses and raise mine in another toast.

"To Upton Sinclair. It's too bad for California he lost the election for governor."

"He had ideas."

"At least he survived."

"You helped save him. He lives to write another day."

"*Et à tes amours…*"

"*À la nôtre, plutôt!*"

"Darling! And you, sweetheart? Which do you find more beautiful—Spring or Fall?"

"*Moi, j'adore le printemps.* I don't like Winter, especially when it insists on lingering. I can't wait for my flowers to return. Can I read you a haiku. I've written you one." Ariane takes a small piece of paper from her pocket, unfolds it, and reads:

A star shaped drop cools
in a green tea aureole—
so whole worlds are formed.

"I think it's beautiful."

"I spilled some tea this morning and it came to me."

The next day, in the stillness before the sun rises, at the time of day when I used to enjoy reading *Genji*, I write a poem emulating Sei Shonagon, the Japanese woman who wrote *The Pillow Book*, a thin volume of poems written in the Heian period at the same time the Lady Murasaki was composing her epic novel.

Things that Can't be Bought or Sold

Paper profits and losses.
An armoire that's too big to wrestle out of the house.
Words never written down.
Heart and soul, time and the tides.
A lost book in a jumbled library.
Penelope and her bed.
The wall paintings of Herculaneum.
Dew on the lotus.
True love.
Fresh tomatoes.
A jade dagger lodged in a bone next to the heart.

That afternoon, I visit Ariane in her bookshop and read her my poem.

Then I ask her if she thinks perhaps we could be true to one another...? When my fortunes change...? When my fortunes change for the better? She gazes upon me with her beautiful green eyes and smiles ever so slightly, ever so wryly. Then she murmurs "*peut-être*" and laughs like a goddess.

"There are book lovers in Los Angeles, too. I can help with your bookstore, while I work to make something better of myself."

"*Oui, mon beau.*"

"We could have a quiet life but an interesting one."

"*Décidement.* That's an ancient Chinese ideal: An uneventful life!"

"*Dès maintenant, au moins!* I've lived several eventful

lives already!"

As I marvel at Ariane's smile and my eyes trace the line of her stockings, I think better of the idea.

"Are weddings too eventful?" I ask quietly.

"*Pas forcément.*"

"*Et des enfants?* Are children too eventful?"

"*Non, mon beau.*"

"What about twins? *Des jumeaux seraient un évènement énorme.*"

She doesn't bat an eye. "*Pas du tout.*"

"*Si. On serait doublement enrichi.* We'd be able to read all those wonderful bedtime stories to them."

"We'll take turns picking our childhood favorites, *n'est-ce pas?*"

"True. And be true."

When we finally go to bed the night of our wedding, the full moon beams through turbulent clouds of shifting and rustling and shimmering silk. Eyes open, we dream of Hokusai, electric shadows ourselves, winds crying and whispering ourselves. Verging on sleep, I feel Ariane blink, her eyelash brushing my shoulder twice. And I ignore everything else, for once forgetting to listen for a knock at the door.

THE END

ABOUT THE AUTHOR

Voorhees has written two novels, many haiku, and several screenplays, as well as a dictionary of *The World's Oldest Professions*. As a journalist, he published countless articles on entrepreneurs, venture capital, economic history, and the global financial markets. He has an English degree from Dartmouth College, graduating Phi Beta Kappa and summa cum laude. He studied film theory and literary criticism at the University of Paris. His documentary, *Proust + Vermeer*, premiered at the De Young Museum in 2013. On Twitter, he tweets haiku @RichVoorhees.

Fic   Voorhees, Richard,
             author
             Shooting Genji

CPSIA information can be obtained at www.ICGtesting.com
Printed in the USA
BVOW04s1725040914

364635BV00002B/3/P